AF757371

PROTEIN BIOCHEMISTRY, SYNTHESIS, STRUCTURE AND CELLULAR FUNCTIONS

PRIONS AND PRION DISEASES

NEW DEVELOPMENTS

PROTEIN BIOCHEMISTRY, SYNTHESIS, STRUCTURE AND CELLULAR FUNCTIONS

Additional books in this series can be found on Nova's website under the Series tab.

Additional e-books in this series can be found on Nova's website under the e-books tab.

PROTEIN SCIENCE AND ENGINEERING

Additional books in this series can be found on Nova's website under the Series tab.

Additional e-books in this series can be found on Nova's website under the e-books tab.

PROTEIN BIOCHEMISTRY, SYNTHESIS, STRUCTURE AND CELLULAR FUNCTIONS

PRIONS AND PRION DISEASES

NEW DEVELOPMENTS

JEAN-MICHEL VERDIER
EDITOR

Nova Science Publishers, Inc.
New York

Copyright © 2012 by Nova Science Publishers, Inc.

All rights reserved. No part of this book may be reproduced, stored in a retrieval system or transmitted in any form or by any means: electronic, electrostatic, magnetic, tape, mechanical photocopying, recording or otherwise without the written permission of the Publisher.

For permission to use material from this book please contact us:
Telephone 631-231-7269; Fax 631-231-8175
Web Site: http://www.novapublishers.com

NOTICE TO THE READER

The Publisher has taken reasonable care in the preparation of this book, but makes no expressed or implied warranty of any kind and assumes no responsibility for any errors or omissions. No liability is assumed for incidental or consequential damages in connection with or arising out of information contained in this book. The Publisher shall not be liable for any special, consequential, or exemplary damages resulting, in whole or in part, from the readers' use of, or reliance upon, this material. Any parts of this book based on government reports are so indicated and copyright is claimed for those parts to the extent applicable to compilations of such works.

Independent verification should be sought for any data, advice or recommendations contained in this book. In addition, no responsibility is assumed by the publisher for any injury and/or damage to persons or property arising from any methods, products, instructions, ideas or otherwise contained in this publication.

This publication is designed to provide accurate and authoritative information with regard to the subject matter covered herein. It is sold with the clear understanding that the Publisher is not engaged in rendering legal or any other professional services. If legal or any other expert assistance is required, the services of a competent person should be sought. FROM A DECLARATION OF PARTICIPANTS JOINTLY ADOPTED BY A COMMITTEE OF THE AMERICAN BAR ASSOCIATION AND A COMMITTEE OF PUBLISHERS.

Additional color graphics may be available in the e-book version of this book.

LIBRARY OF CONGRESS CATALOGING-IN-PUBLICATION DATA

ISBN: 978-1-62100-027-3
LCCN: 2011946079

Published by Nova Science Publishers, Inc. † New York

CONTENTS

PREFACE

Jean-Michel Verdier
Inserm, Montpellier, France; Université Montpellier, Montpellier, France; École Pratique des Hautes Études, Paris, France

Prions, probably the most fascinating proteins ever studied, have been in the spotlight for the last 30 years. However, their history is much older. Indeed, the symptoms of what are now known as prion diseases were first described in Europe in sheep in 1730 and called « scrapie » in England, « vertige » in France and « Traberkrankheit » in Germany. The experimental study of scrapie started in 1936 when two French veterinary doctors of Toulouse, J. CUILLÉ and P.-L. CHELLE, demonstrated that scrapie could be transmitted to healthy goats by intra-ocular injections of spinal cord tissue from infected sheep. Later on, in the 1950s, I.H. PATTISON showed that scrapie had a very long incubation time as transmission of the disease in sheep and goats could take up to 2 - 4 years. In 1960, R.L. CHANDLER demonstrated by infecting mice with brain material from scrapie-affected goats that the disease agent could pass the species barrier. The incubation period in these experiments was reduced to less than one year (about 200 days). The real breakthrough came in 1965 when D.C. GAJDUSEK provided the first medical description of kuru, a neurological disorder specific of the Fore People of New Guinea characterized by symptoms (body tremors) that are strongly reminiscent of what observed in animals with scrapies. He showed that chimpanzees inoculated with brain extracts from Fore patients deceased of kuru developed a disease remarkably similar to scrapie two years after the inoculation. He received the Nobel Prize in Physiology and Medicine in 1976 for establishing that prion disorders are transmissible. The field of these weird "slow virus" diseases, according to the definition by D.C. Gajdusek, was further revolutionized by R.H. KIMBERLIN who showed in 1975 that hamsters injected with brain material from scrapie-infected sheep developed the disease after a much shorter incubation time (i.e., 65 days) in comparison to previous works.

Anyone looking at these results could safely think that prion diseases were due to viruses. However, in 1965, Pattison reported that the scrapie agent was resistant to heat and formaldehyde, two treatments that can inactivate most viruses, thus introducing a reasonable doubt about the nature of the disease agent. Furthermore, in 1967, T. ALPER showed that the agent was also resistant to ionizing radiations and ultraviolet light irradiations that normally inactivate nucleic acids. For the first time, she suggested that:

"the agent of scrapie probably contains no nucleic acid at all!"

J.S. GRIFFITH, a brilliant English theoretical chemist was intrigued by Alper's findings and, in a famous Nature paper in 1967, proposed that the scrapie agent might be a protein that can self-replicate through autocatalytic conformational changes.

Alper's results and Griffith's hypothesis will be confirmed in the 70's by the radiobiologist R. LATARJET, a specialist of ionizing radiation working at the Curie Institute in Paris. Indeed, Latarjet demonstrated that the scrapie agent could be inactivated by radiations that normally destroy proteins, thus suggesting that the infectious agent might be a protein.

With the advent of molecular biology and the arrival on the scene of S.B. PRUSINER and his visionary ideas, a new concept emerged. Against all the patiently built up dogma of biology, Prusiner proposed in 1981 that the infectious agent was a protein:

"Because the novel properties of the scrapie agent distinguish it from viruses, plasmids, and viroids, a new term «prion» is proposed to denote a small *pro*teinaceous *in*fectious particle which is resistant to inactivation by most procedures that modify nucleic acids".

The idea that a protein may act as a virus was unbelievable and he struggled hard to overcome the skepticism of the scientific community. In 1993, he showed that mice in which the gene coding for the prion protein had been genetically ablated were resistant to scrapie inoculation. These outstanding results earned him the Nobel Prize for Physiology and Medicine in 1997.

For the scientific community, the finding that a protein could co-exist in a physiological form (PrP^{c}) and an infectious form (PrP^{Sc}) was shocking. However, when people started to review past work, they found that prion-like propagation had already been described in *Saccharomyces cerevisiae* in the 70's and 80's by F. LACROUTE. More recently, prion generation has been reported in fungi as well (see for instance the work of R.B. WICKNER).

Two effective and necessary steps towards the validation of Prusiner's hypothesis were made recently. First, in 2001, C. SOTO developed the Protein Misfolding Cyclic Amplification (PMCA) method, which mimics PrP^{Sc} propagation by converting PrP^{C} to PrP^{Sc}. Importantly, this method generates infectious PrP^{Sc} that can be indefinitely propagated. Second, G. LEGNAME (see Chapter IV), from Prusiner's group, showed in 2004 that amyloid fibrils generated from recombinant mouse prion proteins can transmit the disease. This work opened new avenues of research on the *de novo* generation of infective prions from recombinant proteins. The finding that prions are infectious proteins was replicated in other models such as hamsters. Altogether, these experiments confirmed that infectious prion proteins, prepared from recombinant proteins, are the sole agent of prion diseases.

Very recently, proteins involved in other neurodegenerative diseases, such as β-Amyloid, Tau or □-Synuclein, have been shown to exhibit prion-like properties. Therefore, the extension of the "prion concept" to other proteins shows that it is a more general concept than expected before, and this will keep researchers busy for at least another 50 years! The main lesson of this extraordinary story is that, in biology, concepts are more important than experiments, as already highlighted by the mathematician R. THOM in the 90's.

The papers gathered in this book provide an update on several aspects of prion studies, going from neuropathology (E. Gelpi) to diagnosis (B. Elmoualij, A. Perret-Liaudet) and therapeutics (V. Perrier) through the nature of the infectious agent (J. Zhang, I. Baskakov), the concept of synthetic prions (G. Legname) and more recent developments in cell biology (H. Abdel-Haq), without forgetting the transmissibility of atypical strains (T. Baron).

I hope this book will stimulate young investigators and convince them that prions still are an extraordinary and challenging research field.

In: Prions and Prion Diseases: New Developments
Editor: Jean-Michel Verdier
ISBN: 978-1-62100-027-3
© 2012 Nova Science Publishers, Inc.

Chapter 1

NEUROPATHOLOGY OF HUMAN PRION DISEASES

Ellen Gelpi*
Neurological Tissue Bank-Biobanc-Hospital Clinic-IDIBAPS, Barcelona, Spain

ABSTRACT

Neuropathology has contributed to the identification and morphological characterization of the different subtypes of human and animal prion diseases and had a hand to the better understanding of pathophysiological aspects of disease. Sporadic, genetic and acquired human disease forms differ in their etiology and in the topographical distribution and severity of spongiform degeneration, neuronal loss, astrogliosis and microglial activation, and amyloid plaque formation. Clinical phenotypes are modulated by the disease subtype and strongly influenced by codon 129 polymorphism and prion protein type. These features will be discussed in this chapter.

INTRODUCTION

It is the intent of this chapter to summarize the most characteristic neuropathological aspects of human prion diseases. In each paragraph, features of sporadic/idiopathic, genetic and acquired forms will be presented, emphasizing differential patterns according to genetic and molecular data. In addition, the relation of each feature with the development of *in vivo* markers is briefly discussed. At the end, a summary of clinical manifestations in relation to the topography of neuropathological changes in the different disease subtypes is presented.

Human prion diseases include:

a) sporadic forms:

- sporadic Creutzfeldt-Jakob disease (sCJD)
- sporadic fatal insomnia (sFI)
- variably protease-sensitive sporadic prionopathy

* elgelpi@clinic.ub.es, ellen.gelpi@gmail.com

b) inherited / genetic forms:

- genetic CJD (gCJD)
- fatal familial insomnia (FFI)
- Gerstmann-Sträussler-Scheinker disease (GSS)

c) acquired forms:

- variant Creutzfeldt-Jakob disease (vCJD)
- iatrogenic Creutzfeldt-Jakob disease (iCJD)
- Kuru

An important effort has been made since the first disease descriptions from Creutzfeldt and Jakob in the 20ies [1,2] and the notion of transmissibility gained from Kuru in the 60ies, to correlate type, topography and severity of disease-related brain alterations with clinical symptoms, prion protein type and host factors.

Initial classifications were based on clinical features and designated human disease forms as amaurotic, myoclonic, transitional, dyskinetic, ataxic and amyotrophic variants [3]. From a topographical point of view, CJD had also been named as cortical, optical, striatal, thalamic, nigral, anterior horn, or panencephalopatic form. Brownell and Oppenheimer used the term ataxic form [4]. One widely accepted classification of sporadic CJD has been proposed by Parchi et al in 1999 in a study on 300 subjects [5]. This molecular classification results from the combination of two factors that have shown to clearly influence susceptibility to disease and the clinical and pathological phenotype: the polymorphism at codon 129 of the prion protein gene *PRNP* (Valine/Valine–VV, Methionine/Methionine-MM or Methionine/ Methionine-MV) and the biochemical properties of the prion protein PrP, known as type 1, type 2A, type 2B according to Western blot results, resulting in the following combinations: MM1, MM2 (further subdivided in MM2T and MM2C), MV1 (identical to MM1), MV2, VV1 and VV2. This nomenclature will be used in this chapter.

In general, there is a good correlation between the molecular subtype, clinical symptoms, results from paraclinical studies such as EEG, MRI and CSF and distribution of neuropathological alterations. According to clinical and paraclinical studies, patients are categorized as possible or probable CJD according to clinical diagnostic criteria [6]. Definite diagnosis relies on neuropathological examination.

The Role of Neuropathology

Definite diagnosis of a prion disorder still requires neuropathological confirmation, usually at autopsy, when the patient passed away. A brain biopsy during life for diagnostic confirmation is not indicated. First, because not all brain areas are equally affected and no lesions might be seen on neuroimaging, the selection of the appropriate region for biopsy might be difficult. In addition, the amount of tissue might not be (representative) enough, and a negative result will not exclude the disease for sure. Secondly, the surgical risk is too high and complications are too serious (e.g. brain hemorrhage or abscess formation) for a disease where there is no treatment. Only when there is a reasonable, potentially treatable condition that has to be excluded, a biopsy can be performed, taking into account all precautionary measures during surgery (see section "Performing the autopsy").

Performing the autopsy is important, even if it is not mandatory, or the disease not reportable in some countries. It is known that at least about 10% of CJD cases may have atypical signs and symptoms that can obscure the clinical diagnosis and this could lead to an underestimation of the true disease rate and impede the recognition of new emerging disease phenotypes, an important issue for Public Health and CJD Surveillance.

Autopsy rates may vary from 40% to more than 90% depending on the countries. Reasons for the low autopsy rates in some countries have been studied by some groups in the United States [7]. The authors reported that most neurologists appeared to be comfortable clinically diagnosing CJD, with more than one third reporting they had never considered pursuing autopsy for CJD cases. In contrast, pathologists appeared to be less comfortable making a histopathological diagnosis, indicating that autopsy performance was limited by infection control concerns (fears about the risk of acquiring CJD from handling contaminated tissue), lack of experience with CJD cases, and institutional restrictions. In addition, escalating cost of autopsy borne by hospitals and county medical examiners, lack of direct reimbursement, fear of litigation, and increasing reliance on modern technology to determine a diagnosis antemortem are other factors that probably contribute to decline of autopsies.

Brain or general autopsy can be performed safely as long as CJD-specific infection control guidelines are strictly followed [8,9]. It can be performed at a Pathology Department and/or Neuropathology Department and/or Prion Disease Referral Centre and/or Brain Bank, depending on the country and facilities. Brain Banks are platforms that collect, handle and store specimens to provide a resource to facilitate high quality and modern clinical and basic neuroscience research of the human brain in health and disease. Brain Banks are getting increasingly important due to the previously mentioned global decline in autopsy rates on the one side, and due to the exponential growth of modern neurobiological techniques that can be applied on human brain tissue on the other side: morphology, molecular biology, neuroanatomy, neurochemistry, tissue culturing, stem cell technologies, genetic studies, etc. [10].

It is also important to use available resources that provide expertise and technical assistance in evaluating CJD such as National Prion Disease Surveillance Centers. Their state-of-the-art diagnostic testing greatly facilitates tissue evaluation with high quality. Such resources are essential for surveillance of CJD and potentially emerging human TSEs, as happened with variant CJD and might happen with potential new human disease forms.

PERFORMING THE AUTOPSY

It is important that the persons who are involved in the autopsy are appropriately informed about the suspicion of a prion disease. Even if prion disease are transmissible but not contagious in the strict sense by natural contacts, they may be transmitted if natural body barriers are broken and infectious tissue is inoculated by "non-natural" routes, as may happen during autopsy. Thus, although the way of transmission and the infectivity titers are probably not sufficient to transmit the disease by any potential exposure during autopsy, precautionary measures have to be taken when handling with infectious tissue, especially due to their resistance to conventional sterilization procedures.

During autopsy, at least 2 persons should be involved to avoid contamination of surfaces and objects. A complete autopsy can be performed, but can be also restricted to brain. In the first case, brain removal should be the final step. Prosector and pathologist should protect themselves with eye, nose and mouth protection, they should wear single-use protective clothes and prevent injuries by wearing Kevlar or chain gloves under latex gloves. Additionally, all local regulatory measures should be taken, as it is done with every infectious disease. During autopsy, it is recommendable to cover the autopsy table with a plastic sheet retaining the corpse in the open body bag to avoid unnecessary contamination of surroundings. It is also recommended to use handsaw to avoid airborne dust and to use absorbent material for fluids. All instruments should be decontaminated after use combining chemical methods (at least 1N NaOH for 1h) followed by 18 minutes autoclaving (porous load, 134°C): this is currently the most accepted decontamination method for instruments. Waste and single-use material should be disposed in special, as "Biohazard" labeled containers for incineration. In case of exposition with intact skin, decontamination with 1 M NaOH or 2.5% NaOCl is needed followed by washing with water. In case of penetrating wound surgical excision should be considered. All potential exposures, especially accidents must be reported to the laboratory supervisor and recorded [11,12].

At least some areas of fresh brain tissue should be frozen for future molecular and genetic testing. Generally, a small fragment of frontal and temporal poles as well as from cerebellum is taken and frozen at -80°C. The rest of the brain can be fixed in 10% buffered formaldehyde solution for 2-4 weeks (still infectious!).

Neuropathological Examination

A.) Macroscopy

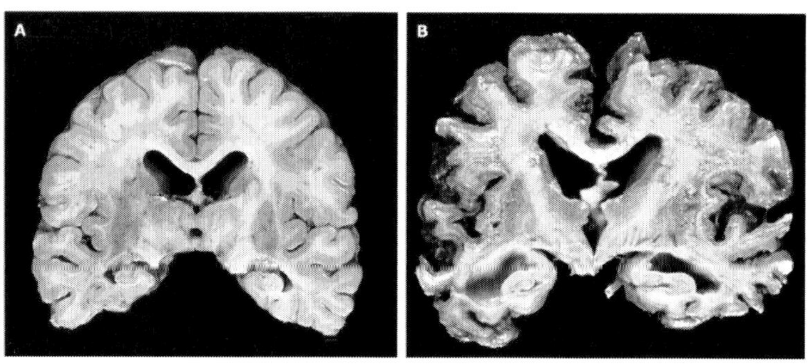

Figure 1. Macroscopical brain appearance of CJD. A: Coronal section at the level of medial thalami with lenticular nucleus and posterior hippocampus at the level of the lateral geniculate body. There is mild ventricular enlargement and relatively normal thickness of the cortical ribbon. White matter seems unremarkable. Hippocampus looks well preserved. This aspect may be observed in MM1-CJD patients with short disease duration of about 4 months. B: Coronal section at the level of the lenticular nucleus, anterior thalamic nuclei and mamillary bodies. There is a severe narrowing of the cortical ribbon with irregular, granular surface, marked atrophy of gyri with enlarged sulci and ventricular enlargement, including the temporal horns. Note also the greyish discoloration of subcortical white matter. This aspect may be observed in MV2-CJD patients, who are usually older, with a long disease of about 20 months (*Figure obtained at the Institute of Neurology, Medical University of Vienna*).

In their classical forms such as MM/MV1, sCJD brains might be macroscopically relatively unremarkable with normal brain weights (1200-1400g) or may show a mild, generalized brain atrophy with cerebellar accentuation, especially in VV2 cases. In patients who presented longer disease duration, such as frequently observed in MV2 cases (> 12 months), the brain may show severe atrophy with reduced brain weight (e.g. 800g) with diffuse narrowing of gyri and of the cortical ribbon, accompanied by severe ventricular enlargement (Figure 1A, B). A brain weight of 560g has been reported in a panencephalopathic sCJD form in Japan. sFI and FFI may show thalamic atrophy and in GSS cortical and/or cerebellar atrophy may be prominent.

B.) Work-Up for Histological Evaluation

For histological evaluation multiple brain areas should be sampled to obtain a detailed mapping of the distribution of disease. Regions of interest include cortex and white matter of all cerebral lobes, caudate, putamen, accumbens, pallidum, n. basalis Meynert, amygdala, thalamus, hypothalamus, hippocampus, cingulate, insula and all brainstem levels including midbrain, pons, medulla oblongata and cervical spinal cord as well as cerebellar vermis, hemisphere and dentate nucleus. Before processing the tissue blocks, fixed tissue in cassettes should be placed in 98% formic acid (FA) for 1h and fixed further in formalin for at least 48h. This procedure is considered to reduce infectivity of tissue to undetectable levels. The rest of the tissue in formaldehyde solution is to be considered still infectious and should be labeled as such and stored in separated cupboards. FA pretreated tissue blocks can be processed normally and cut at the microtome. Referral centers usually have a especially dedicated set for cutting and processing the tissue.

Basic histochemical stains include haematoxilin-eosin, and luxol fast blue for myelin sheaths. PAS and Alcian blue dyes are useful to detect plaques in grey and white matter, when present. Congo red stain allows confirmation of amyloid properties of coarse deposits and plaques, as they stain bright red and show green birefringence under polarized light. In formic acid pretreated tissue blocks Congo red may not react properly. In addition, immunohistochemistry using one or several antibodies recognizing different epitopes of the prion protein after adequate section pretreatment need to be used to confirm the presence of disease-associated PrP (here labeled PrP^{sc}). Additionally, histoblot, paraffin-embedded tissue blot and western blot are further methods that detect protease-resistant fragments of PrP (see section "Detection of PrP).

If it is planned to perform ultrastructural examination, tissue samples should be fixed in glutaraldehyde and embedded in resin (e.g. epoxy resin). From the resin block, semithin sections are cut at 0,5 - 1 μm and are stained with toluidin blue dye. This allows a more detailed evaluation of tissue details. Appropriate blocks are then selected for cutting of thin sections (60nm) that are stained with uranyl acetate and lead citrate, and used for ultrastructural examination with a transmission electron microscope.

C.) Microscopic Assessment

The histological hallmark of prion diseases is that of a spongiform encephalopathy characterized by the classical triad spongiform change, neuronal loss and proliferation of astroglia and microglia [13,14]. This is accompanied by the deposition of the abnormal conformer of the prion protein (PrP^{sc}) in the brain tissue, generally in grey matter, in different patterns. These histopathological changes are the substrate of macroscopic atrophy of specific brain areas and likely of neuroimaging signal alterations. Their topographic distribution also reflects and influences the results of EEG examination and of CSF analysis, being cortical alterations more prone to alter these exams.

The different patterns observed among sporadic CJD subtypes and between acquired and inherited disease forms are influenced by the genotype and the prion protein type and could also reflect their different etiology and site of PrP conversion: primarily in the CNS or spread to the CNS from the periphery via neural or circulatory systems.

In addition, as in other neurodegenerative disorders, in prion diseases, the pattern of cortical degeneration may vary significantly across the different cortical laminae, which might reflect the degeneration of specific anatomical pathways which have their cells of origin or axon terminal within particular cortical laminae [15,16].

Brain pathology is frequently asymmetric, at least in early disease stages, and it is not rare to observe that the same region is much more involved in one hemisphere when compared with the other. Also clinically, a unilateral onset of disease may be seen in about 40%.

I.) Spongiform Change of the Neuropil

Spongiform change or spongiform degeneration is the microscopical designation for a distinct microvacuolation of the neuropil, the felt between neuronal bodies in the grey matter, which is made up by a dense network of neuronal, dendritic processes and their synapses (Scheme 1). Vacuoles are well-delineated, empty holes, and are sometimes referred as opaque vacuoles. They vary in size from 2 to 5, maximal 10 micrometer in their classical forms. Ultrastructural studies have found them in neurites and less frequently in axons, axon terminals and neuronal perikarya, in astrocytes, oligodendrocytes and in myelin. Vacuoles may be surrounded by a membrane in animals, a double membrane or be without membrane delineation [17,18]. It is not clear from which structures they are derived, whether from smooth endoplasmic reticulum or mitochondria or other organelles. Liberski and co-workers have repeatedly reported the presence of 30 to 35nm sized tubulovesicular structures in all forms of human and animal prion diseases and have suggested them as disease-specific structures, but it is still unclear what they represent. What seems to be clear is that they do not contain PrP [19].

The chronology of the triad is of interest: who is first? Some experimental studies have shown that prion replication and infectivity precede spongiform change. Furthermore, there seems to be a spatial correlation between spongiform change and deposition of PrP^{sc}, with spongiform alteration appearing first and PrP depositing later [20,21].

In addition, there are very interesting experiments in which the authors were able to revert spongiform change by depleting endogenous PrP^c by conditional PrP^c knockout mice, preventing neuronal loss and progression to clinical disease [22].

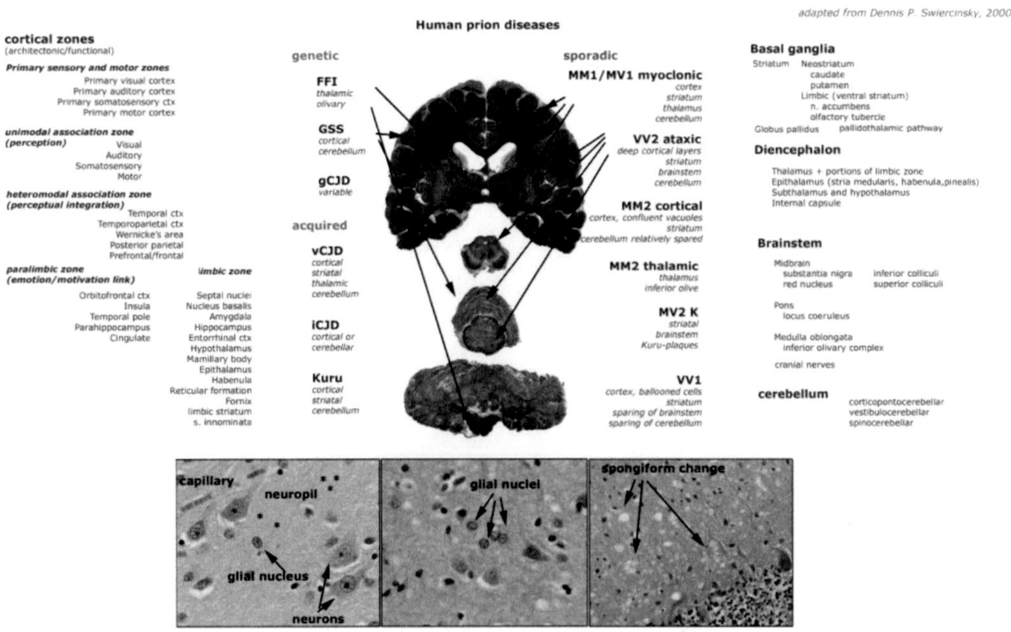

Scheme 1. Schematic illustration of the different forms of human prion diseases and their main topographical distribution of pathology. The histological picture shows the classical triad of a spongiform encephalopathy: spongiform change of the neuropil, neuronal loss and astroglial proliferation. The left microphotograph shows the normal felt-like appearance of neuropil (*), normal pyramidal neurons, a glial cell nucleus and a capillary traversing the neuropil at the left.

Severity, size and distribution of spongiform change differ between sporadic, acquired and genetic subtypes and may also depend on disease duration. In long-lasting disease, the severe degeneration of the neuropil leads to a loss of the well-defined vacuoles that are substituted by a loose glio-fibrillary background, also called status spongiosus (Figure 2A4). This state may be very difficult to differentiate from other, long-lasting neurodegenerative diseases such as advanced Alzheimer's disease, Pick's diseases or other fronto-temporal lobar degenerations as well as metabolic disorders including mitochondrial diseases or even vascular pathology.

a) In Sporadic Forms

In sCJD MM/MV1, vacuoles are small to medium sized, affect preferentially occipital and parietal cortex and less frontal and temporal cortex (Figure 2A1, A2). There is usually prominent involvement of caudate nucleus, more than putamen and pallidum. Thalamus is also frequently affected. Vacuoles are single and not confluent and show even and widespread involvement of the complete cortical thickness, with relative preservation of layers I and II. There is less affection of the limbic system and practically no involvement of brainstem nuclei. In cerebellum, spongiform change is well identifiable in molecular layer, but not in granule cell layer (Figure 4A1, A2).

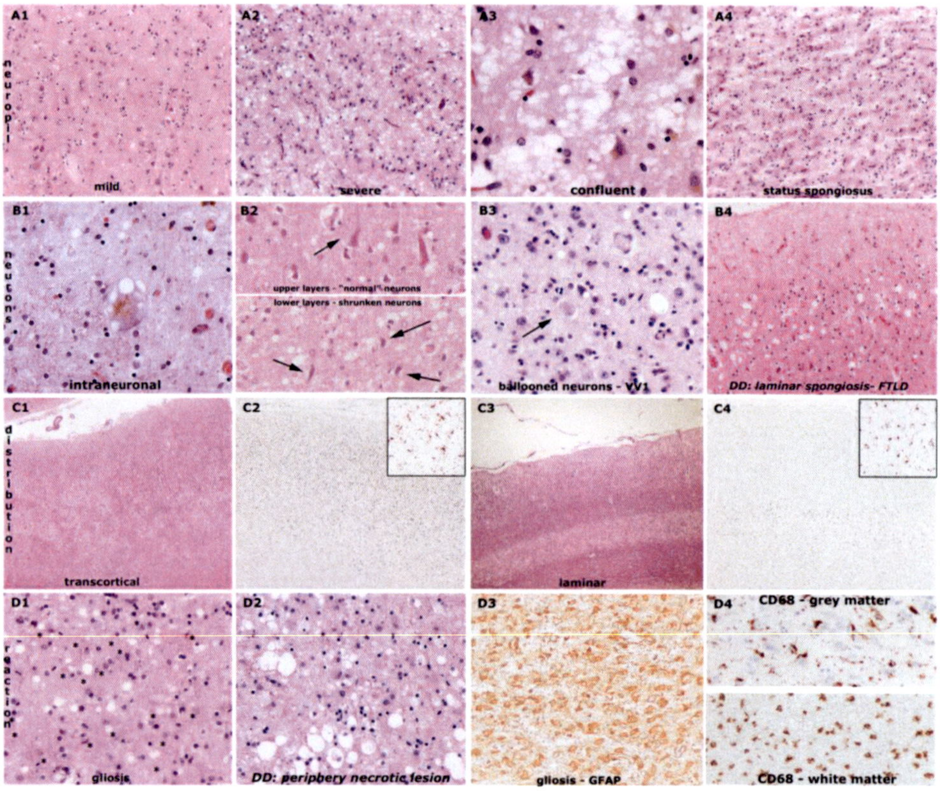

Figure 2. Classical histological features of sporadic CJD. A1-A4 represent different severity grades of spongiform change of the neuropil in frontal cortex ranging from mild (A1) to severe (A2). In some cases such as MM2C, large clusters of grape-like confluent vacuoles may be seen (A3). In long-standing disease and panencephalopathic CJD forms, a nearly complete neuronal loss can be observed, **which has been substituted by a dense mesh of astrocytic processes that induce a "status spongiosus".** Note that the classical spongiform degeneration pattern has been lost. B1-B4 illustrates neuronal changes. Intraneuronal vacuoles in a pigmented neuron of the locus coeruleus in a MV2K patient is shown in B1. This is a rare finding. B2 shows the different sizes of upper and lower laminae neurons in a VV2 cases with a laminar pattern of pathologic changes: lower neurons look shrunken and dark. Ballooned neurons as shown in B3 (arrows) are a frequent finding in most affected cortical brain areas in the rare VV1 subgroup. B4 shows a case with fronto-temporal lobar degeneration with superficial spongiosis of layers I and II, that should be differentiated from spongiform change of the neuropil characteristic of prion disorders. In C1-C4, the differences in the distribution of the pathology throughout the cortex are represented. C1 is the picture that can be observed in MM/MV1 cases (involvement of all cortical layers), whereas VV2 and MV2 cases show usually a laminar or even bilaminar pattern of spongiform neuropil degeneration, neuronal loss and gliosis (preferential involvement of deep layers). Microglial activation (C2, C4 and insets) follows in these cases the same pattern (insets represent higher magnification of activated microglia). D1-D4 show reactive changes in grey matter. Gliosis is usually seen as an increase in naked glial nuclei, although a high density of large, gemistocytic astrocytes is also observed in some cases, here in a VV1 case (D1, asterisks mark the broad eosinophilic cytoplasm typical of gemistocytes). These changes should be interpreted with caution in cases of ischemia or infarcts, where gliosis and vacuolation of parenchyma may be seen due to wallerian degeneration (D2). Gliosis may be well seen by immunohistochemistry using antibodies directed to glial fibrillary acidic protein (GFAP) that highlight astrocytic intermediate filaments in cytoplasm and cell processes (D3). In D4, microglial proliferation with enlarged cells is shown in cortex where abundant ramified processes are observed. In contrast, in severely degenerated white matter their morphology resembles large ameboid cells (microglia/macrophages).

Cortical and basal ganglia spongiform degeneration correlates well with hyperintensities observed in MRI studies in DWI and FLAIR sequences, with normal T1 sequences [23].

In sCJD VV2, vacuoles are somewhat larger but still medium sized, and are characteristically and preferentially observed in deep cortical layers. This is also designated as laminar pattern (Figure 2C3). In this subtype, subcortical involvement is more prominent than in MM/MV1 with severe spongiform degeneration of striatum, thalami, and also brainstem nuclei. In addition, there is a marked involvement of cerebellar granule cells layer and less of molecular layer with medium sized vacuoles (Figure 4A3). Similar distribution is observed in MV2K, but there is much less and different cerebellar involvement (see later on). Hippocampal CA1 sector and subiculum may show marked spongiform change, in contrast to all the other subtypes.

One of the morphological characteristics of MM2C (C = cortical) subtype is the presence of very large and confluent vacuoles, which form figures resembling grapes (Figure 2A3). The most affected brain areas are cortex and striatum, with relative preservation of brainstem and cerebellum. These confluent vacuoles may be seen only focally, intermingled with small and medium sized vacuoles, a feature of the mixed subtypes MM1 + 2C or may clearly predominate the pathology in nearly all cortical layers, the classical MM2C. This subtype is not very frequently encountered (about 2%). MM2T (T = thalamic) is considered by some authors to represent the sporadic form of fatal insomnia (sFI) and shares its lesional pattern and distribution.

The rare VV1 subtype shows widespread cortical and striatal spongiform degeneration with medium sized vacuoles that can show a laminar distribution or involve all laminae including I and II and deep laminae blurring the grey/white matter junction.

The presence of intraneuronal vacuoles is rare in humans, it is more frequently observed in animals in brainstem nuclei (dorsal nucleus of the vagal nerve, vestibular nuclei, locus coeruleus). When present in humans, they may be seen more frequently in MV2 and some VV1 subtypes and may affect pyramidal neurons of cortex and/or hippocampus or neurons of brainstem nuclei (Figure 2B1.). Intraneuronal vacuoles in cortical neurons have been observed in areas where changes were relatively early and neurons were still present, whereas in older lesions neuronal loss and gliosis predominated [24].

In variably protease-sensitive sporadic prionopathy, reported mainly in VV subjects, but also MV and MM cases, lesion profiles have been assessed in several areas including spongiform degeneration, which is described as moderate in major cerebral regions with larger vacuoles than MM1, but smaller than MM2 [25,26].

b.) In Genetic Forms

The neuropathological phenotype varies considerably among genetic cases, depending on the mutation [27]. Some cases may have a pattern of spongiform degeneration undistinguishable from sporadic CJD, as happens with one of the most frequent mutations E200K. In codon 180 mutations, the presence of intraneuronal vacuoles has been reported [24].

Despite the considerable diagnostic significance of spongiform change, it is not invariably present in all disease forms. For example, in FFI, caused by the mutation D178N where the mutated allele carries methionine at codon 129, there is nearly no spongiform degeneration of cortical areas nor cerebellum. Occasionally, it can be found in the presubiculum and focally in the molecular layer of cerebellum. In contrast, when the mutated allele carries valine at codon 129, spongiform neuropil alteration may be exactly the same as in sporadic CJD cases.

In GSS, spongiform degeneration may be focal or widespread, depending on the case and on whether ataxia or cognitive impairment dominates the clinical picture.

c.) In Acquired Forms

In variant CJD, there is severe, even confluent spongiform change of the neuropil, which is most prominent in caudate nucleus, but involves several cortical areas and cerebellum. It shows, in contrast to sCJD, a more patchy distribution. Thalamic nuclei are focally affected and hippocampus is generally devoid of spongiform change [28].

Armstrong and colleagues compared the laminar distribution of pathology between sCJD (MM1) and vCJD (MM2B/MM4) in frontal, temporal, parietal and occipital cortices, and parahippocampal gyrus [29]. The authors analyzed the distribution of the vacuolation, surviving neurons, glial cell nuclei, and PrP^{sc} deposits across the cortical laminae. They observed that the distribution of vacuolation in sCJD and vCJD was similar in many brain areas. Nevertheless, in sCJD there were a higher proportion of brain areas exhibiting vacuolation across all cortical laminae whereas in vCJD, there were a higher proportion of areas in which the vacuolation spared the superficial laminae and the region adjacent to the white matter.

In addition, significant vacuolar degenerative alterations specifically affecting brain macrophages/microglia within the thalamus and, to a lesser extent, within the neocortical grey matter has been described in two cases of vCJD [30]. These changes have been postulated to be related to copper homeostasis, loss of function of cellular prion protein and aberrant lysosomal catabolism within brain macrophages/microglia.

In iatrogenic CJD, spongiform degeneration with small to medium sized vacuoles is observed in cortical areas, in striatum and cerebellum, with relative preservation of brain stem nuclei, similar to sCJD cases.

In Kuru, spongiform change is also present in form of small vacuoles, occasionally confluent. Spongiform change is more significant in caudate nucleus and thalamic nuclei than in cortical areas [31].

Caveats

There are other neurodegenerative diseases that might induce neuropil changes reminiscent of spongiform change. In diffuse Lewy body disease, small vacuoles are frequently observed in entorrhinal and transentorrhinal cortices, that might appear identical to those observed in CJD, but are usually limited to that limbic brain area and do not show the presence of prion protein deposits. Other diseases such as fronto-temporal lobar degeneration may also show cortical spongiosis that usually affects upper cortical layers (layers I and II: also called superficial spongiosis) and is characterized by a looser and more fibrillar background (Figure 2B4). Thus, to avoid any confusion with terminology, the term spongiform change or spongiform degeneration should be only used to designate prion diseases.

In vivo markers of spongiform degeneration are not available: it is discussed whether early signal alteration on serial DWI and FLAIR MRI sequences such as hyperintensities reflect this pathology, considering that in early stages neurons are still viable and that a subsequent DWI pseudonormalization might be related to progressive cell death.

II) Neuronal Death

Neuronal loss is invariably associated to neurodegenerative diseases, and thus, is also observed in human prion diseases. The severity of neuronal loss depends generally on disease duration: the longer the duration the more severe neuronal loss. At early stages in cases with short and fulminant disease duration, spongiform change may predominate over neuronal loss. In addition, depending on the CJD subtype, there is a selective vulnerability of neuronal population of different brain areas, again, depending on codon 129 genotype, PrP type and etiology of the disease. In general, the distribution of neuronal loss parallels that of spongiform degeneration.

By plain histology, neuronal loss is difficult to objectively quantify without applying morphometric methods. For diagnostic purposes it is usually performed on a semiquantitative manner (mild, moderate or severe). Neuronal degeneration may be visualized in form of chromatolysis, rarely neuronophagia and more frequently in form of dark, shrunken and angular neuronal perikarya.

a.) In Sporadic Forms

In sCJD cases with laminar distribution of pathology (e.g. VV2, MV2) it is frequently observed that upper cortical layers show relatively well preserved neurons whereas in deeper layers neurons between vacuoles are darker, angulated and shrunken (Figure 2B2). In cerebellum, neurons of granule cell layer and Purkinje cell layer are more vulnerable to disease in VV2 cases when compared to MM/MV1 and MV2 subtypes. The former show usually marked depletion of granule cells and loss of Purkinje cells with formation of torpedoes (Figure 4A3, B2, B3). This is not seen in MM/MV1, where mainly molecular layer is affected.

In addition, when comparing the distribution of pathology of sCJD with vCJD Armstrong et al. found that in vCJD, the surviving neurons were more frequently evenly distributed across the cortex or exhibited a bimodal distribution in which the size of the upper and lower peaks was similar. By contrast in sCJD, in regions where a bimodal distribution of surviving neurons was present, the density peaks were asymmetric, the larger density peak occurring in the upper laminae [29].

Vital et al studied the nigrostriatal pathway by assessing neuron subtype loss, distribution of prion protein, alpha-synuclein, ubiquitin, and 14-3-3 aggregation, due to the frequent observation of Parkinsonism, chorea, and dystonia in CJD [32]. The authors observed a marked involvement of dopaminergic neurons and striatal outflow neurons with preserved cholinergic interneurons in sCJD. Subjects with chorea or myoclonus showed less presynaptic dopaminergic loss than subjects with Parkinsonism. In 2 vCJD cases with Parkinsonism or chorea, severe cholinergic interneuron loss in the caudate and putamen was found.

b.) In Genetic Forms

In FFI, neuronal loss predominates over spongiform change and is particularly detected in ventral anterior and dorsomedial nuclei of the thalamus as well as in the inferior olivary nucleus of the medulla oblongata (Figure 7B, C). In cortical areas, presubiculum and entorrhinal cortex may be also involved. Other cortical areas may show neuronal loss in cases with long disease duration. In cerebellum, there might be a severe depletion of Purkinje cells in some cases (Figure 4B1).

GSS may show widespread neuronal loss in cortical areas in subjects who suffered from dementia. Hippocampus is relatively well preserved. In the ataxic form there is severe neuronal depletion of all layers of the cerebellar cortex including granule cells and Purkinje cells with formation of torpedoes (Figure 6 A2, A3).

Guentchev et al. showed a uniform and severe loss of parvalbumin immunoreactive neurons in GSS, especially those PV+ neurons surrounded by isolectin-B4 positive perineuronal nets were severely affected. The authors suggested the existence of a factor residing in this type of extracellular matrix around PV+ neurons as modulator for the selective neuronal vulnerability [33].

c.) In Acquired Forms

In vCJD, neuronal loss predominates over spongiform change in posterior thalamic nuclei including the pulvinar. In cortical areas affected by spongiform change, Armstrong et al observed that surviving neurons were more frequently either uniformly distributed or in a bimodal distribution with equal-sized peaks. According to the authors, these results suggest greater neuronal loss in the upper cortex in vCJD and in the lower cortex in sCJD [29].

Proposed Mechanisms of Neuronal Death

It is likely that human brain reacts in front of the disease combining different mechanisms that predominate one over the other in one or other brain area (regional vulnerability) depending on the type, function and age of their neurons (selective neuronal vulnerability), and on other, yet unidentified mechanisms.

Activation of pro- and antiapoptotic elements under stress conditions may contribute to both, neuronal death or cell survival. In CJD, classical apoptotic figures with condensed and fragmented nuclei are difficult to observe by plain histology. Some authors have suggested that this phenomenon might be due to activation, but not completion of apoptotic cascade. Grey et al. and Puig and Ferrer studied mechanisms of cell death by TUNEL-method and cleaved caspase 3 immunohistochemistry in post-mortem brain samples, suggesting that caspase 3 dependent apoptosis may play a role in cell drop out in CJD [34,35].

Recently, the distribution of different apoptosis-related proteins such as PARP (polyADP-ribose polymerase), NF-κB (Nuclear factor), C-Jun, caspase 3 and 9, and BAX has been evaluated systematically by immunohistochemistry in different subtypes of sCJD in different brain regions [36]. The authors observed significant differences in the distribution of apoptosis-related proteins among sCJD subtypes. In MM-1 and MV-1 sCJD, subcortical structures showed more areas with nuclear PARP and/or NF-κB immunoreactivity than cortical and hippocampus regions. In contrast, caspase-3 immunoreactivity was observed more in cortical and hippocampal subregions than in brainstem and cerebellum. In VV-2 sCJD, cytoplasmic BAX predominated in cortical regions, while caspase-3 was present more in subcortical areas. In MV-2 brains, no significant differences between cortical and subcortical subregions were observed.

Expression of nuclear BAX and cytoplasmic caspase 3 was always present in regions with severe loss of neurons and strong PrP immunoreactivity, in contrast with cytoplasmic c-jun and NF-κB expression seen also in relatively preserved areas with mild accumulation of disease-associated PrP. Nuclear PARP and cytoplasmic BAX expression were seen in regions with moderate to severe neuronal loss and PrP deposition.

There was also an inverse correlation between disease duration and the expression of caspase 3, BAX and PARP, i.e. in cases with longer disease duration, less immunoreactive neurons.

Other groups studied mechanisms of phosphorylated RNA-dependent protein kinase (PKR(p))-mediated cell stress by in situ end labeling and immunocytochemistry for PrP, glial fibrillary acidic protein, CD68, activated caspase 3, and phosphorylated PKR (Thr451) in samples of frontal, occipital, and temporal cortex, striatum, and cerebellum from sCJD cases. Their findings suggest that neuronal apoptosis in human CJD may result from PKR(p)-mediated cell stress [36]. In addition, the expression of Fas, Fas ligand (Fas-L), ERK, MEK, Bcl-2, Bax, N-myc, c-myc, and pro-caspase-2, has been analyzed in the cerebellum but no significant modifications in their expression in the granular cell layer have been found.

Nevertheless, there are not so many neurons expressing apoptosis-related proteins in human brains as suggested by experimental studies. Maybe agonal processes in human postmortem brain tissue may act as potential confounding factors [38].

Overactivation of the endosomal-lysosomal system in selective neurons seems to contribute to neuronal dysfunction and finally to neuronal death [39]. An overload of cathepsin D immunoreactive lysosomes indicates altered enzymatic activity and has been correlated with tissue pathology in sCJD. In addition, the TT polymorphism at position 224 in cathepsin D gene seems to be a risk factor for variant CJD but not for sporadic or genetic CJD, although sCJD subjects tended to have a shorter disease duration [40].

In addition, excessive autophagy - a fundamental biological process that implies a cellular homeostasis pathway, whereby cytoplasm portions get sequestered by the membrane into autophagosomes for delivery to lysosomes - has been implicated in programmed cell death type II and has been observed in disease-associated states including neurodegenerative disorders [41] and prion disorders [42,43]. Chaperone-mediated autophagy is another pathway of delivery of cytosolic proteins into the lysosomes through a specific Lamp2 isoform (Lamp2a), assisted by the Hsc70 heat-shock proteins. This process bypasses the entire autophagosomal sequestration stage and, instead, individual proteins are imported directly from the cytosol into the lysosomal lumen.

Autophagy can be explored in human brain tissue by immunohistochemical and ultrastructural studies. Based on experimental models, up to 27 autophagy-related proteins have been described (yeast proteins Atf1-Atf27) and antibodies have been developed to some of them.

Furthermore, the unfolded protein response – UPR, a response of the endoplasmic reticulum in front of the accumulation of unfolded and/or misfolded proteins, by attenuating mRNA translation and increasing transcription of genes encoding ER-resident chaperones, has been suggested to be involved in neurodegeneration in prion diseases, as it has been documented for Alzheimer´s disease. Unterberger et al. addressed this issue in human post-mortem brain tissue of different human prion diseases, AD and control human brains as well as in mouse scrapie and in terminally sick mice infected with sCJD or vCJD by using antibodies directed to phosphorylated forms of the UPR transducer PERK (double-stranded RNA-activated protein kinase [PKR]-like ER kinase) and its downstream effector, the alpha subunit of eukaryotic initiation factor 2 (eIF2alpha) that mediates translation attenuation. In addition, the authors studied the cell stress kinases PKR and p38 MAP (mitogen-activated protein) kinase, which have been also implicated in the pathogenesis of AD. In their study, the authors could not detect a prominent activation of the PERK-eIF2alfa pathway suggesting that in contrast to Alzheimer disease, endoplasmic reticulum stress does not play a crucial role in neuronal death in prion disorders [44].

Synaptic Pathology

It has been described that cellular PrP is located at the synaptic buttons, in brain synapses as well as at the neuromuscular junction. Presynaptic terminals have been observed to be enriched in PrP^{c}. Ferrer et al studied pre and post-synaptic pathology and cell vulnerability in sporadic CJD cases using Golgi methods and parvalbumin immunohistochemistry in cortex and cerebellum [45, 46]. In murine scrapie they observed that synaptic protein loss precedes neuronal loss. In addition to its cellular counterpart, PrP^{sc} has been also found in synapses, in neuronal cytoplasm, dendrites and axons. Intracellularly they may be deposited in endosomal-lysosomal structures. Furthermore, ultrastructural examination of brain biopsies of different forms of disease has shown that autophagic vacuoles were formed in many synapses in all categories of human transmissible encephalopathies. The authors conclude that synaptic autophagy contributes to overall synaptic loss in brains affected in prion diseases [42].

In vivo markers that reflect neuronal loss are 14-3-3 protein, S100, and tau protein in CSF, among others. These are very useful markers during the clinical diagnostic work-up of patients who present a rapid cognitive decline. 14-3-3 has proven to be the most sensitive and specific in the adequate clinical context. It is not a marker of prions, but of neuronal loss and as such has false positive results in other conditions causing neuronal loss: rapidly progressive Alzheimer's disease or other non-prion neurodegenerative disorders, brain tumors, brain hypoxic-ischemic conditions (stroke or hemorrhage), seizures, encephalitis (autoimmune or infectious), metabolic disorders, intoxications, etc. Indirect markers of neuronal loss are brain atrophy observed by neuroimaging and their dysfunction by a reduction of metabolic activities in PET or SPECT scans.

The interest in understanding mechanisms of neuronal death also derives from the possibility of a pharmacological induction of autophagy (e.g. rapamycin) or targeting apoptosis at a therapeutic level.

III.) Astroglial Proliferation

Glial cells are important trophic and supportive elements of neurons. A glial response is present in neurodegenerative diseases including CJD. Astroglial elements (astrocytes) react in front of several stimuli including cellular stress and neuronal loss. In CJD, astrocytes may be responding directly to the presence of PrP within the tissue, rather than to the vacuolar damage to neurons, although the exact timing and trigger of glial activation is not clear.

Gliosis is observed by light microscopy most frequently as a proliferation, enlargement and clearing of glial nuclei that appear naked. Less frequently, large hypertrophic and pleomorphic gemistocytic astrocytes can be seen (Figure 2D1). This might be well visualized by immunohistochemistry using antibodies against glial fibrillary acidic protein (GFAP), a staining that highlights the star-like processes of reactive astrocytes (Figure 2D3).

In general, in all forms of CJD, gliosis accompanies spongiform change and neuronal loss and shares its distribution. Armstrong et al. observed that the laminar distribution of the glial cell nuclei was similar in both, sCJD and vCJD, the gliosis being most prominent in the lower cortex [29]. In FFI, gliosis is mainly restricted to thalamus and inferior olivary nuclei. In iatrogenic CJD due to dura transplantation, more severe pathological changes in regions adjacent to the graft have been described in postmortem studies.

The *panencephalopathic form* of CJD is a disease form that has been more frequently described in Japan [47]. It probably reflects an unspecific end-stage condition of the brain in subjects with an unusually long disease course (more > 24 months). In theses cases the cortex degenerates severely and there is a severe secondary wallerian degeneration of white matter with myelin and axonal loss, abundant macrophages and gliosis (Figure 2D4)

IV.) Microglial Activation

Microglia is the endogenous immune system of the brain and is distributed throughout the CNS. It derives from the reticular-phagocytic system and may react in front of any brain damage. Microglial cells have the capacity to migrate, phagocyte and to induce a inflammatory response releasing several factors that modulate neuronal activity. They can adopt different morphologies according to their activation states: resting or quiescent microglia shows a dense, elongated nucleus with abundant heterochromatin and ramified cytoplasmic processes, activated but not phagocytic microglia gets hypertrophic, with enlarged nucleus and cytoplasm, and finally, activated and phagocytic microglia adopts an ameboid morphology (represent brain macrophages).

This microglial activation associated to neurodegeneration is currently considered "neuroinflammation". The classical concept of inflammation that includes the presence of T-lymphocytes and activated B-lymphocytes is not present in post-mortem human brain tissue of CJD. There are no inflammatory infiltrates, neither in the brain parenchyma, nor around vessels in cuffs. Thus, the term "encephalitis" is not an appropriate term, but encephalopathy should be used.

Initially, microglial activation is a beneficial phenomenon that aims to restore cellular homeostasis and to eliminate damaged or dead neurons. Its overactivation can induce neurotoxicity by excessive production of IL-1a, IL-1b, IL-6, TNF-a and cytotoxic factors such as O2-, nitric oxide (NO) or tumor necrosis factor alpha (TNFalpha).

Experimental studies have shown that macrophages are important in scrapie pathogenesis, as they may take up PrP^{sc}, sequester scrapie infectivity, and impair early scrapie agent replication, or might be vehicles for exporting PrP^{sc} from the brain to the periphery. In addition, perivascular macrophages of the brain have a high rate of turnover by bone marrow-derived blood cells and might represent a pathway for neuroinvasion of vCJD that is alternatively spread along peripheral nerves.

Microglia can be detected by immunohistochemistry using anti HLA-DR or anti-CD68 antibodies (Figure 2C2, C4, D4). Other markers include *Griffonia simplicifolia B4-isoleucine* (mainly for activated and phagocytic, but also quiescent microglia), macrophage markers ED1, ED2 or OX41 (phagocytic state), complement receptors CR3, MHC class I antigens (HLA-DR) or vimentin, common leucocyte antigen and CD4 in activated and phagocytic states.

In sCJD MM1/MV1 cases, microglia is usually diffusely distributed in the cerebral cortex (Figure 2C2) while in VV2 and MV2 cases, it may follow a laminar pattern preferentially involving deep cortical layers, in parallel to spongiform change and gliosis (Figure 2C4). Indeed, van Eitzen et al studied 11 cases of CJD combining immunocytochemistry and computerized image analysis to clarify the relationship between spongiform change and microglial activation [48]. They observed the presence of MHC class II-positive microglia almost exclusively confined to cortical gray matter in a higher proportion of more than 350-fold compared to controls. In cortical regions with a bimodal distribution of spongiform degeneration, the presence of class II-positive microglia correlated well with the presence of vacuolation in layer V, but significantly less with spongiform change in upper layers. In areas where spongiform degeneration affected the entire depth of the cortex, activated microglia were predominantly located in the inner one-half of the cortex or were evenly distributed throughout all cortical laminae. Here, microglia exhibited atypical, tortuous cell processes and occasionally intracytoplasmic vacuoles, suggesting that microglia themselves may become a disease target. The authors suggest that there is no early causative involvement of microglia in the development of spongiform change, but diseased microglia may produce harmful factors, which mediate both astrogliosis and neuronal injury at later stages.

Microglia has been also observed surrounding PrP amyloid plaques, including multicentric plaques of GSS [49].

In vivo markers of microglial activation have recently applied in animal models and humans with different neurological disorders using PET and specific tracers, such as [(18)F]fluoroethyl-DAA1106 [50] or [11C](R)PK11195 [51]. In addition, CSF may be analyzed for the presence of microglial antibodies and several cytokines, as has been studied in other neurodegenerative disorders [52,53].

Elevated levels of prostaglandin E2 were found in the cerebrospinal fluid of subjects affected by sporadic, genetic, or variant CJD [54]. In sCJD patients, higher CSF levels of PGE(2) were associated with shorter survival, suggesting that their levels might represent an important index to predict survival and disease severity. These markers are currently not used for diagnosis but might be helpful when drugs targeting microglial pathology are developed. The interest in neuroinflammation is also based on the experience in Alzheimer's disease, where treatment with non-steroidal anti-inflammatory drugs may reduce the risk of disease.

V.) PrP Amyloid Plaques

PrP plaques are observed in a small subgroup of sporadic, acquired and genetic cases.

a.) In Sporadic Forms

Classical unicentric PrP amyloid plaques, also designated as "Kuru" plaques, are detected mainly in sCJD MV2K subtype. The letter "K" designates the presence of Kuru-plaques. They are most frequently detected in cerebellum, preferentially in granule cell layer, but may also be observed in cerebral cortex. Rarely, some MM1 cases with unusual long disease duration have been reported to present abundant unicentric plaques not only in grey matter but also in white matter [55]. Plaques are relatively easily seen by plain histology on HE stains. They are PAS positive and stain also with Alcian blue, are congophilic and show green birefringence when observed under polarized light (can be altered in formic acid pretreated tissue). Unicentric plaques have radially oriented processes and a fringed outline (Figure 4C1). Ultrastructurally, they appear as stellate arrangements of amyloid bundles emanating from densely interwoven center. A proportion of kuru plaques form very dense stars, reminiscent of sea urchins in shape. Others present a looser pattern. Amyloid stars are enveloped by astrocytic processes. High-power electron micrographs reveal that amyloid bundles are concealed within grooves of obscure cellular origin [56,57].

Variably protease-sensitive sporadic prionopathy is also characterized by the presence of microplaques that are seen as small homogeneous formations in HE stains in molecular layer of cerebellum.

b.) In Genetic Forms

In GSS disease, in most of the mutations (e.g. P102L, P105L, A117V, F198S, Q217R), unicentric plaques tend to group in clusters and form large aggregates of plaques that are designated "multicentric plaques". The term "cluster plaques" refers to clusters of small plaques or focal accumulations of dense PrP deposits. Their size and extent can vary. They are observed in all cortical areas (Figure 6B1, C1), in basal ganglia and in cerebellar molecular layer, more than in granule cell layer or Purkinje cell layer (Figure 6A1, A2; Figure 4C2, C3). They are also PAS positive, congophilic and green birefringent under polarized light, i.e. they feature amyloid characteristics. Ultrastructurally, they have similar characteristics as unicentric plaques, and are surrounded by dystrophic neurites filled with abnormal organelles such as electron-dense bodies, multi-vesicular bodies and multilamellar bodies and are indistinguishable from those seen in scrapie and CJD or Alzheimer's disease, except that they do not contain paired helical filaments [57]. This is also observed by silver stains and immunohistochemistry, where argyrophilic, ubiquitinated and tau-immunoreactive dystrophic neurites surround multicentric plaques (Figure 6C2, C3).

Insertional mutations are also frequently characterized by the presence of coarse and plaque-like aggregates as well as plaques reminiscent of multicentric plaques in cerebellum and other brain areas. Some cases are morphologically so similar to GSS (e.g. 192 bpi) that are included under the term GSS syndrome, although their clinical presentation might be very different. In other insertional mutations, like 144 bpi, grape like clusters of aggregates may be focally found in molecular layer and subiculum (Figure 5F, case from reference 60) [58-60].

c.) In Acquired Forms

In variant CJD, the hallmark of disease is the presence of "florid plaques". They can measure up to 150 micrometer. The core of the florid plaques shares morphological and tinctorial features with unicentric PrP plaques but show more radiating fibrils and are additionally surrounded by a collar of vacuoles. Due to their similarities to a flower, they have also been named daisy plaque (Figure 8A). Unicentric Kuru plaques are also observed in vCJD. Ultrastructurally, florid plaques are made up by broad bundles of amyloid and are highly neuritic. This feature makes them more similar to neuritic plaques of Alzheimer´s disease than "kuru-type plaques". Dystrophic neurites surrounding the plaque contain lysosomal electron-dense bodies or vesicles. Microglial cells have been found within florid plaques with occasional amyloid fibrils in membrane-bound pockets of microglial cells. Significant tau immunoreactivity in DNs around florid plaques is observed, more than in sCJD, GSS and kuru [57,61]. Florid plaques involve nearly all brain areas layers, mainly occipital and cerebellar cortices [62].

Using fluorescent molecular-imaging probes, Bresjanac and co-workers showed that FDDNP (2-(1-[6-[(2-fluoroethyl)(methyl)amino]-2-naphthyl]ethylidene) malononitrile reliably identifies all prion plaques, including small cluster-plaques in vCJD [63].

In iatrogenic CJD (mainly after implantation of dura mater grafts, but also after treatment with pituitary hormones, use of contaminated instruments or cornea transplants), the presence of rare plaques that are identical to florid plaques has been reported in a subgroup of patients from Japan, France and Germany [64,65]. Also microplaques in white matter have been described.

Yamada et al have analyzed clinical, pathological, and molecular features in 74 patients with dura-related iCJD. They could classify them into two distinct clinico-pathological phenotypes: a non-plaque type (two thirds), showing typical features identical with those of classic CJD and having MM genotype except for one case and PrP^{sc} type 1; and a plaque type (one third), characterized by atypical clinical features, and plaque formation in the brain, and having MM genotype and an intermediate PrP^{sc} type between 1 and 2. These data make the authors suggest a contamination of the dura mater grafts with different prion strains [66]. In addition, codon 219-lysine allele may influence the clinico-pathological features and PrP profiles in this subtype [67].

In Kuru, besides spongiform change, the presence of amyloid plaques was described in the mid 50ies and from this observation derived the term "infectious amyloidosis".

The term "plaque-like" refers to the results of PrP immunohistochemistry and reflects coarse PrP deposits that are not seen in HE sections, but only by immunohistochemistry.

It is interesting to observe that most acquired prion diseases have plaques: strain of agent, route of infection and host genotype influence the disease phenotype. As vCJD and Kuru may share a presumptive route of infection, Mc Lean et al compared the pathologic profiles and genotypes of variant CJD and kuru. The authors observed distinct lesional differences particularly in the PrP load and distribution as seen by immunohistochemistry. According to their results, the authors postulate that clinico-pathologic phenotypes and the genotypes of these two diseases are sufficiently different to suggest that the strain of agent may play a greater role than any possible common route of peripherally acquired infection [68,69].

Richard and co-workers analyzed the presence and distribution of 14.3.3 zeta protein by immunohistochemistry in different types of amyloid plaques in human prion diseases. The authors observed that, in contrast to beta-amyloid plaques of Alzheimer's disease and multicentric plaques from GSS, Kuru plaques from MV2 sCJD, plaque-like deposits from VV2 sCJD and florid plaques from vCJD showed PrP^{sc} and 14.3.3 zeta deposits in the same plaques, suggesting that 14.3.3 zeta could interact with PrP or other components of abnormal PrP^{sc} deposits in CJD [70].

In vivo markers that reflect the presence of PrP amyloid plaques are used in experimental and also clinical setting by fluorescent molecular imaging probes such as FDDNP or [(11)C]BF-227 PET [63,71], but not by 11C-PiB PET [72].

VI.) Cerebellar Pathology

The cerebellum is invariably involved in most CJD cases, sporadic, genetic and acquired cases and deserves special attention. Because the pattern and severity of cerebellar pathology may vary significantly among subtypes, its evaluation may be very useful to infer to the CJD subtype relatively rapidly. In addition, due to its connections to cerebral cortex via brainstem nuclei and spinal cord, entry of pathology via trans-synaptic spread and retrograde transport has been proposed for acquired forms of the disease [73].

The normal cerebellar cortex is constituted by three layers: stratum moleculare or molecular layer where we find few neuronal nuclei of basket cells, star cells and golgi cells (inhibitory interneurons) as well as of glial cells; but it is mostly composed of fibers: the axons of granule cells in form of parallel fibers and the complex dendritic arborization of Purkinje cells. The middle layer is also called stratum ganglionare and is made by Purkinje cells (GABAergic). Perikarya of Purkinje cells are surrounded by the cellular processes of the basket cells and lay on a monolayer of larger glial cells or Bergman glia. Purkinje cells and their processes are surrounded by climbing fibers that come from the olivary complex from the medulla oblongata. Purkinje cells axons contact with neurons of the dentate nucleus in deep cerebellar white matter. In the lower layer, stratum granulosum, there is the highest neuronal density (95% of cerebellar neurons) and synaptic concentration and is made of small nuclei of granular neurons (glutamatergic) that receive inputs from all afferent fibers through the mossy fibers and project their axons to the molecular layer where they make synapsis with the apical dendrites of Purkinje cells. In addition, larger Golgi type II neurons are also found (Figure 4A1).

a.) In Sporadic Forms

Molecular layer is usually affected by spongiform change and gliosis. Its severity varies among sCJD subtypes [5,74] from mild in early MM/MV1 cases to severe in advanced disease stages or in MM2C, where the largest vacuoles can be observed (Figure 4A1, A2). Purkinje cells are relatively preserved in MM/MV1 and MM2 cases, but are severely affected in VV2. In VV2 there is additionally a severe depletion of granule cells (Figure 4A3) with a severe depletion of parallel fibers of molecular layer. When Purkinje cells are lost, torpedoes or axonal swellings can be observed in granule cell layer and are well visualized with silver stains or antibodies directed against neurofilaments (Figure 4B1-B3). When Purkinje cells disappear, empty baskets are frequently detected by silver stains. In addition, the complex arborization of apical dendrites as seen by calbindin-immunohistochemistry is lost in molecular layer. Their degeneration induces also axonal degeneration and as such, gliosis of adjacent white matter. VV1 rarely affects cerebellum. Unicentric PrP amyloid plaques or Kuru-type plaques are detected mainly in granule cell layer in MV2K subtype (Figure 4C1).

In variably protease-sensitive sporadic prionopathy, cerebellar molecular layer shows small formations of characteristic compact granular and plaque-like PrP deposits [25].

b.) In Genetic Forms

The detection of large multicentric plaques predominantly in molecular layer is the main characteristic of GSS (Figure 4C2). There can be also unicentric Kuru-plaques in granule cell layer (Figure 4C3). Focal spongiform change or severe Purkinje cell loss may be observed in some FFI cases (Figure 4B1). Abnormal PrP patterns such as grape-like, coarse or strip-like deposits resembling the arborization of climbing fibres may suggest a *PRNP* mutation, including insertional ones (Figure 5H).

c.) In Acquired Forms

In vCJD, cerebellum is also involved and shows large and clusters of unevenly distributed vacuoles in molecular layer, marked loss of Purkinje cells and florid plaques in molecular and granule cell layer. Recently, a quantitative study on the pathology of cerebellum has been performed in vCJD [73]. The authors analyzed the distribution of pathology among laminae, the spatial topography along foliae, spatial correlations between pathological changes and compared these alterations with sCJD MM1. They observed that in vCJD, all laminae were affected by disease, but the most severely affected was granule cell layer. Pathology was distributed along the foliae, especially in Purkinje cell layer and molecular layer. The authors postulate that pathology might spread along anatomical connections between cerebellum, thalamus, cerebral cortex and pons. The distribution of pathology differed from classical MM1 sCJD.

In vCJD it has been suggested that vacuolation of molecular layer may occur after loss of Purkinje cell perikarya and may precede PrP^{sc} deposition. The vacuoles may form in relation to the dendritic trees of the Purkinje cells. The same authors have observed positive spatial correlation between the vacuolation and PrP^{sc} plaque, suggesting that both pathological features may develop more or less simultaneously within a lamina and in relation to the same clusters of degenerating neurons. In contrast, pathological features in molecular layer were not spatially correlated with those in the granular layer, suggesting that pathology in these layers may develop more or less independently [73].

In dura mater related iCJD and after administration of human pituitary-derived hormones, an important cerebellar involvement has been described with the presence of amyloid plaques, including PrP miniplaques in cerebellar white matter.

In Kuru, spongiform degeneration of the molecular layer may be mild. The granule cell layer is usually relatively well preserved and here, unicentric amyloid plaques - Kuru plaques - are detected in variable amount.

RELATIVE RESISTANCE OF HIPPOCAMPUS IN CJD

In contrast to Alzheimer's diseases where impaired memory is one of the leading clinical symptoms and hippocampus is one of the early involved vulnerable brain areas, in human prion diseases, hippocampal formation is usually relatively preserved. Cornu Ammonis (CA) sectors CA1 to CA4 and granular neurons of dentate gyrus do not show marked neuronal loss nor spongiform change in the most frequent sporadic CJD subtypes MM1/MV1, independently of disease duration. In VV2, MV2 and VV1 there might be spongiform change in all sectors, but mainly in CA1 that increases in severity associated to neuronal loss and gliosis in subiculum and entorrhinal area. Spongiform change is in some cases relatively prominent in stratum moleculare of dentate gyrus. Subiculum and entorrhinal cortex might also be one of the few areas involved in FFI by spongiform degeneration, preserving CA4-CA1 sectors. These observations might indicate that cognitive decline and memory impairment in CJD are probably not related to hippocampal damage [75].

In infrequent subtypes such as VV1, MV2K/MV2K+2C and some genetic cases (e.g. 96 bpi) an increased number of partially bizarre appearing Hirano bodies have been described [76,77]. Their presence seems not to be related to age or other concomitant neurodegenerative diseases. Their significance, especially in young VV1 sCJD subjects and in other rare subtypes without hippocampal involvement is unclear and might be partly related to cellular stress and failure of clearance systems.

VII.) Detection of PrP

VIIa.) By Immunohistochemistry

PrP immunohistochemistry on paraffin sections using different antibodies demonstrates in most of the cases the presence of aggregates of the abnormal prion protein conformer (here termed PrP^{sc} for practical reasons).

Several monoclonal antibodies have been developed. Even if antibodies directed to the aggregated synthetic prion protein peptides selectively recognize disease-associated prion protein from human brain specimens [78], most of the antibodies currently used for diagnostic purposes are directed against the cellular PrP [79,80]. Thus, tissue sections need to be submitted to special pretreatments to denaturate physiological PrP for demonstrating only the resistant, disease associated protein. Some centers digest the sections with proteinase K, which hampers morphological evaluation due to the tissue digestion. Other centers use a combination of a 3 tiered tissue pretreatment protocols, including 10 minutes hydrated autoclaving at 121°C, 5 minutes 96% formic acid, and 2 hours 4M guanidine thiocyanate at 4°C prior to anti-PrP antibody incubation or 30 minutes hydrated autoclaving at 121°C, and 5 minutes 96% formic acid without further treatments. These protocols preserve brain morphology and eliminate PrP^c. The staining quality will additionally depend on the tissue itself, on the primary antibody and on the antigen retrieval procedures used [81].

In a multicenter study, 10 different monoclonal antibodies were compared to assess the reliability of their application for the definitive diagnosis of different human prion disease subtypes [82]. The authors compared the following antibodies that recognize different epitopes: antibody/epitope/isotype/supplier/dilution/immunogen

FH11/23-85/IgG2b/TSE Resource Centre, Birkett CR, Compton, U.K./ 1:1000/ Sheep recPrP, BG4/23-85/IgG2b/TSE Resource Centre, Birkett CR, Compton, U.K. / 1:1000/ Cow recPrP, 8G8/95-110/IgG2a/CEA, Service de Pharmacologie et d'Immunologie, Saclay, France/ 1:500 / Human recPrP, 3F4/109-112/IgG2a/SENETEK, Maryland Heights, MO, USA/ 1:300/ Hamster SAF, 6H4/144-152/IgG1/Prionics, Zürich, Switzerland/ 1:500/ Cow recPrP, 12F10/142-160/IgG2a/CEA, Service de Pharmacologie et d'Immunologie, Saclay,

France / 1:1000/ Human recPrP, SAF54/142-160 / IgG2b / CEA, Service de Pharmacologie et d'Immunologie, Saclay, France / 1:1000 / Hamster SAF, L42/141-159/IgG1/FRC for Virus Diseases of Animals, Dr. M.H. Groschup, Tübingen, Germany/ 1:300/ Sheep recPrP, KG9/140-180/IgG1/TSE Resource Centre, Birkett CR, Compton, U.K./ 1:1000/ Cow recPrP, DF7/140-180/IgG2b/TSE Resource Centre, Birkett CR, Compton, U.K./ 1:2000/ Cow recPrP.

Strong immunoreactivity is usually observed when using antibodies directed against the mid part of the prion protein, such as 3F4, 6H4, 12F10, SAF54, KG9, DF7. In contrast, antibodies directed to the N-terminus rarely show this staining intensity such as FH11, BG4, 8G8. These usually stain well coarser aggregates and plaques, probably reflecting a higher accessibility of the flexible N-terminal end in the amyloid and pre-amyloid states (e.g. patchy/perivacuolar or plaque-like deposits and PrP plaques). No antibody labels exclusively one CJD subtype.

PrP Deposition Patterns in the CNS

a.) In Sporadic Forms

The molecular subtype of CJD influences not only the severity and distribution of spongiform change and gliosis, but also the distribution and deposition pattern of PrP^{sc} [5].

Diffuse synaptic pattern refers to the fine dotted immunoreactivity observed in grey matter that is very similar to synaptic stains such as synaptophysin (Figure 3A1, A2). This type of deposit is generally related to PrP^{sc} type 1 according to western blot studies. PrP^{sc} type 1 is more prone to form fine, diffuse aggregates. MM/MV1 sCJD cases show this type of deposits in cortical and subcortical grey matter and in cerebellar cortex. In cerebellum, molecular layer shows besides the diffuse staining frequently a pattern that follows parallel fibers (Figure 5A1, A2). In granular layer, deposits are coarser and detectable in the glomerula (Figure 5A3). In spinal cord, fine synaptic deposits are mainly detected in substantia gelatinosa. In VV1, diffuse synaptic deposits are also observed throughout the grey matter, but are extremely faint and sometimes difficult to detect.

In contrast, PrP^{sc} type 2 is more prone to aggregate in coarse, *plaque-like* (focal) deposits and *plaques* with amyloid characteristics: congophilia and green birefringence when visualized under polarized light. Especially in VV2 cases, PrP^{sc} delicately surround neuronal perikarya and processes preferentially in deep cortical layers (laminar pattern) in a *perineuronal* and *periaxonal* staining pattern (Figure 3B1, B2), and rarely intraneuronal (Figure 3A3). In addition, in VV2 cases coarse and focal *plaque-like* deposits, are frequently seen in grey and also in white matter and along white matter tracts in basal ganglia, thalamus, hippcampus and cerebellar white matter (Figure 3B3). These deposits are not detectable in routine HE stains. In addition, brainstem nuclei including colliculi, periaqueductal grey matter, nuclei pontis, substantia nigra, inferior olives and dentate nucleus show diffuse synaptic PrP^{sc} deposits in VV2 cases. When large, dense and coarse aggregates are seen around large and confluent vacuoles, the pattern is designated as *patchy perivacuolar* or *morula* type. This pattern is mainly observed in MM2C subtype (Figure 3C2). This subtype also shows a laminar PrP^{sc} deposition pattern in cortical areas and plaque-like aggregates in grey and white matter. PrP^{sc} amyloid plaques are easily detected by most of the antibodies in form of unicentric plaques in MV2K subtype, mainly in granular layer of cerebellum but also in some cortical areas (Figure 5D1, D2). Vascular PrP amyloid has been rarely described in sCJD co-localizing with beta-amyloid angiopathy [83] and in a stop codon 145 *PRNP* mutation [84].

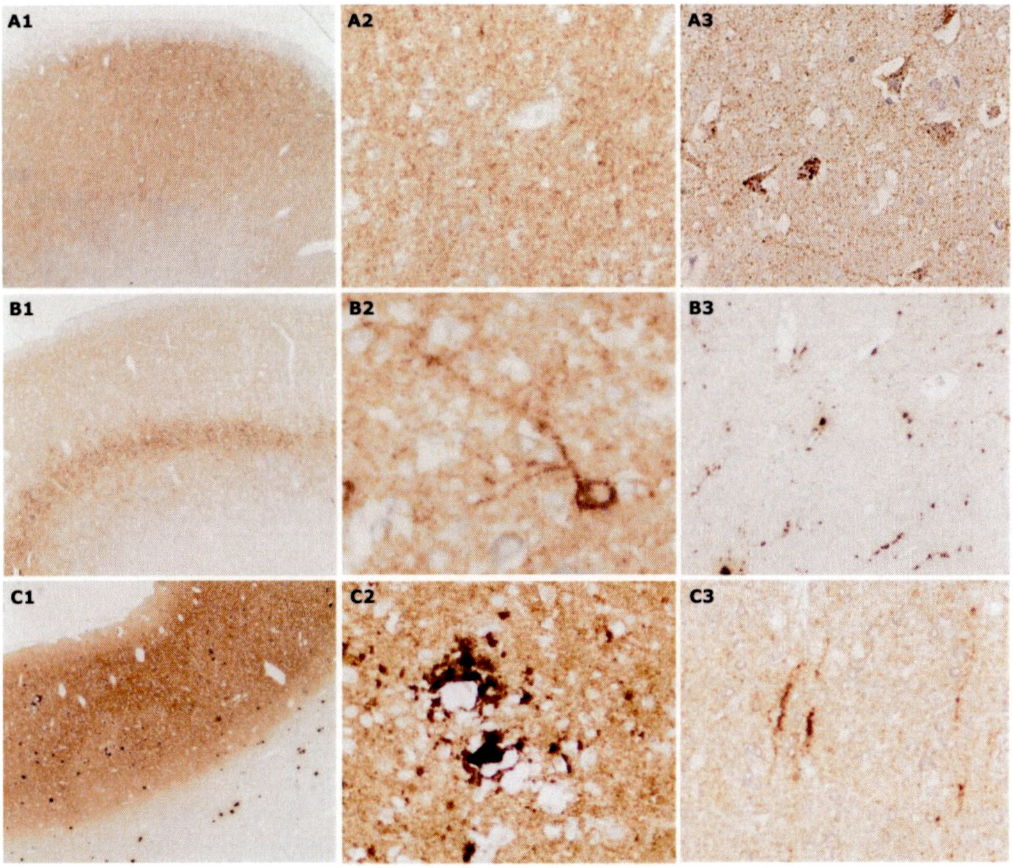

Figure 3. PrP^{sc} immunohistochemical deposition patterns in CJD. A1 and A2 show the classical diffuse, fine punctate PrP^{sc} aggregates in grey matter designated as *diffuse synaptic* pattern, which is observed in MM/MV1 sCJD cases and in some genetic cases, such as E200K mutation. Very rarely, dot-like *intraneuronal* deposits may be seen in some *PRNP* mutation carriers. B1-B3 illustrate the *laminar pattern* observed in VV2 and MV2 sCJD cases with clear accentuation of deep cortical layers. At higher magnification (B2) a coarser *perineuronal pattern* surrounding perikarya and neuronal processes is frequently seen. In addition, *plaque-like aggregates* in basal ganglia, thalami, brainstem and cerebellar white matter (B3) are characteristically detected in VV2. In C1-C3, coarse aggregates as observed in MM2C in form of large patches surrounding large confluent vacuoles are designated as patchy/perivacuolar deposits. These aggregates may be seen focally and combined with a diffuse synaptic staining pattern in mixed MM1+2C cases (C2). In C3, coarser longitudinal aggregates are shown in grey matter.

Variably protease-sensitive sporadic prionopathy shows in addition to fine synaptic and coarser dots a *target-like* pattern in cerebrum and *microplaques* in cerebellum in its more frequent VV form [25,26]. In the MV genotype, the target-like pattern seems to be less recognizable and the molecular layer of cerebellum shows a more plaque-like immunostaining pattern. MM subjects show a predominant plaque-like immunostaining pattern in cerebrum and small plaque-like formations in cerebellum.

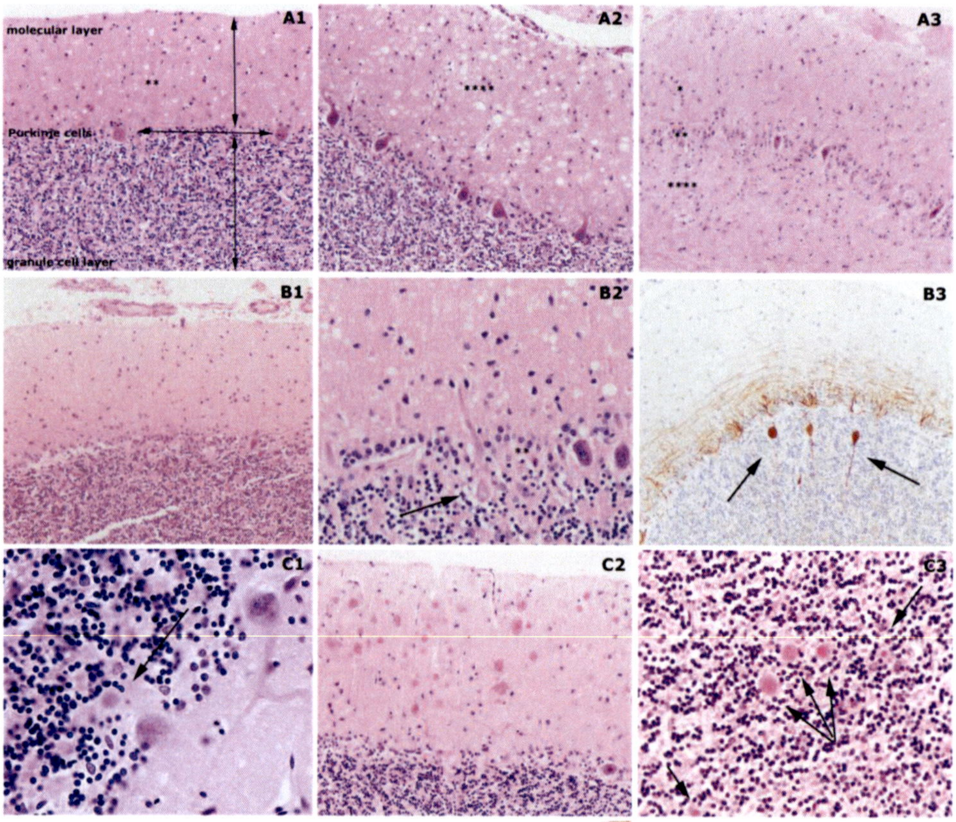

Figure 4. Cerebellar pathology. A1: The cerebellar cortex has three layers, the outer molecular layer, the intermediate Purkinje cell layer and the inner granule cell layer. These layers are differently affected in human prion disorders. In A1 mild, and in A2 marked spongiform change of molecular layer is depicted. This is frequently observed in MM/MV1 sCJD. Large vacuoles may be also seen in MM2C cases. In both images, Purkinje and granule cells look relatively well preserved. In contrast, A3 shows severe and nearly complete depletion of granule cell layer (***) and segmental loss of Purkinje cells (**), whereas molecular layer shows only minimal changes (*). When Purkinje cells are lost (B1, a case of FFI), there is a proliferation of Bergmann glia at the level where Purkinje cells had been. In subacute Purkinje cell damage, their axonal swellings can be detected in granule cell layer as round or tear-like homogeneous, pale-eosinophilic structures (B2, arrow). They should not be confounded with amyloid plaques. They are much more easily seen by silver stains or by immunohistochemistry (B3) using antibodies to e.g. neurofilaments (arrows).

Concomitant deposits of both PrP^{sc} types (1+2) such as clusters of confluent vacuoles with patchy-perivacuolar PrP^{sc} pattern together with diffuse synaptic pattern is the morphological substrate of currently considered *mixed* phenotypes (Figure 3C1, C2; Figure 5B). Mixed patterns can be detected if multiple WB studies are performed in multiple brain areas in around 30% of cases [85,86]. Small foci of clustered vacuoles may be missed in WB, thus extensive neuropathological work-up might be more sensitive for detecting some mixed cases. The regional PrP^{sc} immunostaining pattern correlates well with the PrP^{res} type detected by WB in that region [86]. Also in variant CJD a lower level presence of type 1 PrP^{sc} exists [87].

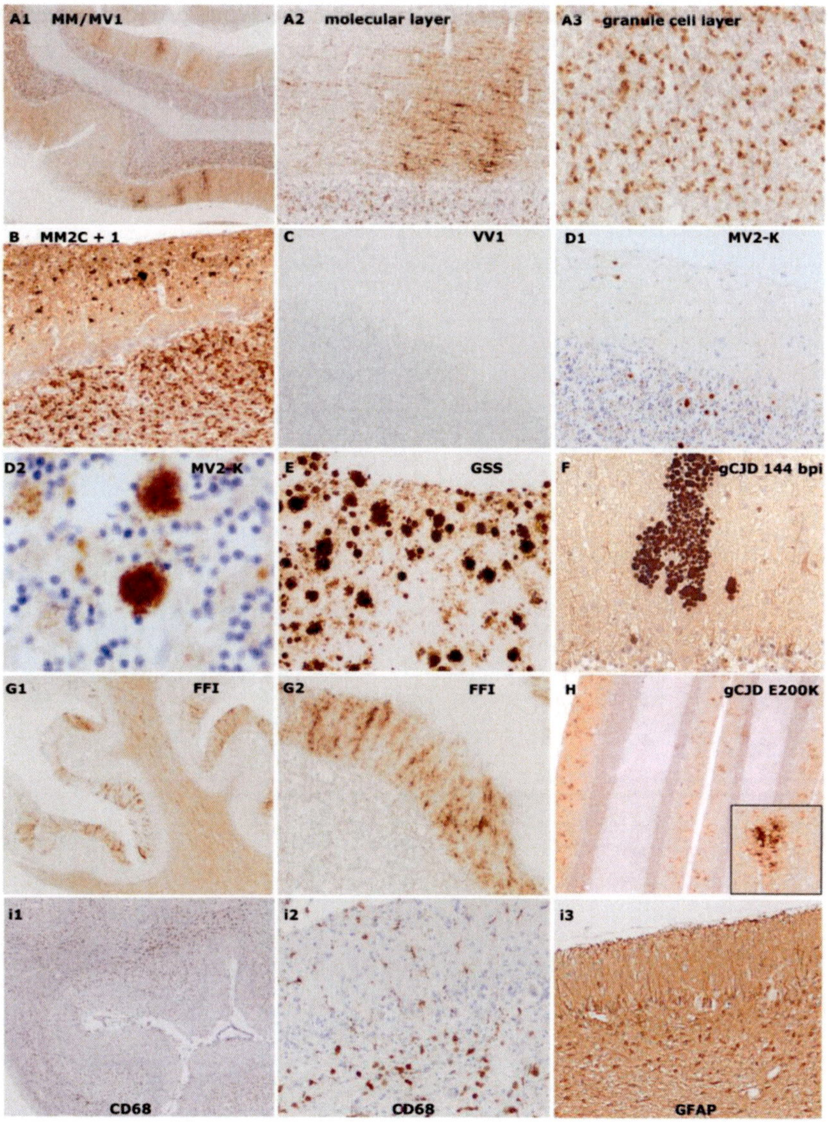

Figure 5. PrP^{sc} immunohistochemical deposition patterns in cerebellum. A1 to A3 illustrates the most characteristic PrP^{sc} deposition patterns observed in cerebellar cortex in sCJD MM/MV1. In molecular layer (A2) a diffuse synaptic pattern is generally observed with focal areas of denser aggregates following parallel fibers. In granule cell layers, coarse aggregates in cerebellar glomerula complete the classical picture (A3). B: Some cases may show in addition to the synaptic PrP^{sc} deposition pattern, coarse aggregates in molecular layer, as seen in MM2C or mixed cases. In contrast, VV1 cases may show very faint or even absent PrP^{sc} aggregates (C). The sCJD MV2K subtype (D1) is characterized by the presence of unicentric PrP amyloid or Kuru-plaques, which are more frequently encountered in granule cell layer (D2) than in molecular layer. In contrast, in GSS (E), multicentric plaques are typically seen in molecular layer. When unusual PrP^{sc} aggregates in form of coarse, plaque-like or grape-like globules are observed in molecular layer, the suspicion of *PRNP* mutation / base-pair insertion (bpi) can be raised, as seen in a 144 bpi case (F). In other genetic cases such as FFI (G1-G2) or E200K mutation (H), a stripe-like pattern may be detected in molecular layer. i1-i3 illustrate reactive changes of cerebellum when it is severely affected by a prion disease, such as intense microglial activation (i1 and i2 – immunohistochemistry for CD68) and intense astrogliosis (i3 – immunohistochemistry for GFAP).

Diffuse synaptic deposits have been detected in neurohypophysis. In the eye, PrP^{sc} has been detected in the synaptic layers of the retina and in lower levels in the optic nerve, in both, sCJD and vCJD [88]. Even if by immunohistochemistry it is difficult to observe, PrP^{sc} has been reported to accumulate in astrocytes, microglia and macrophages. PrP^{sc} hasn't been described in oligodendrocytes, myelin sheaths or ependymal cells. In choroid plexus, some focal immunoreactivity has been detected with some antibodies. In areas devoid of PrP^{c}, e.g. due to an old infarction of grey matter, no PrP^{sc} aggregates will be detected in that area in contrast to the presence of abundant aggregates in adjacent, non-infarcted areas (H. Budka).

b.) In Genetic Forms

In GSS, PrP^{sc} aggregates in form of *multicentric plaques* in cortical areas and also in cerebellum, here preferentially in molecular layer whereas unicentric plaques predominate in granule cell layer (Figure 5E). In addition, a diffuse synaptic staining pattern can be observed as a background staining of cerebral and cerebellar cortices and deep grey matter (Figure 6B2, B3).

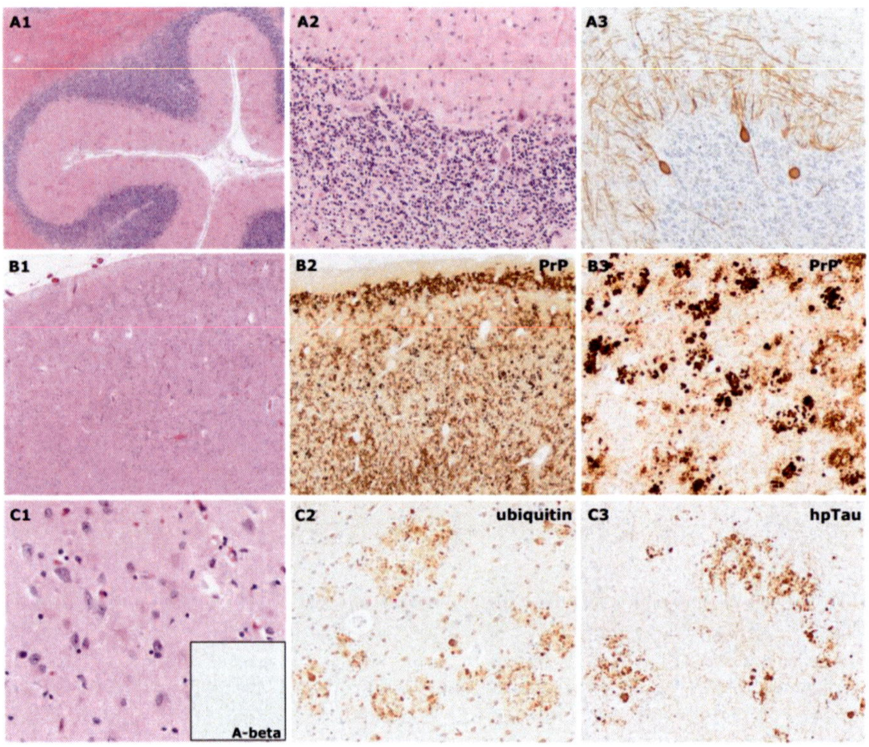

Figure 6. Neuropathological features of Gerstmann-Sträussler-Scheinker disease – GSS. The histopathological hallmark of GSS is the presence of multicentric PrP^{sc} amyloid plaques. These are already visible on HE stained sections in molecular layer of cerebellum (A1, A2) and throughout the cerebral cortex (B1 and C1). In cerebellum, they may also induce a segmental Purkinje cell loss with formation of torpedoes (A2) in granule cell layer that are highlighted by immunohistochemistry with anti-neurofilament antibodies (A3). In granule cell layers, unicentric plaques are also frequently observed. Multicentric plaques are strongly immunolabeled by anti-PrP antibodies (B2 and B3) where amorphous and synaptic aggregates are also observed between the plaques. The plaques are highly neuritic and neurites immunoreact with ubiquitin (C2) and hyperphosphorylated tau (C3, AT8).

In contrast, in FFI PrP^{sc} deposits may be undetectable or only focally observed as diffuse synaptic deposits in subiculum/entorrhinal cortex or may be focally detected in molecular layer of the cerebellum (Figure 5G1, G2). Here the pattern is different to that observed in sCJD cases, showing more linear deposits perpendicular to the surface. Additionally, fine dotted intraneuronal aggregates may be observed in residual neurons of the inferior olives.

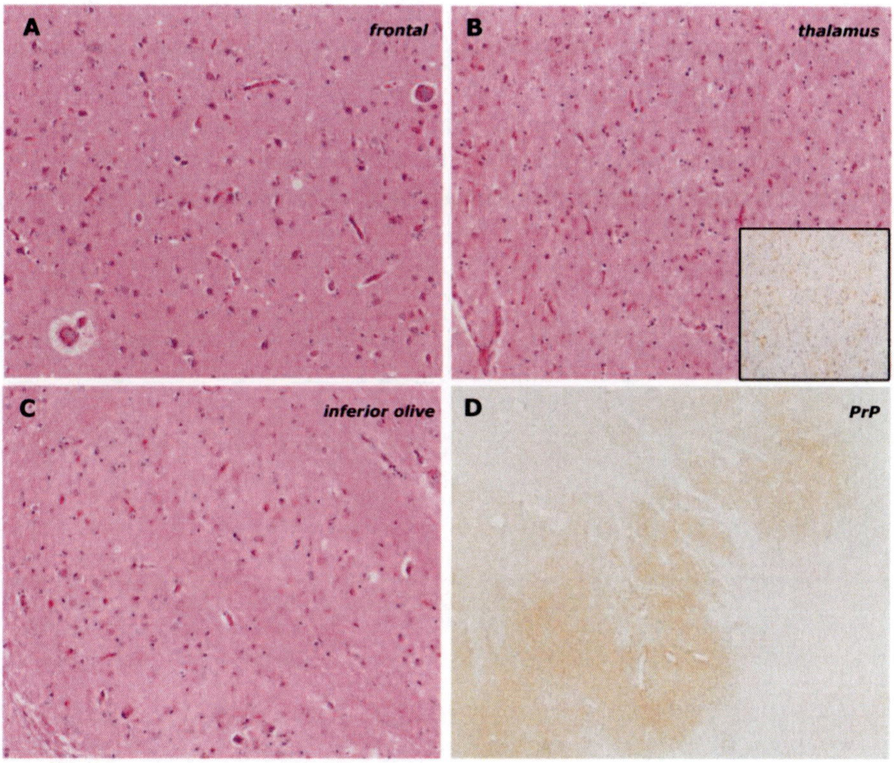

Figure 7. Neuropathological features of fatal familial insomnia – FFI. FFI differs from other human prion disease by its paucity of spongiform change in cortical areas (A), basal ganglia or even cerebellum. In some cases, focal spongiform degeneration of subiculum and entorrhinal cortex can be observed. In contrast, neuronal loss and gliosis of thalamus (B, inset: immunohistochemistry for GFAP showing large star-like reactive astrocytes), subiculum and entorrhinal cortex, and inferior olivary nucleus (C) is a characteristic finding. In cerebellum there might be a segmental Purkinje cell loss. PrP^{sc} deposits may be undetectable or faint in inferior olives and focal in cerebellar molecular layer following an unusual deposition pattern (see also Figure 5 "Cerebellar pathology").

E200K mutation in gCJD shows in addition to a diffuse synaptic pattern in cerebral cortex and basal ganglia, a special pattern in molecular layer with characteristic strips perpendicular to the surface, also called stripe-like, that seems to follow climbing fibers (Figure 5H) [89].

In insertional mutations it has been postulated that the longer the bpi the higher the tendency of PrP to aggregate and to show proteinase K resistance. By PrP immunohistochemistry coarse and patchy, plaque- or grape-like as well as globular deposits especially in molecular layer of cerebellum are a frequent feature (Figure 5F) [58,59,60].

Vascular PrP amyloid has been also described as an isolated or predominant pattern in a genetic disease form caused by a stop codon mutation at codon 145. It is usually accompanied by neurofibrillary pathology [84].

c.) In Acquired Forms

In vCJD, cores of florid plaques are strongly stained and well visualized by immunohistochemistry. In addition, "fine feathery diffuse deposits" or "fine diffuse plaques" are also observed and are weakly stained, less aggregated and amorphous deposits that lack the dense central core of florid plaques (Figure 8B) [73]. There are also irregular pericellular deposits around small neurons (Figure 8B inset) as well as a diffuse synaptic PrP^{sc} deposition pattern in diencephalon and brainstem. Furthermore, a "leopard skin-like" immunostaining pattern has been described in the molecular layer of cerebellum [90].

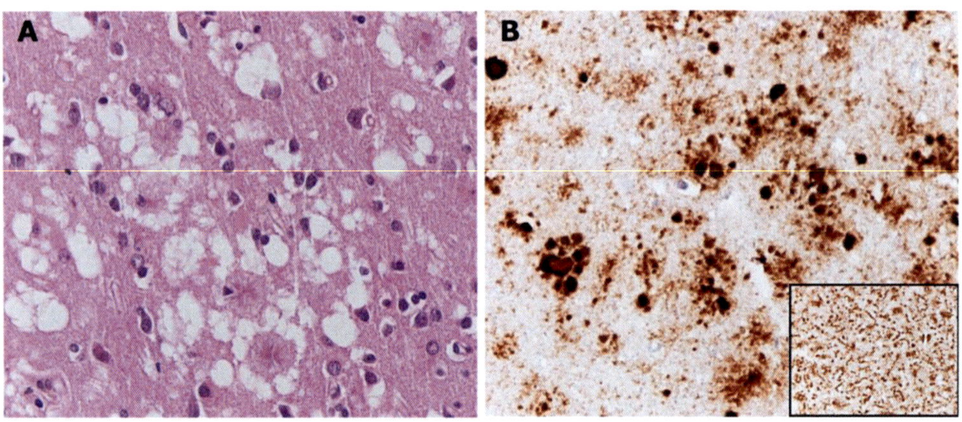

Figure 8. Neuropathological features of variant CJD. *Figure kindly provided by Dr. Alberto Rábano, Director of the Neuropathology Unit and Brain Bank, Research Institute Fundación Cien, Madrid, Spain.* A: The hallmark of vCJD is the presence of florid plaques that consist of a central fibrillar plaque surrounded by a collar of vacuoles. B: PrP^{sc} immunohistochemistry showing plaques, amorphous PrP aggregates and pericellular and perivascular deposits (inset).

In the eye, PrP^{sc} has been detected in the synaptic layers of the retina and in lower levels in the optic nerve [88].

Armstrong et al. observed significant differences in the distribution of the PrP^{sc} deposits in sCJD and vCJD [73]. The diffuse and florid PrP^{sc} deposits were more frequently distributed in the upper cortex in vCJD while the synaptic deposits were predominantly distributed in the lower cortex in sCJD.

In Kuru, cortical areas may show diffuse synaptic PrP^{sc} deposits when present at low levels; at higher density PrP^{sc} may form dense plaques that vary from small dense granules to plaques of up to 30 mm in diameter [31].

McLean et al. have compared neuropathological features of Kuru and vCJD brains and observed distinct differences, particularly in the immunohistochemical PrP deposition pattern. In vCJD they observed a much greater PrP^{sc} load in all brain areas than in Kuru, except in granule cell layer of cerebellum. This was better visualized using 12F10 antibody than 3F4.

PrP patterns also varied. The authors summarize that Kuru pathology resembles more MV2 sCJD cases [69].

The distribution of the normal, cellular PrP^c has been studied in other neurodegenerative diseases such as Alzheimer´s disease, Lewy-body disease, PSP, MSA, and motoneuron disease [91]. Fibrillar inclusions did not show immunoreactivity for PrP^c but in early, cytoplasmic lesions an overlap of hpTau or alpha-synuclein and PrP^c was observed. The authors also observed a loss of PrP^c immunoreactivity in motor neurons in ALS, suggesting in all that PrP^c may react unspecifically to cellular stress, independently of the underlying protein aggregation. Non-specific immunoreactivity may be observed in the absence of a prion disease; for example in the core or at the periphery / neuritic component of senile plaques of Alzheimer's disease, but not in neurofibrillary tangles or other intraneuronal inclusion bodies of other neurodegenerative diseases. In beta-amyloid plaques PrP immunoreactivity is considered to represent most likely a co-aggregation of the cellular PrP in the plaque. Thus, any PrP immunoreactivity has to be interpreted with caution and experience and appropriate controls should be used.

VIIb.) By histoblot and Paraffin-Embedded Tissue Blot

Paraffin-embedded tissue (PET) blot is a very useful tool when unfixed tissue is not available for Histoblot or Western blot studies to analyze the protease resistant core of PrP. It allows the study of PrP^{res} on formalin-fixed and paraffin embedded tissue blocks. Paraffin sections are placed onto nitro-cellulose membrane for detection of PrP^{sc} using a monoclonal antibody (e.g. 3F4) after proteinase K digestion [92].

Patterns are comparable to those observed by immunohistochemistry, i.e. diffuse granular or synaptic pattern, coarse or patchy/perivacuolar deposits and different types of plaques. The most affected area observed in the neuropathological study should be ideally used for these studies.

VIId.) By Western blot

Whenever frozen tissue is available, Western blot analysis for typing of the prion protein should complement the neuropathological study and should be carried out at a micro-biological containment level 3 facility, adhering to safety protocols.

A brain homogenate is usually made from frozen tissue and is cleared by low speed centrifugation. The supernatant is then digested with proteinase K. The protease resistant fragments are separated by SDS-PAGE and transferred to nitrocellulose or PVDF membranes. For its detection, a monoclonal anti-PrP antibody (e.g. 3F4) together with a horseradish peroxidase conjugated secondary antibody and an enhanced chemiluminiscence system is used.

Depending on the glycosylation pattern, conformation and degree of resistance to protease digestion different subtypes of PrP^{res} have been described and can co-exist in the same brain. These types correlate well with clinical and neuropathological features of disease. According to the electrophoretic mobility of the proteinase K resistant core fragment, two major types are described: type 1 (21 kDa and primary cleavage site at residue 82) and type 2 (19 kDa and primary cleavage site at residue 97). Both types are seen in all subtypes of CJD, independently of their etiology, and may even co-exist in the same brain (mixed subtypes). According to their glycosylation, type 1 and type 2 can be further subdivided in pattern A when the monoglycosylated form predominates and type B, where the fully glycosylated form is present. The only disease form that shows PrP^{res} type 2B is variant CJD.

The London classification describes also four PrP^{res} types, but are labeled as PrP^{res} type 1 to 4 [93,94].

Recently, a variably protease-sensitive sporadic prionopathy has been described in which Western blot studies showed 5 major bands with the antibody 1E4 migrating at approximately 26kDa, 23kDa, 20kDa, 17kDa, and 7kDa, in contrast to other CJD forms with the classical pattern of 3 bands migrating at 32/30kDa, 28/26kDa, and 21/19kDa [25].

In vivo, when the suspicion of variant CJD is raised, some peripheral tissues can be biopsied and are informative enough on the presence of PrP^{res} by Western blot and/or immunohistochemistry, e.g. lymphoid tissues, being the palatine tonsils the most accessible. A positive biopsy is used as a diagnostic criterium for probable vCJD when other clinical signs are present and complementary paraclinical examinations support the clinical suspicion.

Extraneural PrP Deposition

a.) In Sporadic Forms

Deposition of PrP^{sc} is not restricted to the central nervous system and has been also detected in peripheral nervous system, including autonomic ganglia, in all forms of disease [95,96]. Glatzel et al analyzed the presence of PrP^{sc} in extraneural tissues of patients with sporadic CJD [97]. A part from brain, they found PrP^{sc} in 10/28 spleens and 8/32 skeletal muscle samples using a three times more sensitive Western blot technique by differential precipitation with sodium phosphotungstic acid. The levels of PrP^{sc} were much lower than those of the brain by a factor of 1:10-4 and were not detectable by standard plain Western blot analyses. Patients with extraneural PrP^{sc} (around one third) had a significantly longer duration of disease and were more likely to have uncommon molecular variants of sporadic Creutzfeldt–Jakob disease such as MM2C and MV2. Due to the longer disease duration, it has been suggested that a protracted disease course may increase the probability of central PrP^{sc} to spread to the periphery.

It has been also suggested that conditions that induce an overexpression of PrP^{c}, such as chronic inflammation, may increase the chance of conversion of PrP^{c} to PrP^{sc}. Indeed, PrP^{sc} has been detected in granulomatous inflammatory processes and in the muscle of a patient with sCJD and concomitant inclusion body myositis [98].

Furthermore, PrP^{sc} has been focally detected in the walls of intracerebral and extracerebral arteries such as basilar artery and/or branches of circulus Willisi, extracranial segments of carotid artery and/or ascending aorta by immunohistochemistry and PET-blot in sporadic and in variant CJD [99]. PrP^{sc} deposits were mainly detected in the tunica media of deep perforating and occasionally of meningeal and basal arteries and in small parenchymal vessels, rarely in the intima. There was no correlation between the presence of vascular PrP and the amount of PrP^{sc} deposits in the brain parenchyma. By double immunofluorescence, the authors observed that PrP^{sc} deposits were in HLA-DR and S100 positive elements of the vascular-associated dendritic cell network, and in macrophages of intima and media, suggesting that these elements may be involved in the spread of PrP^{sc} and possibly also of infectivity.

b.) In Genetic Forms

A stop mutation of *PRNP* at codon 145 induces typically a PrP amyloid angiopathy and has been called vascular variant of CJD with abundant tangles [84].

c.) In Acquired Forms

In variant CJD, it was considered that due to the oral route of prion infection, tissues and organs outside the CNS could be affected. Indeed, lymphoreticular organs such as lymph nodes, spleen, appendix, and tonsils, as well as colon, ileum, jejunum, rectum borne PrP^{sc}, and have been detected by both, western blot and immunohistochemical studies and some, but not all, by bioassays or transmission studies. In addition, adrenal gland, autonomic ganglia, spinal ganglia, trigeminal ganglia, peripheral nerves, and skeletal muscle have shown PrP^{sc}. Recently, Notari et al described multiorgan distribution of PrP^{sc} in a vCJD case with long disease duration (32 months) and found PrP^{sc} not only in lymphoreticular system, pituitary and adrenal glands, and gastrointestinal tract, but also in the dura mater, liver, pancreas, kidney, ovary, uterus, and skin using highly sensitive immunoblot and higher tissue concentrations [90].

Head et al. investigated the presence of PrPres in oral and dental tissues of vCJD subjects. Trigeminal ganglion, alveolar nerve, dental pulp, gingiva, salivary gland, tongue and tonsils were studied by Western blot, PET blot and immunocytochemistry [100]. Disease-associated PrP was only detected in the brain, trigeminal ganglia and tonsils. The same group also investigated the presence of PrP^{sc} in the eyes of sCJD and vCJD. They detected PrP^{sc} accumulation throughout the synaptic layers of the retina in sCJD and vCJD [88]. The levels of PrP^{sc} found in the retina were comparable with those found in the brain. Lower levels of PrP^{sc} could be found in the optic nerve, but no PrP^{sc} was detectable in other ocular tissues. The glycoform ratio of PrP^{sc} in the retina did not correspond to that found in the brain.

Koperek et al also described the presence of PrP^{sc} in the vessel walls of intracerebral and extracranial arteries in vCJD [99].

In addition, peripheral blood is considered to harbor infectivity. Isolated cases of secondary vCJD transmission after blood donation from preclinial vCJD donors caused disease in blood recipients [101]. Infectivity is most likely caused by the migration of cellular elements of the lymphoreticular system carrying PrP^{sc} to and from the blood.

In Kuru, no abnormal PrP deposition has been detected in heart, pericardium, lung, muscle, thymus, dura and cranial nerves by immunohistochemistry. By highly sensitive Western blots no PrP^{sc} could be detected in spleen or in distal ileum [31]. Negative tonsil biopsy has been also reported [102]. These findings are of great interest, because the probably common peripheral route of exposure with vCJD has raised the hypothesis that involvement of peripheral tissues would be comparable to that of vCJD. This may thus indicate that characteristic peripheral pathogenesis of vCJD is probably more likely defined by prion strain type rather than route of infection [31].

In vivo detection of PrP^{sc} is still under investigation. There are no methods to detected pathological PrP in blood or CSF with sufficient specificity, as currently available methods are too sensitive and also seem to detect cellular PrP.

VIII.) Co-deposition of other Abnormal Protein Aggregates in CJD

It is increasingly suggested that in neurodegenerative diseases several proteins such as amyloid beta, tau and alpha-synuclein interact synergistically, promoting the aggregation, phosphorylation and accumulation of each other, and thus accelerating cellular dysfunction and disease progression. Since cellular PrP has been involved in the resistance to oxidative stress, it is possible that PrP with an abnormal conformation may also contribute to the pathogenesis of other neurodegenerative diseases. PrP^c overexpression has been shown experimentally to inhibit the beta-secretase cleavage of APP reducing amyloid-beta formation while its depletion increased amyloid-beta peptides.

Based on these observations, it is important to perform additional immunohistochemical stains when diagnosing a prion disease to evaluate the presence of concomitant abnormal protein aggregates that characterize neurodegenerative diseases. The most frequently used stains include silver stains (e.g. Gallyas or modified Bielschowsky) and immunohistochemistry using antibodies directed against *ubiquitin, p62, beta-amyloid* (for Alzheimer's disease and cerebral amyloid angiopathy), *hyperphosphorylated tau* (AT8) and its *3- and 4-repeat isoforms* (e.g. for Alzheimer's disease and tauopathies such as corticobasal degeneration, progressive supranuclear palsy, argyrophilic grain disease, atypical forms, Pick's disease), *alpha-synuclein* (for Parkinson's disease, Lewy body dementia and multiple system atrophy), *alpha-internexin* (for neuronal intermediate filament inclusion disease), and TAR-DNA binding protein *TDP43* and fused in sarcoma protein *FUS* (both for a subgroup of fronto-temporal lobar degeneration and amyotrophic lateral sclerosis).

a) In Sporadic Forms

Indeed, concomitant deposition of tau, alpha-synuclein and amyloid-beta has been reported in human prion disease. Hainfellner et al observed Alzheimer type pathology in 30% of sCJD cases, but in their series the authors conclude that it might have been more related to ageing [103]. The presence of concomitant Alzheimer-type pathology may be influenced by the ApoE carrier status, ε4 carriers having the higher risk of AD pathology [104]. Recently, "minimal change" multiple system atrophy with alpha-synuclein immunoreactive glial cytoplasmic inclusions has been described in the brain of an otherwise typical MM1 CJD subject [105] who also showed moderate Alzheimer-type pathology. We have also observed a MV2 cases with abundant alpha-synuclein Lewy bodies and neurites in brainstem nuclei and limbic areas corresponding to Braak stage 4 of Parkinson's disease related pathology. Vital et al have also reported a 79 year old sCJD MV1 patient with long disease duration (> 2 years) who showed in addition to spongiform encephalopathy, neurofibrillary pathology in the neocortex, marked beta amyloid cerebral angiopathy and several Lewy bodies in brainstem nuclei and in cortical neurons [106].

Frequently, fine hpTau immunoreactive cell processes are found surrounding vacuolar change in cortical areas, independently of the presence of Alzheimer´s disease related pathology. Additionally, granular alpha-synuclein deposits have been observed in sCJD, iCJD and vCJD, mainly in cases with longer disease duration.

In a study by Vital et al. of the nigrostriatal pathway the authors found alpha-synuclein, ubiquitin, and 14-3-3 aggregation coexisting with prion protein aggregation, thereby generating mixed pathological features, suggesting a possible pathophysiological overlap of abnormal protein aggregation in CJD and Parkinson disease [32].

b) In Genetic Forms

A systematic clinical, neuropathological and biochemical study of 39 CJD subjects carrying the E200K *PRNP* mutation, revealed parenchymal amyloid-beta deposition in 53%, beta-amyloid angiopathy in 23.1%, phospho-tau immunoreactive neuritic profiles in 92.3%, neurofibrillary degeneration in 38.45%, new types of tau pathology in 33.3% and Lewy-type alpha-synuclein pathology in 15.4% [107].

In GSS, abundant hpTau-immunoreactive neurofibrillary pathology has been described, in both, surrounding multicentric plaques and diffusely distributed in limbic areas, generally without amyloid beta deposits [108,109]. Plaques are also usually accumulating ubiquitin, a essential molecule that targets abnormal proteins to be degraded by the ubiquitin-proteasome system. (Figure) In FFI, concomitant alpha-synuclein positive Lewy body pathology has been also described [110].

c) In Acquired Forms

In iCJD, concomitant Alzheimer-type pathology has been detected in a 28-year old patient. The authors postulated that traumatic brain injury that lead to dura transplant at the age of 4 years might have triggered AD-pathology [111].

IX.) Differential Diagnoses from Autopsy Series

Rapidly progressive cognitive decline with additional neurological symptoms that might suggest a prion disease may be caused by other conditions. Alternative neuropathological diagnoses include Alzheimer's disease, rapidly progressive diffuse Lewy-body disease, corticobasal degeneration, vascular encephalopathy, metabolic encephalopathy, limbic or other type of encephalitis (viral or autoimmune / paraneoplasic), primary brain tumors (e.g. lymphoma), leptomeningeal carcinomatosis [110,112].

X.) Neuronal Systems and Their Clinico-Pathological Correlates

As observed in most neurological disorders, it is generally the alteration of neuronal systems that leads to clinical symptoms. Basic behavioral and cognitive domains of human beings are regulated by functional pathways that interconnect cortical areas with basal ganglia, diencephalic, brainstem and cerebellar structures and spinal cord (scheme 1).

When disease involves primary sensory and/or motor areas, there will be an alteration of the somatosensory perception of face, trunk, upper and lower extremities and/or a dysfunction of the motor system of head, hands and arms, feet and legs, as well as coordination and equilibrium. In addition, there might be a dysfunction of the visual/auditory sensory and oculomotor systems, olfaction, taste and even autonomic and endocrine functions, as reported in some dura-related iatrogenic CJD cases [113].

For example, the frequent involvement of occipital cortex including primary visual area (Brodmann Area A17) leads to the classical *cortical blindness* observed in MM/MV1 sCJD subtype, that has been also called amaurotic subtype or Heidenhain variant.

The frequently observed *myoclonus* is considered to have a cortical origin and is most likely caused by a dysfunction of the sensorimotor cortex. Additionally, in conditions associated with cortical myoclonus the cerebellar system has been involved, emphasizing the association of myoclonus with degeneration of the olivodentatorubral system, with or without involvement of the dentate nucleus, loss of Purkinje cells, and Bergmann gliosis in the cerebellar cortex, preferentially affecting the vermis and superior lobes or the lateral cerebellar hemispheres [114].

Parkinsonism is probably caused by severe spongiform degeneration, neuronal loss and gliosis of caudate and putamen, inducing a post-synaptic parkinsonism (striatal alteration), as well as by a loss and dysfunction of dopaminergic neurons of substantia nigra causing a pre-synaptic parkinsonism, as observed in Parkinson's disease, or a combination of both. Dysfunction of other brainstem nuclei involved in circuits for motor and sensorimotor integration (including spinal cord, brainstem, cerebellum, basal ganglia and cortex) may induce dystonia. Infrequent presentations include bulbar dysfunction that can be diagnosed as motor neuron disease or Miller Fisher variant of Guillain-Barré syndrome [115]. In some patients, paraspastic gait has been described as be an unusual presenting symptom and has been related with bilateral parietal edge syndrome—that is, first motoneuron dysfunction in the leg areas of both precentral gyri [116].

Ataxia is a prominent symptom in several disease forms and is caused by cerebellar degeneration. Vermal atrophy induces truncal ataxia and hemispheric involvement more limb ataxia. In addition, cerebellar pathology may be involved in myoclonus, dysartrhia and periodic alternating nystagmus.

Thalamic degeneration and hypothalamic dysfunction as observed in FFI may induce alterations of circadian rhythm, insomnia, and autonomic dysregulation. Alteration of the function of the serotoninergic system might mediate, at least in part, the fluctuating attention and arousal observed in some patients. *Sensory symptoms* appear in around two thirds of vCJD patients and may present as limb pain (63 %, often non-specific and poorly localized), cold feelings (25 %), dysaesthesia (28 %), paraesthesia (31 %) and numbness (25 %) [117]. These symptoms are also considered to have a thalamic origin, as neuropathological changes in the thalamus show marked astrocytosis and neuronal loss. Indeed, MRI shows a very characteristic alteration in the form of symmetric hyperintensity in the pulvinar thalami.

Alterations of *cognitive domains* are a key feature in several neurodegenerative diseases including CJD. Affected fields can be any of those involved in attention and concentration, working memory, implicit and explicit memory, written and oral aspects of language, calculation, tactile and visual-spatial perception, imagery, reasoning, auditory discrimination, and several praxiae (ambulatory, ideomotor, ideational and constructional). Also, abstraction, sequencing and planning, insight, mood-state or affect, thought process and contents as well as behavior may be altered [118].

Thus, in prion disorders, a broad spectrum of complex neurological symptoms and signs may appear. Depending on the CJD subtype, celerity of disease progression varies from a mean of 4 months in MM/MV1 subtypes, 6,5 months in VV2, 17 months in MV2 and more than 15 months in MM2 and VV1 subjects. Clinically, CJD is suspected when a combination of these symptoms appears rapidly in few months and other diseases have been excluded. Prion diseases lead invariably to death, generally in less than 2 years, mainly due to respiratory or systemic infection.

The rapid evolution of the disease and the fact that clinical diagnosis is usually made after excluding all known treatable diseases - which may take several months and frequently different medical visits since the beginning of the symptoms - as well as the concept of transmissibility, makes these diseases difficult to cope with by family members, caregivers and physicians.

CONCLUSION

There are still several intriguing features of human prion disease, not only the nature of the disease agent but also the relatively characteristic brain degeneration pattern and the extremely rapid, probably trans-synaptic degeneration of several, interconnected neuronal systems leading to complex neurological symptoms and signs. Furthermore, the lack of a definite *in vivo* disease marker and of effective treatment strategies makes prion research still necessary. Neuropathological studies are still essential and serve as complementary elements that support and contribute to the efforts made by clinical and basic neuroscientists to better understand prion diseases, in both, human and animal fields.

ACKNOWLEDGMENTS

To all brain donors and relatives for their interest in research, to the Neurological Tissue Bank of the Biobanc-HC-IDIBAPS and to the Institute of Neurology, Medical University of Vienna, especially to Prof. Herbert Budka and Prof. Gabor Kovacs for their support during so many years.

REFERENCES

[1] Creutzfeldt HG. *Z Neurol Psychiatr* (1920)

[2] Jakob A. *Z Neurol Psychiatr* (1921)

[3] Alema G, Bignami A. *Riv Sper Freniatr Med Leg Alien Ment.* 83, Suppl:1485-1623 (1959).

[4] Brownell B, Oppenheimer Dr. *J Neurol Neurosurg Psychiatry.* 28, 350-361 (1965)

[5] Parchi P, Giese A, Capellari S, Brown P, Schulz-Schaeffer W, Windl O, Zerr I, Budka H, Kopp N, Piccardo P, Poser S, Rojiani A, Streichemberger N, Julien J, Vital C, Ghetti B, Gambetti P, Kretzschmar H. *Ann Neurol*; 46, 224-233 (1999)

[6] Zerr I, Kallenberg K, Summers DM, Romero C, Taratuto A, Heinemann U, Breithaupt M, Varges D, Meissner B, Ladogana A, Schuur M, Haik S, Collins SJ, Jansen GH, Stokin GB, Pimentel J, Hewer E, Collie D, Smith P, Roberts H, Brandel JP, van Duijn C, Pocchiari M, Begue C, Cras P, Will RG, Sanchez-Juan P. *Brain.* 132, 2659-2668 (2009)

[7] Lillquist PP, Thomas N, Belay ED, Schonberger LB, Morse D. *Neuroepidemiology*. 26, 207-211 (2006)

[8] Budka H, Aguzzi A, Brown P, Brucher JM, Bugiani O, Collinge J, Diringer H, Gullotta F, Haltia M, Hauw JJ. *Brain Pathol*. 5, 319-322 (1995)

[9] Bell J, Ironside. *J Neuropathol Appl Neurobiol*. 23, 281–288 (1997)

[10] Bell JE, Alafuzoff I, Al-Sarraj S, Arzberger T, Bogdanovic N, Budka H, Dexter DT, Falkai P, Ferrer I, Gelpi E, Gentleman SM, Giaconne G, Huitinga I, Ironside JW, Klioueva N, Kovacs GG, Meyronet D, Palkovits M, Parchi P, Patsouris E, Reynols R, Riederer P, Roggendorf W, Seilhean D, Schmitt A, Schmitz P, Streichenberger N, Schwakber A, Kretzschmar H. *Acta Neuropathol* 115, 497–507 (2008)

[11] WHO infection control guidelines for transmissible spongiform encephalopathies (1999) Available from: *http://www.who.int/emcdocuments/ tse/whocdscsraph2003c.html*

[12] Questions and answers regarding Creutzfeldt-Jakob disease infection- control practices (2003) Available from: *http://www.cdc.gov/ncidod/diseases/cjd/cjd_inf_ ctrl_qa.htm*

[13] Budka H, Aguzzi A, Brown P, Brucher JM, Bugiani O, Gullotta F, Haltia M, Hauw JJ, Ironside JW, Jellinger K. *Brain Pathology*. 5, 459–466 (1995)

[14] Budka H. *Br Med Bull*. 66, 121-130 (2003)

[15] Armstrong RA. *Patholog Res Int*. 2011, 236346 (2010)

[16] De Lacoste M. C. and White C. L.. *Neurobiology of Aging*. 14, 1–16 (1993).

[17] Liberski PP, Sikorska B, Hauw JJ, Kopp N, Streichenberger N, Giraud P, Boellaard J, Budka H, Kovacs GG, Ironside J, Brown P. *Ultrastruct Pathol*. 34, 351-361 (2010)

[18] Liberski PP, Brown P, Xiao SY, Gajdusek DC. *J Comp Pathol*. 105, 377-386 (1991)

[19] Liberski P. *Acta Neurobiol Exp (Wars)*. 68, 113-121 (2008)

[20] Masters C. L. and Richardson E. P.. *Brain*. 101, 333–344 (1978)

[21] Armstrong R. A.. *Current Neurovascular Research*. 6, 239–245 (2009)

[22] Mallucci G, Dickinson A, Linehan J, Klöhn PC, Brandner S, Collinge J. *Science* 302, 871-874 (2003)

[23] Meissner B, Kallenberg K, Sanchez-Juan P, Collie D, Summers DM, Almonti S, Collins SJ, Smith P, Cras P, Jansen GH, Brandel JP, Coulthart MB, Roberts H, Van Everbroeck B, Galanaud D, Mellina V, Will RG, Zerr I. *Neurology*. 72, 1994-2001 (2009)

[24] Kobayashi S, Saito Y, Maki T, Murayama S. *Clin Neurol Neurosurg*. 112, 520-523 (2010)

[25] Zou WQ, Puoti G, Xiao X, Yuan J, Qing L, Cali I, Shimoji M, Langeveld JP, Castellani R, Notari S, Crain B, Schmidt RE, Geschwind M, Dearmond SJ, Cairns NJ, Dickson D, Honig L, Torres JM, Mastrianni J, Capellari S, Giaccone G, Belay ED, Schonberger LB, Cohen M, Perry G, Kong Q, Parchi P, Tagliavini F, Gambetti P. *Ann Neurol*. 68, 162-172 (2010)

[26] Gambetti P, Puoti G, Zou WQ. *J Mol Neurosci*. May 17 (2011)

[27] Kovacs GG, Trabattoni G, Hainfellner JA, Ironside JW, Knight RS, Budka H. *J Neurol* 249, 1567-1582 (2002)

[28] Ironside J. W.. *Archives of Virology*. Suppl 16, 143–151 (2000)

[29] Armstrong RA, Lantos PL, Ironside JW, Cairns NJ. *J Neural Transm*. 110, 130313-11 (2003)

[30] Rezaie P, Al-Sarraj S. *Acta Neuropathol.* 114, 651-658 (2007)
[31] Brandner S, Whitfield J, Boone K, Puwa A, O'Malley C, Linehan JM, Joiner S, Scaravilli F, Calder I, P Alpers M, Wadsworth JD, Collinge J. *Philos Trans R Soc Lond B Biol Sci.* 363, 3755-3763 (2008)
[32] Vital A, Fernagut PO, Canron MH, Joux J, Bezard E, Martin-Negrier ML, Vital C, Tison F. *J Neuropathol Exp Neurol.* 68, 809-815 (2009)
[33] Guentchev M, Wanschitz J, Voigtländer T, Flicker H, Budka H. *Am J Pathol.* 155, 1453-1457 (1999)
[34] Puig B, Ferrer I. *Acta Neuropathol.* 102, 207-215 (2001)
[35] Gray F, Chrétien F, Adle-Biassette H, Dorandeu A, Ereau T, Delisle MB, Kopp N, Ironside JW, Vital C. *J Neuropathol Exp Neurol.* 58, 321-328 (1999)
[36] Kovacs GG, Budka H. *Brain Res.* 1323, 192-199 (2010)
[37] Paquet C, Bose A, Polivka M, Peoc'h K, Brouland JP, Keohane C, Hugon J, Gray F. *J Neuropathol Exp Neurol.* 68, 190-198 (2009)
[38] Ferrer I. *Acta Neuropathol.* 97, 5-12 (1999)
[39] Kovács GG, Gelpi E, Ströbel T, Ricken G, Nyengaard JR, Bernheimer H, Budka H. *J Neuropathol Exp Neurol.* 66, 628-636 (2007)
[40] Kovacs GG, Sanchez-Juan P, Ströbel T, Schuur M, Poleggi A, Nocentini S, Giannattasio C, Belay G, Bishop M, Capellari S, Parchi P, Gelpi E, Gal A, Bakos A, Molnar MJ, Heinemann U, Zerr I, Knight RS, Mitrova E, van Duijn C, Budka H. *Alzheimer Dis Assoc Disord.* 24, 104-107 (2010)
[41] Deretic V. *Trends in Immunology* 26, 523-528 (2005)
[42] Sikorska B, Liberski PP, Giraud P, Kopp N, Brown P. *Int J Biochem Cell Biol.* 36, 2563-2573 (2004)
[43] Liberski, P.P., Sikorska, B., Bratosiewicz-Wasik, J., Gajdusek, D.C., Brown, P. *Int J Biochem Cell Biol.* 36, 2473–2490 (2004)
[44] Unterberger U, Höftberger R, Gelpi E, Flicker H, Budka H, Voigtländer T. *J Neuropathol Exp Neurol.* 65, 348-357 (2006)
[45] Ferrer I. *Cerebellum.* 1, 213-222 (2002)
[46] Ferrer I, Puig B, Blanco R, Martí E. *Neuroscience.* 97, 715-726 (2000)
[47] Mizutani T. *Acta Pathologica Japonica*, 31, 903–922 (1981)
[48] von Eitzen U, Egensperger R, Kösel S, Grasbon-Frodl EM, Imai Y, Bise K, Kohsaka S, Mehraein P, Graeber MB. *J Neuropathol Exp Neurol*, 57, 246–256 (1998)
[49] Barcikowska M, Liberski PP, Boellaard JW, Brown P, Gajdusek DC, Budka H. *Acta Neuropathol.* 85, 623-627 (1993)
[50] Higuchi M. *Curr Alzheimer Res.* 6, 137-143 (2009)
[51] Ramlackhansingh AF, Brooks DJ, Greenwood RJ, Bose SK, Turkheimer FE, Kinnunen KM, Gentleman S, Heckemann RA, Gunanayagam K, Gelosa G, Sharp DJ. *Ann Neurol.* 70, 374-383 (2011)
[52] McRae A, Dahlström A, Polinsky R, Ling EA. *Behav Brain Res.* 57, 225-234 (1993)
[53] Mattsson N, Tabatabaei S, Johansson P, Hansson O, Andreasson U, Månsson JE, Johansson JO, Olsson B, Wallin A, Svensson J, Blennow K, Zetterberg H. *Neuromolecular Med.* 13, 151-159 (2011)
[54] Minghetti L, Pocchiari M. *Int Rev Neurobiol.* 82, 265-275 (2007)
[55] Kobayashi A, Arima K, Ogawa M, Murata M, Fukuda T, Kitamoto T. *Acta Neuropathol.* 116, 561-566 (2008)

[56] Liberski PP. *Folia Neuropathol.* 42 Suppl B:109-119 (2004)
[57] Sikorska B, Liberski PP, Sobów T, Budka H, Ironside JW. *Neuropathol Appl Neurobiol.* 35, 46-59 (2009)
[58] Capellari S, Vital C, Parchi P, Petersen RB, Ferrer X, Jarnier D, Pegoraro E, Gambetti P, Julien J. *Neurology*, 49, 133-141 (1997)
[59] Collinge J, Brown J, Hardy J, Mullan M, Rossor MN, Baker H, Crow TJ, Lofthouse R, Poulter M, Ridley R, et al. *Brain*, 115, 687-710 (1992)
[60] Gelpi E, Kovacs GG, Ströbel T, Koperek O, Voigtländer T, Liberski PP, Budka H. *Acta Neuropathol.* 110, 513-519 (2005)
[61] Liberski P. P., Ironside J, McCardle L, and Sherring A. *Folia Neuropathologica*, 38, 167–170 (2000)
[62] Armstrong R. A., Lantos P. L., Ironside J. W., and Cairns N. J.. *Clin Neuropathol.* 22, 209–214 (2003)
[63] Bresjanac M, Smid LM, Vovko TD, Petric A, Barrio JR, Popovic M. *J Neurosci.* 23, 8029-8033 (2003)
[64] Shimizu S, Hoshi K, Muramoto T, Homma M, Ironside JW, Kuzuhara S, Sato T, Yamamoto T, Kitamoto T. *Arch Neurol.* 56, 357-362 (1999)
[65] Kretzschmar HA, Sethi S, Földvári Z, Windl O, Querner V, Zerr I, Poser S. *Brain Pathol.* 13, 245-249 (2003)
[66] Yamada M, Noguchi-Shinohara M, Hamaguchi T, Nozaki I, Kitamoto T, Sato T, Nakamura Y, Mizusawa H. *Neuropathology.* 29, 609-618 (2009)
[67] Ikawa M, Yoneda M, Matsunaga A, Nakagawa H, Kazama-Suzuki A, Miyashita N, Naiki H, Kitamoto T, Kuriyama M. *J Neurol Sci.* 285, 265-267 (2009)
[68] McLean CA, Ironside JW, Alpers MP, Brown PW, Cervenakova L, Anderson RM, Masters CL. *Brain Pathol.* 8, 429-437 (1998)
[69] McLean CA. *Phil. Trans. R. Soc. B.* 363, 3685–3687(2008)
[70] Richard M, Biacabe AG, Streichenberger N, Ironside JW, Mohr M, Kopp N, Perret-Liaudet A. *Acta Neuropathol.* 105, 296-302 (2003)
[71] Okamura N, Shiga Y, Furumoto S, Tashiro M, Tsuboi Y, Furukawa K, Yanai K, Iwata R, Arai H, Kudo Y, Itoyama Y, Doh-ura K. *Eur J Nucl Med Mol Imaging.* 37, 934-941 (2010)
[72] Hyare H, Ramlackhansingh A, Gelosa G, Edison P, Rudge P, Brandner S, Brooks DJ, Collinge J, Mead S. *J Neurol Neurosurg Psychiatry.* Apr 8 (2011)
[73] R. A. Armstrong, J. W. Ironside, P. L. Lantos, and N. J. Cairns. *Neuropathol Appl Neurobiol.* 35, 36–45 (2009).
[74] W. J. Schulz-Schaeffer, A. Giese, O. Windl, and H. A. Kretzschmar. *Clin Neuropathol.* 15, 353–357 (1996)
[75] Masullo C, Macchi G. *Clin Neuropathol.* 16, 37-44 (1997)
[76] Cartier L, Gálvez S, Gajdusek DC. *J Neurol Neurosurg Psychiatry* 48, 234–238 (1985)
[77] Martinez-Saez E, Gelpi E, Rey M, Ferrer I, Ribalta T, Botta-Orfila T, Nos C, Yagüe J, Sanchez-Valle R. *Neuropathol Appl Neurobiol.* Jul 5 (2011)
[78] Jones M, Wight D, McLoughlin V, Norrby K, Ironside JW, Connolly JG, Farquhar CF, MacGregor IR, Head MW. *Brain Pathol.* 19, 293-302 (2009).
[79] S. Krasemann, M. H. Groschup, S. Harmeyer, G. Hunsmann, and W. Bodemer. *Molecular Medicine*, 2, 725–734 (1996)
[80] Bodemer W. *Naturwissenschaften* 86, 212- 220 (1999)

[81] Hegyi I, Hainfellner JA, Flicker H, Ironside JW, Hauw JJ, Tateishi J, Haltia M, Bugiani O, Aguzzi A, Budka H. *Clin Neuropathol.* 16, 262-263 (1997)
[82] Kovács GG, Head MW, Hegyi I, Bunn TJ, Flicker H, Hainfellner JA, McCardle L, László L, Jarius C, Ironside JW, Budka H. *Brain Pathol.* 12, 1-11 (2002)
[83] Paquet C, Privat N, Kaci R, Polivka M, Dupont O, Haik S, Laplanche J.L., Hauw J.J., Gray F. *Acta Neuropathol.* 116, 567-573 (2008)
[84] Ghetti, B.; Piccardo, P.; Spillantini, M.G.; Ichimiya, Y.; Porro, M.; Perini, F.; Kitamoto, T.; Tateishi, J.; Seiler, C.; Frangione, B.; Bugiani, O.; Giaccone, G.; Prelli, F.; Goedert, M.; Dlouhy, S.R.; Tagliavini, F. *Proc. Natl. Acad. Sci. USA.* 93, 744-748 (1996)
[85] Polymenidou M, Stoeck K, Glatzel M, Vey M, Bellon A, Aguzzi A. *Lancet Neurol.* 4, 805-814 (2005)
[86] Parchi P, Strammiello R, Notari S, Giese A, Langeveld JP, Ladogana A, Zerr I, Roncaroli F, Cras P, Ghetti B, Pocchiari M, Kretzschmar H, Capellari S. *Acta Neuropathol.* 118, 659-671 (2009)
[87] Yull HM, Ironside JW, Head MW. *Biologicals.* 37, 210-5 (2009)
[88] Head MW, Northcott V, Rennison K, Ritchie D, McCardle L, Bunn TJ, McLennan NF, Ironside JW, Tullo AB, Bonshek RE. *Invest Ophthalmol Vis Sci.* 44, 342-346 (2003)
[89] Jarius C, Kovacs GG, Belay G, Hainfellner JA, Mitrova E, Budka H. *Acta Neuropathologica* 105, 449-454 (2003)
[90] Notari S, Moleres FJ, Hunter SB, Belay ED, Schonberger LB, Cali I, Parchi P, Shieh WJ, Brown P, Zaki S, Zou WQ, Gambetti P. *PLoS One.* 5, e8765 (2010)
[91] Kovacs GG, Zerbi P, Voigtländer T, Strohschneider M, Trabattoni G, Hainfellner JA, Budka H. *Neurosci Lett.* 329, 269-272 (2002)
[92] Schulz-Schaeffer WJ, Tschoke S, Kranefuss N, Drose W, Hause-Reitner D, Giese A, Groschup MH, Kretzschmar HA. *Am J Pathol* 156, 51-56 (2000)
[93] Collinge, J., Sidle, K. C. L., Meads, J., Ironside, J. & Hill, A. F. *Nature* 383, 685–690 (1996)
[94] Hill, A. F., Joiner, S., Wadsworth, J. D. F., Sidle, K. C., Bell, J. E., Budka, H., Ironside, J. W. & Collinge, J. *Brain.* 126, 1333-1346 (2003)
[95] Hainfellner JA, Budka H. *Acta Neuropathol.* 98, 458-460 (1999)
[96] Lee CC, Kuo LT, Wang CH, Scaravilli F, An SF. *J Neuropathol Exp Neurol.* 64, 716-721 (2005)
[97] Glatzel M, Abela E, Maissen M, and Aguzzi A. *N Engl J Med.* 349, 1812-1820 (2003)
[98] Kovacs GG, Lindeck-Pozza E, Chimelli L, Araújo AQ, Gabbai AA, Ströbel T, Glatzel M, Aguzzi A, Budka H. *Ann Neurol.* 55, 121-125 (2004)
[99] Koperek O, Kovács GG, Ritchie D, Ironside JW, Budka H, Wick G. *Am J Pathol.* 161, 1979-1984 (2002)
[100] Head MW, Ritchie D, McLoughlin V, Ironside JW. *Br Dent J.*195, 339-343 (2003)
[101] Llewelyn CA, Hewitt PE, Knight RS, Amar K, Cousens S, Mackenzie J, Will RG. *Lancet.* 363, 417-421 (2004)
[102] Collinge J, Whitfield J, McKintosh E, Frosh A, Mead S, Hill AF, Brandner S, Thomas D, Alpers MP. *Philos Trans R Soc Lond B Biol Sci.* 363, 3725-39 (2008)
[103] Hainfellner JA, Wanschitz J, Jellinger K, Liberski PP, Gullotta F, Budka H. *Acta Neuropathol* 96, 116-122 (1998)
[104] Van Everbroeck B, Croes EA, Pals P, Dermaut B, Jansen G, van Duijn CM, Cruts M, Van Broeckhoven C, Martin JJ, Cras P. *Neurosci Lett.* 313, 69-72 (2001)

[105] Rodriguez-Diehl R, Rey MJ, Gironell A, Martinez-Saez E, Ferrer I, Sánchez-Valle R, Jagüe J, Nos C, Gelpi E. *Neuropathology*. doi: 10.1111/j.1440-1789.2011.01232.x. (2011)

[106] Vital A, Canron MH, Gil R, Hauw JJ, Vital C. *Neuropathology*. 27, 273-277 (2007)

[107] Kovacs GG, Seguin J, Quadrio I, Höftberger R, Kapás I, Streichenberger N, Biacabe AG, Meyronet D, Sciot R, Vandenberghe R, Majtenyi K, László L, Ströbel T, Budka H, Perret-Liaudet A. *Acta Neuropathol.* 121, 39-57 (2011).

[108] Amano N, Yagishita S, Yokoi S, Itoh Y, Kinoshita J, Mizutani T, Matsuishi T. *Acta Neuropathol.* 84, 15-23 (1992)

[109] Ghetti B, Dlouhy SR, Giaccone G, Bugiani O, Frangione B, Farlow MR, Tagliavini F. *Brain Pathol.* 5, 61-75 (1995)

[110] Gelpi E, Heinzl H, Hoftberger R, Unterberger U, Strobel T, Voigtlander T, Drobna E, Jarius C, Lang S, Waldhor T, Bernheimer H, Budka H. *Neuroepidemiology*. 30, 215-221 (2008)

[111] Preusser M, Ströbel T, Gelpi E, Eiler M, Broessner G, Schmutzhard E, Budka H. *J Neurol Neurosurg Psychiatry* 77, 413-416 (2006)

[112] Gaig C, Valldeoriola F, Gelpi E, Ezquerra M, Llufriu S, Buongiorno M, Rey MJ, Martí MJ, Graus F, Tolosa E. *Mov Disord.* 26, 1316-1323 (2011)

[113] Meissner B, Kallenberg K, Sanchez-Juan P, Ramljak S, Krasnianski A, Heinemann U, Eigenbrod S, Gelpi E, Barsic B, Kretzschmar HA, Schulz-Schaeffer WJ, Knauth M, Zerr I. *J Neurol.* 256, 355-363 (2009)

[114] Tijssen M.A.J., Thom M, Ellison D.W., Wilkins P, Barnes D, Thompson P.D., and Brown P. *Neurology* 54, 1350–1356 (2000)

[115] Mittal M, Hammond N, Husmann K, Lele A, Pasnoor M. *Muscle Nerve.* 42, 833-855 (2010)

[116] Furtner M, Gelpi E, Kiechl S, Knoflach M, Zangerl A, Gotwald T, Willeit J, Maier H, Ströbel T, Unterberger U, Budka H. *J Neurol Neurosurg Psychiatry* 79, 229-231 (2008)

[117] Macleod MA, Stewart GE, Zeidler M, Will R and Knight R, 249, 706-711 (2002)

[118] 2000, Dennis P. Swiercinsky, Ph.D. *Basic Functional Neuroanatomy Brain Map*

In: Prions and Prion Diseases: New Developments
Editor: Jean-Michel Verdier
ISBN: 978-1-62100-027-3
© 2012 Nova Science Publishers, Inc.

Chapter 2

THE NATURE OF THE INFECTIOUS AGENTS: PRP MODELS OF RESISTANT SPECIES TO PRION DISEASES (DOG, RABBIT AND HORSES)

Jiapu Zhang*
Centre for Informatics and Applied Optimization &
Graduate School of Sciences, Information Technology and Engineering,
The University of Ballarat, Victoria, Australia

Abstract

Prion diseases are invariably fatal and highly infectious neurodegenerative diseases affecting humans and animals. The neurodegenerative diseases such as Creutzfeldt-Jakob disease, variant Creutzfeldt-Jakob diseases, Gerstmann-Sträussler-Scheinker syndrome, Fatal Familial Insomnia, Kuru in humans, scrapie in sheep, bovine spongiform encephalopathy (or mad-cow disease) and chronic wasting disease in cattle etc belong to prion diseases. By now there have not been some effective therapeutic approaches to treat all these prion diseases. In 2008, canine mammals including dogs (canis familials) were the first time academically reported to be resistant to prion diseases (Vaccine 26: 2601–2614 (2008)). Rabbits are the mammalian species known to be resistant to infection from prion diseases from other species (Journal of Virology 77: 2003-2009 (2003)). In 2010 horses were reported to be resistant to prion diseases too (Proceedings of the National Academy of Sciences USA 107: 19808–19813 (2010)). By now all the NMR structures of dog, rabbit and horse prion proteins had been released into protein data bank respectively in 2005, 2007 and 2010 (Proceedings of the National Academy of Sciences USA 102: 640–645 (2005), Journal of Biomolecular NMR 38:181 (2007), Journal of Molecular Biology 400: 121-128 (2010)). Thus, at this moment it is very worth studying the NMR molecular structures of horse, dog and rabbit prion proteins to obtain insights into their immunity prion diseases.

This article reports the findings of the molecular structural dynamics of wild-type horse, dog, and rabbit prion proteins. The dog and horse prion proteins have stable molecular structures whether under neutral or low pH environments. Rabbit prion protein has been found having stable molecular structures under neutral pH environment, but without structural stability under low pH environment. Under low pH environment,

*E-mail addresses: jiapu_zhang@hotmail.com, j.zhang@ballarat.edu.au, Phone: 61-423 487 360

the salt bridges such as D177–R163 were broken and caused the collapse of the stable α-helical molecular structures. The contribution of D177–R163 salt bridge was confirmed by the recent experimental results on the X-ray and NMR structures of rabbit prion protein (Proceedings of National Academy of Sciences USA 107: 19808-19813 (2010), Journal of Biological Chemistry 285 (41), 31682–31693 (2010), Journal of Molecular Biology 400: 121-128 (2010)). This salt bridge might have a value to the scientific community in its drive to find treatments for prion diseases.

Keywords: Prion diseases; Immunity; Rabbit, dog, and horse prion proteins; Molecular dynamics.

1. Introduction

Prion diseases, including Creutzfeldt-Jakob disease (CJD), variant Creutzfeldt-Jakob diseases (vCJD), Gerstmann-Sträussler-Scheinker syndrome (GSS), Fatal Familial Insomnia (FFI), Kuru in humans, scrapie in sheep, bovine spongiform encephalopathy (BSE or 'mad-cow' disease) and chronic wasting disease (CWD) in cattle, etc., are invariably fatal and highly infectious neurodegenerative diseases affecting humans and animals. However, for treating all these diseases, there is no effective therapeutic approach [Aguzzi et al. 2006, Prusiner 1998, Weissmann 2004].

Fortunately, dogs, rabbits, and horses have been reported to be the few mammalian species being resistant to infection from prion diseases. Their NMR molecular structures were released into the Protein Data Bank [Berman et al., 2000] in the years 2003, 2005, 2010 respectively. The N-terminal residues of prion proteins are unstructured and not included in this study. The C-terminal residues are well structured, with 3 α-helices, 2 short anti-parallel β-sheets, and a disulfide bond between the 2nd and 3rd α-helix (residues number 178 and number 213). The infectious prion (PrP^{Sc}) is an abnormally folded form of the normal cellular prion (PrP^{C}) and the conversion of PrP^{C} to PrP^{Sc} is believed to involve conformational change from a predominantly α-helical protein (42% α-helix, 3% β-sheet) to a protein rich in β-sheets (30% α-helix, 43% β-sheet).

Rabbits are one of the few mammalian species reported to be resistant to infection from prion diseases isolated from other species [Vorberg et al., 2003]. Recently, the NMR molecular structures of wild-type, mutant S173N and mutant I214V rabbit prion proteins (124-228) were released into the Protein Data Bank [Berman et al., 2000] with PDB ID codes 2FJ3, 2JOH, 2JOM respectively. Zhang (2010a) studied these NMR structures by MD simulations and simulation results at *450 K* under low and neutral pH environments confirmed the structural stability of wild-type rabbit prion protein. However, the previous MD simulation results at *500 K* under neutral pH environment showed that wild-type rabbit prion protein (124-228) does not have a structural stability [Zhang 2009]. At *450 K*, Zhang (2011a) also studied the molecular dynamics of NMR structures of human and mouse prion proteins (1QLX.pdb and 1AG2.pdb respectively) to make comparisons with that of rabbit prion protein [Zhang 2011a]. The comparisons show that the enhanced stability of the C-terminal ordered region especially helix 2 through the D177-R163 salt-bridge formation renders the rabbit prion protein stable, the salt bridge D201-R155 linking helices 3 and 1 and the hydrogen bond H186-R155 also contribute to the structural stability of rabbit prion protein; however, the human and mouse prion protein structures were not affected by the removing these two salt bridges.

Dogs (canis familials, canine mammals) were the first time academically reported in 2008 to be resistant to prion diseases [Polymenidoua et al. 2008]. Zhang et al. (2011) studied the molecular dynamics of dog prion protein (1XYK.pdb) at *450 K* and found that the dog prion protein has stable molecular structures whether under neutral or low pH environments [Zhang 2011b].

Horses were academically reported to be resistant to prion diseases recently [Perez et al. 2011]. Zhang (2011) studied the molecular dynamics of horse prion protein (2KU4.pdb) at *450 K* and found that the dog prion protein has stable molecular structures whether under neutral or low pH environments [Zhang 2011c]. Molecular dynamics results show that the strong salt bridge ASP177–ARG163 contributes to the structural stability of horse prion protein [Zhang 2011c].

All the above molecular dynamics simulations done for rabbit, dog and horse prion proteins are at *450 K* and *300 K* under neutral and low pH environments. The simulations done at room temperature *300 K* whether under neutral or low pH environment display very little fluctuation for rabbit, dog, horse, human and mouse prion proteins. The common result for rabbit, dog and horse prion proteins found at *450 K* is: there is a strong bridge ASP177–ARG163 (like a taut bow string) keeping the $\beta 2$-$\alpha 2$ loop of prion proteins linked. The finding agrees with the recent experimental results on the $\beta 2$-$\alpha 2$ loop [Bett et al., 2012, Lin et al. 2011, Fernandez-Funez et al. 2011, Perez et al. 2011, Khan et al. 2010, Sweeting et al. 2009, Wen et al. 2010a, Wen et al. 2010b], which plays an important role to stabilize the structural stability of prion proteins.

This Chapter reports the molecular dynamics simulation results done for rabbit, dog and horse prion proteins are at *350 K* under neutral and low pH environments. Molecular dynamics results agree with the results found at *450 K*. The stable α-helical secondary structure of rabbit prion protein collapses under low pH environment. The strong bridge ASP177–ARG163 (like a taut bow string) keeping the $\beta 2$-$\alpha 2$ loop of prion proteins linked contributes to the structural stability of rabbit, dog and horse prion proteins. This salt bridge might be a potential drug target and have a value to the scientific community in its drive to find treatments for prion diseases. The rest of this article is arranged as follows. The molecular dynamics simulation materials and methods are introduced in Section 2. Section 3 mainly gives molecular dynamics simulation results and their discussions. Concluding remarks are given in the last Section.

2. Materials and Methods

The molecular dynamics simulation materials and methods for horse, dog and rabbit prion proteins are completely same as the ones of [Zhang 2010]. Simulation initial structure for the dog and rabbit prion proteins were built on HoPrP^{C}(119-231) (PDB entry 2KU4), DoPrP^{C}(121-231) (PDB entry 1XYK) and RaPrP^{C}(124-228) (PDB entry 2FJ3), respectively. Simulations were done under low pH and normal pH environments respectively. All the simulations were performed with the AMBER 11 package [Case et al. 2010], with analysis carried out using functionalities in AMBER 9 [Case et al. 2006] and AMBER 7

CARNAL [Case et al. 2002]. Graphs were drawn by XMGRACE of Grace 5.1.21, DSSP [Kabsch et al. 1983].

All simulations used the ff03 force field of the AMBER 11 package, in neutral and low pH environments (where residues HIS, ASP, GLU were changed into HIP, ASH, GLH respectively by the XLEaP module of AMBER 11 in order to get the low pH environment). The systems were surrounded with a 12 angstrom layer of TIP3PBOX water molecules and neutralized by sodium ions using XLEaP module of AMBER 11. The solvated proteins with their counterions were minimized mainly by the steepest descent method and then a small number of conjugate gradient steps were performed on the data, in order to remove bad hydrogen bond contacts. Then the solvated proteins were heated from *100* to *300 K* during 1 ns (with step size 1 fs) and from *300* to *350 K* during 1 ns (with step size 2 fs). The thermostat algorithm used is the Langevin thermostat algorithm in constant NVT ensembles. The SHAKE algorithm and PMEMD algorithm with nonbonded cutoffs of 12 angstrom were used during the heating. Equilibrations were done in constant NPT ensembles under Langevin thermostat for 2 ns. After equilibrations, production MD phase was carried out at *350 K* for 30 ns using constant pressure and temperature ensemble and the PMEMD algorithm with nonbonded cutoffs of 12 angstrom during simulations. Step size for the production runs is 2 fs. The structures were saved to file every 1000 steps.

3. Results and Discussion

At *350 K* there are fluctuation and variation among rabbit, dog and horse prion proteins, but their backbone atom RMSDs (root mean square deviations) respectively calculated from their minimized structures and their radii of gyrations do not have great difference even under low pH environment. Their secondary structures under neutral pH environment at *350 K* do not change very much either. However, the secondary structures under low pH environment at *350 K* have great differences between rabbit prion protein and dog and horse prion proteins (Figure 1): the α-helices of rabbit prion protein were completely unfolded and began to turn into β-sheets but those of dog and horse prion proteins were not changed very much. These results indicate the C-terminal region of $RaPrP^C$ has lower thermostability than that of $DoPrP^C$ and $HoPrP^C$. Under the low pH environment, the important salt bridges such as D177-R163, D201-R155 were removed (thus the free energies of the salt bridges changed the thermostability) so that the structure nearby the central helices 1-3 was changed for rabbit prion protein.

There always exists a strong salt bridge (where the oxygen-nitrogen distance cut-off calculated for the salt bridges is 3.2 angstroms) between D177-R163 for rabbit prion protein, and D178-R164 for dog and horse prion proteins (Figure 2) under neutral pH environment at *300 K*, *350 K*, and *450 K*. We can see in Figure 2 that this salt bridge is just like a taut bow string linking β2-sheet and α2-helix. It contributes to the structural stability of all these prion proteins. Thus, the region of $\beta 2$–$\alpha 2$ loop should be a potential drug target region according to recent reports on the $\beta 2$–$\alpha 2$ loop of prion proteins [Bett et al., 2012, Lin et al. 2011, Fernandez-Funez et al. 2011, Perez et al. 2011, Khan et al. 2010, Sweeting et al. 2009, Wen et al. 2010a, Wen et al. 2010b].

Lastly, we compare rabbit with dog and horse prion proteins through the pairwise sequence and structure alignments. We find that there are more identities and similarities be-

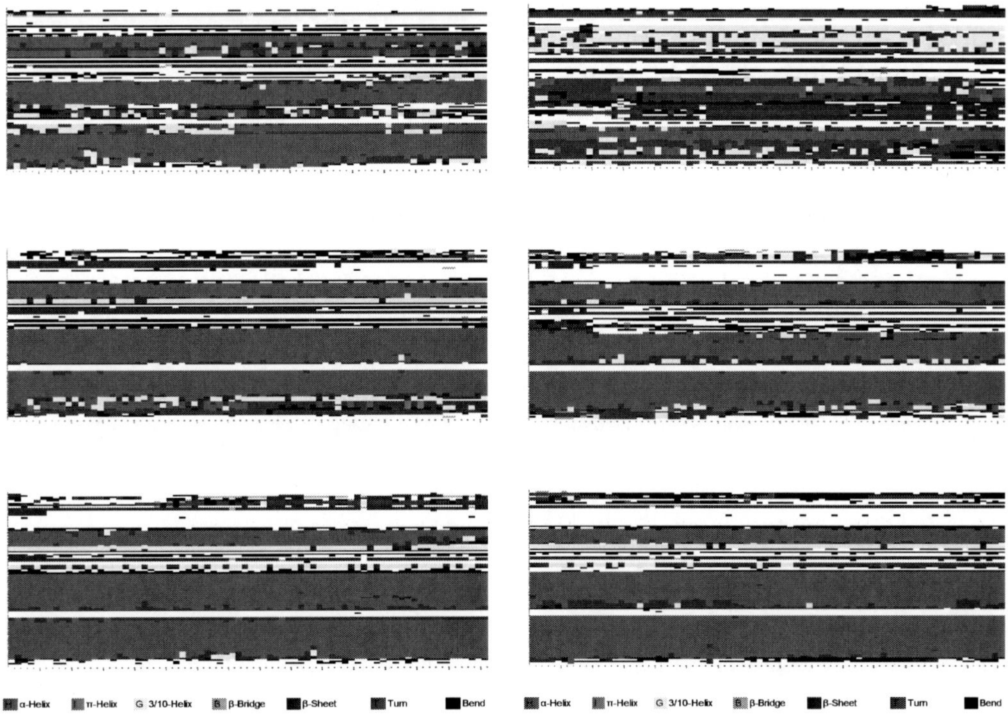

Figure 1. Secondary structures of rabbit, dog and horse prion proteins (from up to down) at *350 K* under neutral to low pH environments (from left to right) (X-axis: 0 ns - 30 ns (from left to right), Y-axis: residue numbers 124 - 228 / 121 - 231 / 119 - 231 (from up to down)).

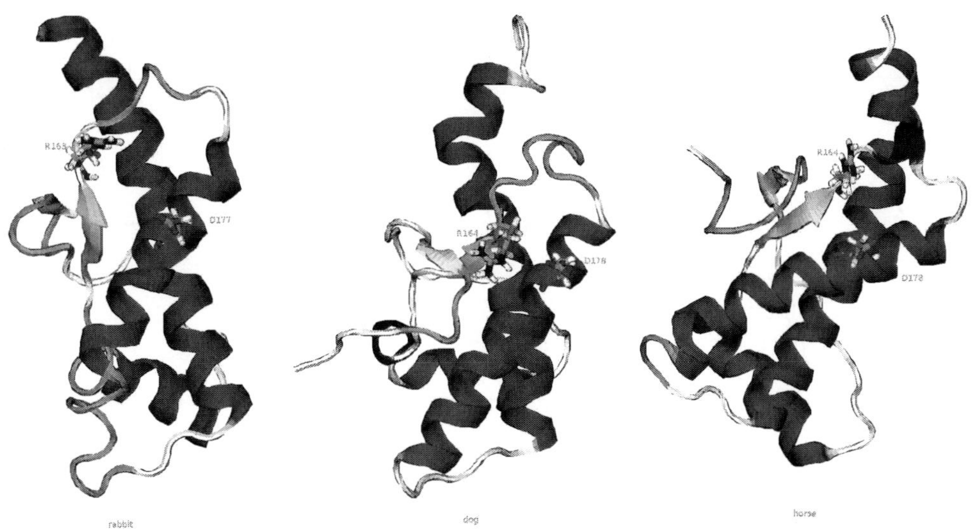

Figure 2. The salt bridge D177-R163 of rabbit prion protein, D178-R164 of dog and horse prion proteins.

tween horse and dog prion proteins, compared with the identities and similarities between dog and rabbit prion proteins, and between horse and rabbit prion proteins. This point can be furthermore confirmed by the following data of the Needleman-Wunsch or Smith-Waterman Pairwise Sequence Alignment and the jCE algorithm or jCE Circular Permutation Pairwise Structure Alignment. (1) For dogs and horses, the Identities are 89.38 % (query) and 90.99 % (subject) and the Similars are 93.81 % (query) and 95.50 % (subject) for the Sequence Alignment, and the Identity is 89.11% and the Similarity is 93.07% for the Structure Alignment. (2) For dogs and rabbits, the Identities are 90.09 % (query) and 72.46 % (subject) and the Similars are 95.95 % (query) and 77.18 % (subject) for the Sequence Alignment, and the Identity is 92.93 % and the Similarity is 98.99 % for the Structure Alignment. (3) For horses and rabbits, the Identities are 87.61 % (query) and 71.74 % (subject) and the Similars are 93.81 % (query) and 76.81 % (subject) for the Sequence Alignment, and the Identity is 71.72% and the Similarity is 77.78% for the Structure Alignment. This might explain the reasons why rabbit prion protein differs very much from dog and horse prion proteins in secondary structures under low pH environment [Zhang 2011b, Zhang 2011c].

4. Conclusion

The paper is a straight forward molecular dynamics simulation study of rabbit, dog and horse prion proteins which apparently resist the formation of the scrapie form. The analyses of molecular dynamics results confirmed the structural stability of rabbit prion protein under neutral pH environment, and of dog and horse prion proteins under neutral and low pH environments. The main point is that the enhanced stability of the C-terminal ordered region especially helix 2 through the D177-R163 (D178-R164) salt-bridge formation renders the rabbit, dog and horse prion proteins stable. This salt bridge might be a potential drug target for prion diseases. Zhang (2011) systemically analyzes this salt bridge in [Zhang 2011d] and, like GN8 of [Kuwata et al., 2007], fixing the distance between D177 and R163 to form a salt bridge distance might be able to design a drug for treating prion diseases.

Acknowledgments

This research has been supported by a Victorian Life Sciences Computation Initiative (VLSCI) grant number VR0063 on its Peak Computing Facility at the University of Melbourne, an initiative of the Victorian Government.

References

[Aguzzi et al. 2006] Aguzzi A., Heikenwalder M., 2006. Pathogenesis of prion diseases: current status and future outlook. Nat. Rev. Microbiol. 4, 765–775.

[Berman et al., 2000] Berman H.M., Westbrook J., Feng Z., Gilliland G., Bhat T.N., Weissig H., Shindyalov I.N., Bourne P.E., 2000. The protein data bank. Nucleic Acids Res. 28, 253–242.

[Bett et al., 2012] Bett C., Fernndez-Borges N., Kurt T.D., Lucero M., Nilsson K.P., Castilla J., Sigurdson C.J., 2012. Structure of the $\beta 2$-$\alpha 2$ loop and interspecies prion transmission. FASEB J. 2012 Apr 9, PMID: 22490928.

[Case et al. 2002] Case D.A., Pearlman J.W., Caldwell T.E., Cheatham III, Wang J., Ross W.S., Simmerling C.L., Darden T.A., Merz K.M., Stanton R.V., Cheng A.L., Vincent J.J., Crowley M., Tsui V., Gohlke H., Radmer R.J., Duan Y., Pitera J., Massova I., Seibel G.L., Singh U.C., Weiner P.K., Kollman P.A., 2002. AMBER 7, University of California: San Francisco.

[Case et al. 2006] Case D.A., Darden T.A., Caldwell T.E., Cheatham III, Simmerling C.L., Wang J., Duke R.E., Luo R., Merz K.M., Pearlman D.A., Crowley M., Walker R.C., Zhang W., Wang B., Hayik S., Roitberg A., Seabra G., Wong K.F., Paesani F., Wu X., Brozell S., Tsui V., Gohlke H., Yang L., Tan C., Mongan J., Hornak V., Cui G., Beroza P., Mathews D.H., Schafmeister C., Ross W.S., Kollman P.A., 2006. AMBER 9, University of California: San Francisco.

[Case et al. 2010] Case D.A., Darden T.A., Cheatham T.E., Simmerling III C.L., Wang J., Duke R.E., Luo R., Walker R.C., Zhang W., Merz K.M., Roberts B.P., Wang B., Hayik S., Roitberg A., Seabra G., Kolossváry I., Wong K.F., Paesani F., Vanicek J., Liu J., Wu X., Brozell S.R., Steinbrecher T., Gohlke H., Cai Q., Ye X., Wang J., Hsieh M.-J., Cui G., Roe D.R., Mathews D.H., Seetin M.G., Sagui C., Babin V., Luchko T., Gusarov S., Kovalenko A., Kollman P.A., 2010. AMBER 11, University of California, San Francisco.

[Fernandez-Funez et al. 2011] Fernandez-Funez P., Zhang Y., Sanchez-Garcia J., Jensen K., Zou W.Q., Rincon-Limas D.E., 2011. Pulling rabbits to reveal the secrets of the prion protein. Commun. Integr. Biol. 4(3), 1–5.

[Kabsch et al. 1983] Kabsch W., Sander C., 1983. Dictionary of protein secondary structure: pattern recognition of hydrogen-bonded and geometrical features. Biopolymers 22, 2577–2637.

[Khan et al. 2010] Khan M.Q., Sweeting B., Mulligan V.K., Arslan P.E., Cashman N.R., Pai E.F., Chakrabartty A., 2010. Prion disease susceptibility is affected by β-structure folding propensity and local side-chain interactions in PrP. Proc. Natl. Acad. Sci. USA 107(46), 19808–19813.

[Kuwata et al., 2007] Kuwata K, Nishida N, Matsumoto T, Kamatari YO, Hosokawa-Muto J, Kodama K, Nakamura HK, Kimura K, Kawasaki M, Takakura Y, Shirabe S, Takata J, Kataoka Y, Katamine S, 2007. Hot spots in prion protein for pathogenic conversion. Proc. Natl. Acad. Sci. USA 104(29), 11921–11926.

[Lin et al. 2011] Lin D.H., Wen Y., 2011. Progresses on prion proteins. SCIENTIA SINICA Chimica 41(4), 683–698 (in Chinese).

[Perez et al. 2011] Perez D.R., Damberger F.F., Wuthrich K., 2010. Horse prion protein NMR structure and comparisons with related variants of the mouse prion protein. J. Mol. Biol. 400(2), 121–128.

[Polymenidoua et al. 2008] Polymenidoua M., Trusheimb H., Stallmacha L., Moosa R., Julius J.A., Mielea G., Lenzbauerb C., Aguzzia A., 2008. Canine MDCK cell lines are refractory to infection with human and mouse prions. Vaccine 26, 2601–2614.

[Prusiner 1998] Prusiner S.B., 1998. Prions. Proc. Natl. Acad. Sci. USA 95, 13363–13383.

[Sweeting et al. 2009] Sweeting B., Brown E., Chakrabartty A.,Pai E.F., 2009. The structure of rabbit PrP^{C}: clues into species barrier and prion disease susceptibility. Canadian Light Source 28:
http://www.lightsource.ca/science/pdf/activity_report_2009/28.pdf

[Vorberg et al., 2003] Vorberg I., Martin H.G., Eberhard P., Suzette A.P., 2003. Multiple amino acid residues within the rabbit prion protein inhibit formation of its abnormal isoform. J. Virol. 77, 2003–2009.

[Weissmann 2004] Weissmann C., 2004. The state of the prion. Nat. Rev. Microbiol. 2, 861–871.

[Wen et al. 2010a] Wen Y., Li J., Yao W.M., Xiong M.Q., Hong J., Peng Y., Xiao G.F., Lin D.H., 2010. Unique structural characteristics of the rabbit prion protein. J. Bio. Chem. 285(41), 31682–31693.

[Wen et al. 2010b] Wen Y., Li J., Xiong M.Q., Peng Y., Yao W.M., Hong J., Lin D.H., 2010. Solution structure and dynamics of the I214V mutant of the rabbit prion protein. PLoS One 5(10): e13273.

[Zhang 2009] Zhang J.P., 2009. Studies on the structural stability of rabbit prion probed by molecular dynamics simulations. J. Biomol. Struct. Dyn. 27, 159–162.

[Zhang 2010] Zhang J.P., 2010. Studies on the structural stability of rabbit prion probed by molecular dynamics simulations of its wild-type and mutants. J. Theor. Bio. 264, 119–122.

[Zhang 2011a] Zhang J.P., 2011. Comparison studies of the structural stability of rabbit prion protein with human and mouse prion proteins. J. Theor. Bio. 269, 88–95.

[Zhang 2011b] Zhang J.P., 2011. Molecular dynamics studies on the structural stability of wild-type dog prion protein. J. Biomol. Struct. Dyn. 28(6), 861–869.

[Zhang 2011c] Zhang J.P., 2011. Molecular Dynamics Studies on the Structural Stability of Wild-type horse prion protein. J. Biomol. Struct. Dyn. 29(2), 369–377.

[Zhang 2011d] Zhang J.P., 2011. Molecular Dynamics - Practical Application - Mechanism underlying the resistance to prion diseases in rabbits: a technology review from MIT and in 7 languages, LAP Academic Publishing, ISBN 978-3-8465-4843-1, 164 pages.

In: Prions and Prion Diseases: New Developments
Editor: Jean-Michel Verdier
ISBN: 978-1-62100-027-3
© 2012 Nova Science Publishers, Inc.

Chapter 3

INDUCING TRANSMISSIBLE PRION DISEASES WITH RECOMBINANT FIBRILS: A NEW CONCEPT ON GENESIS AND EVOLUTION OF INFECTIOUS PRIONS

Ilia V. Baskakov
Center for Biomedical Engineering and Technology,
and Department of Anatomy and Neurobiology,
University of Maryland School of Madicine, MD, US

ABSTRACT

Prion diseases are fatal neurodegenerative disorders that can be sporadic, inherited or infectious in origin. The transmissible agent of prion disease consists of a prion protein in its abnormal, β-sheet rich state (PrP^{Sc}), which is capable of replicating itself according to the template-assisted mechanism. This mechanism postulates that the folding pattern of a newly recruited polypeptide chain accurately reproduces that of a PrP^{Sc} template. This chapter summarizes our current knowledge about synthetic prions and introduces the new hypothesis that transmissible prion diseases can be induced by prion protein structures substantially different from that of authentic PrP^{Sc}. We suggest that a new mechanism for triggering PrP^{Sc} formation different from classical templating exists. This new mechanism designated as "deformed templating" postulates that prion protein cross-β structures can induce or template conformationally different cross-β structures typical for PrP^{Sc}, and that such templating involves a switching from one folding pattern present in rPrP fibrils to a significantly different folding pattern, the one specific for PrP^{Sc}. The possibilities that a similar mechanism of deformed templating account for prion adaptation to new hosts are discussed. The current chapter offers new mechanistic insight into genesis and evolution of mammalian prions and the etiology of transmissible neurodegenerative diseases.

INTRODUCTION

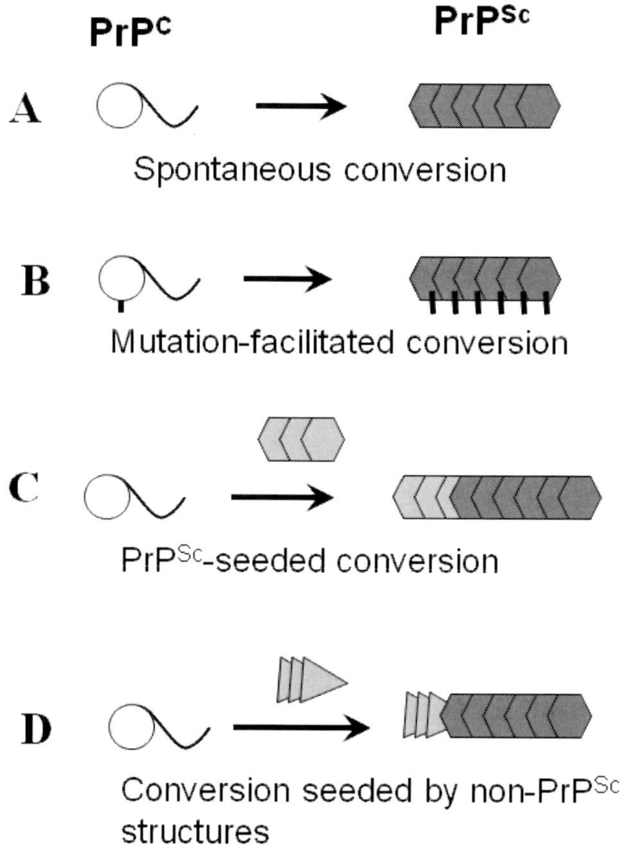

Figure 1. Four mechanisms for PrP^{Sc} formation. (A) Spontaneous conversion of PrP^{C} into PrP^{Sc} is believed to underlie the sporadic forms of the prion diseases. (B) Disease-related mutations in prion protein can facilitate the conversion of PrP^{C} into PrP^{Sc}. (C) The template-assisted model postulates that PrP^{Sc} replicate its pathogenic structure by recruiting and converting PrP^{C}. According to this model, the folding pattern of a newly recruited polypeptide chain accurately reproduces that of a PrP^{Sc} template. (D) A new mechanism referred to as deformed templating postulates that the formation of PrP^{Sc} *de novo* can be triggered by abnormal PrP structures substantially different from that of authentic PrP^{Sc}. A transformation from one cross-β folding pattern present in a template to a significantly different folding pattern, the one specific for PrP^{Sc}, occurs during deformed templating.

Prion diseases, or transmissible spongiform encephalopathies, are fatal neurodegenerative disorders that can be sporadic, inherited or infectious in origin. Misfolding and aggregation of the normal, cellular form of the prion protein (PrP^{C}) into an abnormal β-sheet rich, disease-related conformation (PrP^{Sc}) underlies the pathogenic mechanisms of the prion diseases for all three origins (*1*). Spontaneous conversion of PrP^{C} into PrP^{Sc} is believed to underlie the sporadic forms of prion diseases (Figure 1). On average, one person per million succumb each year to sporadic disease. This low occurrence rate is likely to reflect the extremely low probability of spontaneous conversion of PrP^{C} into PrP^{Sc}. Inherited forms of the disease have been linked to a number of single point mutations, truncation or octarepeat expansion mutations in the *PRNP* gene (a gene that encodes prion protein), with more than 20 disease-inducing mutations identified so far (*2*). In addition to sporadic and inherited origins, prion diseases can be also acquired via transmission, just like other infectious diseases. The "protein only" hypothesis postulates that the transmissible agent of prion disease consists of a prion protein in its abnormal, β-sheet rich, disease-related state (PrP^{Sc}), which is capable of propagating its abnormal conformation in an autocatalytic manner by recruiting and converting PrP^{C} (*3, 4*). According to the classical templating mechanism, during PrP^{Sc}-seeded conversion, the folding pattern of a newly recruited polypeptide chain accurately replicates that of a PrP^{Sc} template (Figure 1). As a result, the PrP^{Sc}-specific folding pattern can be amplified endlessly and with a high precision, when homologous PrP^{C} molecules are provided.

This Chapter introduces the new hypothesis that transmissible prion diseases can be induced by cross-β PrP structures substantially different from that of authentic PrP^{Sc} (Figure 1). This hypothesis suggests that a new templating mechanism (referred to as "deformed templating") different from the classical templating exists. Deformed templating involves a switching from one cross-β folding pattern present in a template to a significantly different folding pattern, the one specific for PrP^{Sc}. The studies on synthetic prions conducted in the past decade strongly support this hypothesis. This Chapter summarizes our current knowledge about synthetic prions. It also offers a new mechanistic insight into genesis, evolution and adaptation of transmissible prion structures.

GENERATING TRANSMISSIBLE PRION DISEASES *DE NOVO*

The recent years witnessed a number of studies, where transmissible prion diseases were generated in animals *de novo* by inoculating prion infectious material produced *in vitro* (*5-11*). All studies on generating prion infectivity could be divided into two large groups, where the material for inoculating animals was produced either using (i) serial Protein Misfolding Cyclic Amplification (sPMCA) (*9-11*), or (ii) *in vitro* fibrillation protocols that utilized recombinant PrP (rPrP) (*5-8*).

In the studies that employed the first approach, the application of sPMCA accomplished two purposes: (i) generating PrP^{Sc} particles *de novo* and (ii) amplification of newly formed PrP^{Sc} to the amounts that can effectively produce clinical disease in wild type animals with 100% success rate (*9-11*). *De novo* formation of PrP^{Sc} in PMCA showed stochastic behavior, i.e. less than 100% of the sPMCA reactions were positive, while the number of sPMCA rounds required for amplification of the newly formed PrP^{Sc} to the amount detectible by Western blot was variable even within the same experimental conditions. Therefore, it remains unclear whether the substantial infectivity produced after multiple rounds of sPMCA was a result of amplification of a few or even a single PrP^{Sc} particle.

The second approach involved conversion of rPrP into amyloid fibrils *in vitro* without application of sPMCA (*5-8*). In these studies, transmissible diseases were generated either in transgenic animals with high levels of PrP^{C} expression or in wild type animals (*5-8*). In transgenic animals, the disease was produced with 100% success rate in the first passage, although, after relatively long incubation time (*5, 6, 8*). In wild type animals, the disease was induced with less than 100% success rate, while two serial passages required for appearance of clinical symptoms (*7*). Critical concerns that rPrP amyloid fibrils did not induce the disease *de novo* but only accelerated an on-going pathogenic process have been raised regarding the studies performed on transgenic mice (*12-14*). Indeed, the mice that overexpress PrP^C were found to develop a neurological disorder that was accompanied by PrP aggregation, though, these disorders were not transmissible in serial passages (*8*). In contrast to sporadic formation of non-transmissible PrP aggregates, inoculation of rPrP fibrils triggered formation of authentic PrP^{Sc} that can transmit disease, a process that appears to compete with aggregation of non-transmissible PrP.

The experiments conducted on wild type animals provided strong evidence that rPrP fibrils can induce transmissible prion disease *de novo* (*7*). However, when triggered by rPrP fibrils, only a small fraction of animals showed signs of infection. Furthermore, the clinical disease was observed only at the second serial passage. Less than a 100% success rate and long clinically silent stage raised a number of questions regarding the molecular mechanism underlying the genesis of transmissible prions. The question of great interest is how rPrP amyloid fibrils triggered formation of transmissible PrP^{Sc}? In the prevailing opinion, the preparations of rPrP amyloid fibrils must contain minuscule amounts of PrP^{Sc} or particles with the structure of PrP^{Sc}, and that this tiny sub-fraction was responsible for the disease.

THE MECHANISM OF TRIGGERING PRION DISEASE BY RPRP AMYLOID FIBRILS

Before discussing models on triggering transmissible prion diseases by rPrP fibrils, it is useful to briefly review the data on the structure of rPrP fibrils and PrP^{Sc}. Several recent studies presented strong evidence that the structures of rPrP amyloid fibrils are fundamentally different from those of authentic PrP^{Sc}, which was either isolated from scrapie-infected animals or produced via sPMCA *in vitro* (*15-17*). X-ray diffraction experiments revealed substantial differences in equatorial diffraction patterns collected from rPrP fibrils and PrP^{Sc} purified from scrapie brain, illustrating that their folding patterns were significantly different (*15, 16*). The results of X-ray diffraction analysis was consistent with the FTIR data, which also pointed to significant differences in conformations of PrP^{Sc} and rPrP fibrils (*18, 19*). Depending on the prion strain, the maxima of the β-sheet absorption collected for PrP^{Sc} isolates varied between 1625 and 1637 cm^{-1} (*18*), whereas the maxima of β-sheet absorption for rPrP fibrils was found to be at 1614 and 1626/28 cm^{-1} under the same solvent conditions (*16, 19*). Distinct positions in absorption maxima illustrate the differences in cross β-sheet folding patterns in PrP^{Sc} and rPrP fibrils. Furthermore, as judged from AFM and EM imaging, PrP^{Sc} produced *in vitro* displayed a spherical but not the elongated shape typical for amyloid fibrils (*17*). rPrP fibrils were not capable of seeding PrP^{Sc} formation in sPMCA further supporting the view that the structures of PrP^{Sc} and rPrP fibrils are different (*20*). How can rPrP fibrils seed PrP^{Sc} *in vivo* and trigger transmissible prion disease, if their structure is fundamentally different prom that of PrP^{Sc}?

Bearing the results on structural studies in mind, two alternative models could be put forward. According to the first model, the preparations of rPrP amyloid fibrils contain very small amounts of PrP^{Sc} or particles with a structure similar to authentic PrP^{Sc} (Figure 2A). If this is correct, then the low success rate in infecting the animals and the long clinically silent stage can be attributed to the miniscule amounts of PrP^{Sc} in preparation of the fibrils. The second model proposes that formation of PrP^{Sc} and transmissible prion diseases in wild type animals are triggered by rPrP seeding material that lacks PrP^{Sc} (Figure 2B). Despite substantial differences in folding patterns, rPrP fibrils are capable of triggering formation of PrP^{Sc}. Because of the structural differences, rPrP fibril-induced seeding of PrP^{Sc} is not efficient, which explains the low rate of infection in the first passage. For the same reasons, transformation of rPrP amyloid structure into PrP^{Sc} structure might involve several steps before fully infectious, authentic PrP^{Sc} emerges, which explains the long silent stage to clinical disease.

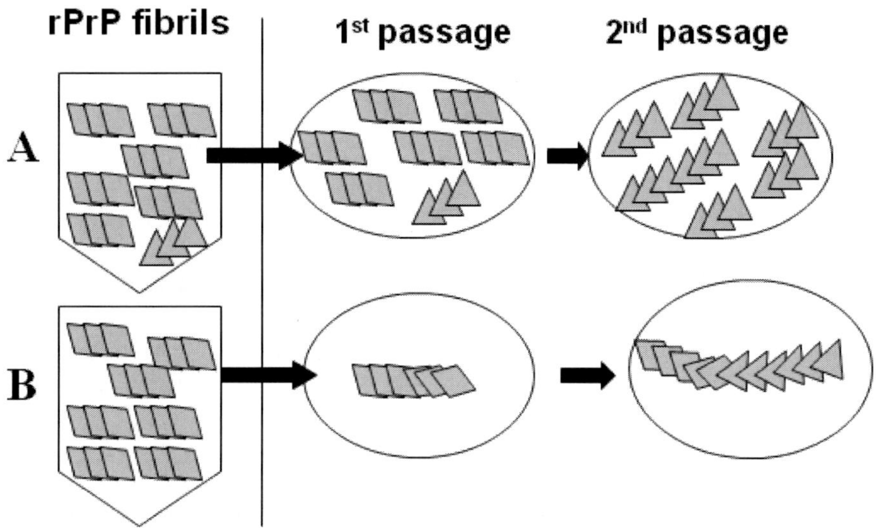

Figure 2. Schematic representation of two mechanisms responsible for generating transmissible prion diseases *de novo*. According to the first mechanism (A), the preparations of rPrP amyloid fibrils contain very small amounts of PrP^{Sc}. The silent stage of the disease is attributed to the long time required for amplification of this extremely small amount of PrP^{Sc}. A second mechanism referred to as deformed templating postulates that there are no PrP^{Sc} particles in the preparations of amyloid fibrils (B). Instead, when inoculated into animals, amyloid fibrils can seed conversion of PrP^{C} into PrP^{Sc}-like structures, although with a low efficiency. The process of transformation of rPrP fibrils into PrP^{Sc} is accompanied by a long clinically silent stage before authentic PrP^{Sc} emerges..

Experimental Evidence Support the Second Model

Experimental data accumulated to date strongly support the second model. First, no PrP^{Sc} could be detected in the preparations of rPrP amyloid fibrils in the sPMCA format that detects single PrP^{Sc} particles (Makarava & Baskakov, personal communication). If one assumes that the first model is correct, the amount of infectivity in 50 μl of inoculum should be equivalent to approximately 0.5-1 infectious dose to account for the less than 100% infection rate in the first passage. This amount of infectivity is equivalent to ~10,000-100,000 PrP molecules or to ~100-1000 PrP^{Sc} particles, assuming that an average PrP^{Sc} particle consists of ~100 PrP molecules (*21*). This amount of PrP^{Sc} was well above the detection limits of sPMCA, and should have been easily detected if present in preparations of rPrP fibrils.

Second, the experimental protocol used for producing rPrP amyloid fibrils employs denaturants (a mixture of 1M GdnHCl and 3M urea) - the solvent conditions under which PrP^{Sc} undergoes denaturation. Because rPrP fibrils are much more stable than PrP^{Sc} (*7, 22, 23*), rPrP fibrils can be formed under solvent conditions where PrP^{Sc} is largely denatured. Furthermore, formation of authentic PrP^{Sc} *in vitro* requires RNA and lipids (*10, 11*), whereas rPrP amyloid fibrils were formed in the absence of any cellular co-factors. Therefore, it is highly unlikely that PrP^{Sc} particles with authentic structures could be formed during preparation of rPrP fibrils conducted in the absence of co-factors essential for authentic PrP^{Sc} structures and under solvent conditions that promote PrP^{Sc} denaturation.

Third, when transmissible prion disease is triggered by rPrP amyloid fibrils, a decrease in PrP^{Sc} conformational stability was observed during serial passages of synthetic prions (*7, 24*). Similar dynamics in PrP^{Sc} conformational stability was observed regardless of whether transgenic mice or Syrian hamsters were inoculated with rPrP fibrils, suggesting that a common pathway in genesis and evolution of infectious structures might exist (*7, 24*). Observed changes in physical properties illustrate that the PrP^{Sc} structure undergoes transformation during serial transmission providing a direct support for the second model.

Fourth, in recent studies on synthetic prions, a strong correlation between conformational stability of rPrP amyloid fibrils, the stability of PrP^{Sc} produced in animals upon inoculating rPrP fibrils, and the incubation time to disease were described (*6*). If a miniscule fraction in the preparation of rPrP fibrils is responsible for the disease, the correlation between stability of rPrP amyloid, which is a bulk property of fibril preparation, and PrP^{Sc} would be challenging to explain. Again, these results provide a strong support toward the second model.

Fifth, as judged from the clinical and neuropathological features, the synthetic strain generated in Syrian hamsters by rPrP fibrils was remarkably different from all previously known rodent strains including those generated by sPMCA (*7, 9-11*). Among the most distinguishing features were slow progression of clinical disease, accumulation of large plaques in subpial and subependymal areas, distinctive lesion and PrP immunoreactivity profiles, and unusual clinical phenotype (obesity, hair loss) (*7*). The fact that rPrP fibrils produced a disease phenotype remarkably different from the phenotype expressed by strains generated in sPMCA or isolated from animals is consistent with the hypothesis that rPrP fibrils gave rise to PrP^{Sc} with unique physical and biological features.

THE HYPOTHESIS OF DEFORMED TEMPLATING

All the data on synthetic prions accumulated to date support the hypothesis that transmissible prion diseases can be triggered by PrP structures substantially different from that of authentic PrP^{Sc} (Figure 2B). This hypothesis assumes that only partial overlap or distant similarities in structures of fibrillar rPrP and PrP^{Sc} are sufficient for triggering transmissible prion diseases. While the precise mechanistic details for inducing PrP^{Sc} formation by conformationally different PrP structures are not known, the model of conformational switching provides one possible explanation of how such transformation occurs (*25, 26*) (Figure 3). According to this model, the global folding pattern of PrP molecules within amyloid fibrils and PrP^{Sc} are different, yet nevertheless, they share a common structural motif. For instance, a common β-strand that can link two structures provides opportunity for limited templating. This model is consistent with experimental observations that the global structures of PrP^{Sc} and rPrP fibrils are different (*15-17, 27*), while it explains a correlation between conformational stability of two structures (*6*). Because there is only partial overlap between two structures, the seeding of PrP^{Sc} by rPrP fibrils is not efficient, which explains the low infection rate in the first passage. Previous studies on molecular imaging of single amyloid fibrils provided a proof of principle that the conformational switching between two alternative PrP folding patterns can occur within an individual PrP fibril or particle (*25*).

The work on synthetic prions suggests that a new mechanism designated as "deformed templating" that is different from the classical templating might exist (Figure 1 C,D). In classical templating, the folding pattern of a newly recruited polypeptide chain accurately reproduces that of a template. In deformed templating, while the template provides limited seeding, a newly recruited polypeptide chain acquires a new folding pattern which only partially overlaps with the folding pattern of a template. Two glycosyl groups and GPI anchor present in PrP^{C} might impose steric constraints on the spectrum of folding patterns available to PrP^{C} (*28*), thus providing a driving force behind switching the recruited PrP folding pattern from rPrP fibril-specific to PrP^{S}-specific.

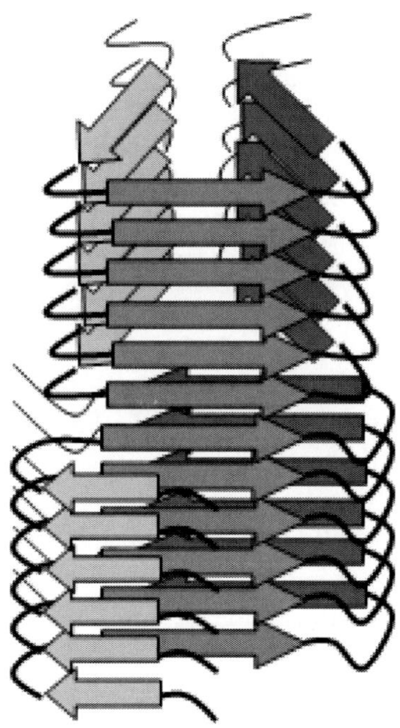

Figure 3. A schematic diagram illustrating conformational switch within individual fibril. The hybrid fibril consists of two segments with different global folding pattern. In both segments, common β-strand structure is formed within the same PrP region that links two segments together. This diagram does not intend to model PrP folding pattern within amyloid fibrils or PrP^{Sc}.

If the hypothesis that the fibril-specific PrP folding pattern can template a folding pattern typical for authentic PrP^{Sc} is correct, one can assume that the opposite reaction, i.e. the seeding of rPrP fibrils by PrP^{Sc} is also possible. Indeed, several assays exploited the phenomenon of PrP^{Sc}-seeded conversion of α-rPrP into amyloid fibrils for detecting miniscule amounts of PrP^{Sc} (*29, 30*). Interestingly, the structure of rPrP fibrils produced as a result of seeding by PrP^{Sc} only distantly resembled those of authentic PrP^{Sc} structure and had limited infectivity (*31*).

Conformational Switching Within Individual Amyloid Fibrils and Strain Adaptation Phenomenon

According to the prevailing view, multiple amyloid structures could be produced within the same amino acid sequence (*19, 32*). However, the folding pattern of a polypeptide chain within individual amyloid fibrils or PrP^{Sc} particles is believed to be uniform. In amyloid fibrils or PrP^{Sc} particles, β-strands are arranged perpendicularly to the axis of the cross-β spine (*15, 16*) and their individual, strain-specific folding pattern provide a template for recruiting and converting a monomeric precursor at the growing edge. Faithful templating of cross-β structures is based on self-complementation of a polypeptide chain involved in cross-β assembly (*33*). Self-complementation can be achieved through several mechanisms including tight complementarity of amino acid side chains in the steric zippers of the cross-β spine; the stacking of side chains in so-called "polar zippers", where the side chain hydrogen bonds are formed between β-strands along the fibrilar axis; or domain swapping (*33*).

The recent studies that employed single-fibril microscopy imaging revealed that the elongation of fibrils does not always support uniformity in cross-β structures within individual fibrils (*25, 34*) (Figure 3). The cross-seeding reaction, where hamster rPrP fibrils were used as seeds while mouse rPrP was used as a substrate, was shown to produce hybrid fibrils consisted of two segments, one composed of hamster and another mouse rPrP (*25*). Most important, within individual fibrils, the folding pattern within the mouse segment was considerably different from that within the hamster segment. The switch from hamster- to mouse-specific folding patterns within hybrid fibrils occurred presumably because the amino acid sequence of mouse rPrP was not compatible with the hamster-specific folding pattern. In addition to species-specific variations in amino acid sequence within prion-folding C-terminal domain, a deletion of a few N-terminal amino acid residues outside of the prion-folding domain can dramatically alter the folding pattern of the prion-folding domain (*35*).

The question of how cross-β folding patterns change without interrupting fibril continuity is not trivial. We proposed that within a hybrid fibril, two segments have different global folds while sharing common local motifs that account for the integrity of the hybrid structure (Figure 3) (*26*). To satisfy this requirement, the same polypeptide region must adopt the identical parallel β-strand conformation within two fundamentally different folding structures. Because the region that acquires the common β-strand conformation is connected by hydrogen bonds to the same region in the polypeptide molecules along the cross-β spine, the parallel β-sheet propagates along the whole length of the fibril despite being part of two different global folds. Hydrogen bonds running up and down the common β-sheet provide conformational stability for the whole hybrid structure. This model proposes that the catalytic activity in recruiting and converting monomeric precursors into an alternative cross-β folding pattern is due to partial overlap in folding patterns.

The observation of a conformational switch within individual fibrils highlights high adaptation potential for amyloid structures. Adaptive conformational switching allows recruitment of non-identical but homologous polypeptide molecules which otherwise are not compatible with the existing structure. Adaptive conformational switching within individual fibrils may provide a mechanistic explanation for modification, adaptation, or emergence of new prion strains, a phenomenon that has been frequently observed upon transmission of prions across species (*36-38*). Notably, the process of triggering transmissible disease by rPrP fibrils displays features typical for the process of prion adaptation to a new host. Both processes are characterized by a long clinically silent stage (*39-41*), a transformation in the physical properties of PrP^{Sc} (*36*), and sometimes, a change in the accumulation pattern of PrP^{Sc} during serial transmission (*42*). Therefore, both phenomena, prion adaptation to a new host and generating transmissible disease by rPrP fibrils, might share a common mechanism.

The studies on interspecies transmission using PMCA reactions or bioassays revealed that prion strains have variable adaptation potential. Some strains are capable of maintaining their individual strain-specific properties within a range of PrP amino acid sequences, whereas other strains can faithfully replicate only within a single or closely homologous PrP sequence (*36, 36-38, 43*). The work on cross-seeding of rPrP amyloids provided direct illustration that self-replicating amyloid structures are not equally selective with respect to the amino acid sequence of the substrate molecules that can be recruited for their replication (*34*). This difference in selectivity between amyloid strains specifies a direction in which adaptation or evolution of amyloid structures or prion strains occurs upon interspecies transmission. Conformational adaptation is expected to proceed from highly selective or species-specific structures toward promiscuous ones. A switch from a species-specific to promiscuous strain presumably occurs when a species-specific strain faces a heterologous substrate that is not compatible with the conformation of the original strain. Therefore, one can predict that inter-species transmissions could lead to formation of new promiscuous strains.

Cross-Talk Between Amyloidogenic Proteins

The hypothesis that transmissible prion diseases can be triggered by cross-β PrP structures substantially different from that of authentic PrP^{Sc} has large implications for understanding the ethiology of prion and other neurodegenerative diseases. A growing number of studies have documented that amyloid forms of several proteins linked to neurodegenerative diseases were capable of seeding their own aggregation in a prion-like manner in a cell and spreading from cell to cell through the nervous system (reviewed in (*44-46*). One recent study provided strong evidence that pathological changes associated with non-prion neurodegenerative diseases could be induced or transmitted through inoculation of the aggregated forms of non-prion proteins such as Aβ (*47*). Furthermore, recent study illustrated that amyloids can template structures different from their own (*25*). It is generally assumed that self-perpetuating aggregation requires identity in amino acid sequence between seeds and substrate. Recent work, however, suggested the possibility of cross-talk between non-related amyloidogenic proteins (*48-50*). *In vivo,* amyloidosis of one protein was found to be triggered by fibrils of an unrelated protein in a manner similar to cross-seeded polymerization (*48-50*). Cross-talk between several yeast prion proteins provides another example of how direct interactions between newly forming and pre-existing heterologous fibrils might take place in a cell (*51-53*). Moreover, pathological studies revealed that protein aggregates produced from two different proteins or peptides, including PrP, Aβ, α-synuclein, immunoglobulin light chain λ, and β_2 microglobulin often co-localize within the same amyloid plaque in a variety of organs or tissues (*54-58*). The promiscuous nature of the propagating activity of amyloid structures can lead to devastating consequences for cellular health. For instance, the cross-talk between non-related amyloidogenic proteins may offer a possible explanation for the development of age-related conformational disorders that are considered to be sporadic. In future studies, it would be interesting to define the spectrum of structures and sequences capable of triggering the PrP^C to PrP^{Sc} conversion and inducing transmissible prion diseases.

REFERENCES

[1] S. B. Prusiner, in *Viral Pathogenesis*, N. Nathanson *et al.*, Eds. (Raven Press, New York, 1996), pp. 855-911.

[2] S. B. Prusiner, M. R. Scott, *Annu. Rev. Genet.* 31, 139 (1997).

[3] S. B. Prusiner, *Science* 216, 136 (1982).

[4] J. S. Griffith, *Nature* 215, 1043 (1967).

[5] G. Legname *et al.*, *Science* 305, 673 (2004).

[6] D. W. Colby *et al.*, *Proc. Acad. Natl. Sci. U. S. A.* 106, 20417 (2009).

[7] N. Makarava *et al.*, *Acta Neuropathol.* 119, 177 (2010).

[8] D. W. Colby *et al.*, *PLoS Pathogen* 6, e1000736 (2010).

[9] M. A. Barria, A. Mukherjee, D. Gonzalez-Romero, R. Morales, C. Soto, *PLOS Pathog.* 5, e1000421 (2009).

[10] N. R. Deleault, B. T. Harris, J. R. Rees, S. Supattapone, *Proc. Acad. Natl. Sci. U. S. A.* 104, 9741 (2007).

[11] F. Wang, X. Wang, C.-G. Yuan, J. Ma, *Science* 327, 1132 (2010).

[12] B. Caughey, G. S. Baron, B. Chesebro, M. Jeffrey, *Annu. Rev. Biochem.* 78, 177 (2009).

[13] B. Caughey, G. S. Baron, *Nature* 443, 803 (2006).

[14] C. Soto, *Trends Biochem. Sci* 36, 151 (2011).

[15] H. Wille *et al.*, *Proc. Acad. Natl. Sci. U. S. A.* 106, 16990 (2009).

[16] V. G. Ostapchenko *et al.*, *J. Mol. Biol.* 400, 908 (2010).

[17] J. R. Piro *et al.*, *Biochemistry* 50, 7111 (2011).

[18] S. Spassov, M. Beekes, D. Naumann, *Biochim Biophys Acta* 1760, 1138 (2006).

[19] N. Makarava, I. V. Baskakov, *J. Biol. Chem.* 283, 15988 (2008).

[20] N. R. Deleault, R. Kascsak, J. C. Geoghegan, S. Supattapone, *Biochemistry* 49, 3928 (2010).

[21] P. Saa, J. Castilla, C. Soto, *J. Biol. Chem.* 281, 35245 (2006).

[22] D. Peretz *et al.*, *Protein Sci.* 10, 854 (2001).
[23] Y. Sun *et al.*, *J. Biol. Chem.* 282, 9090 (2007).
[24] G. Legname *et al.*, *Proc. Natl. Aca. Sci. USA* 102, 2168 (2005).
[25] N. Makarava, V. G. Ostapchenko, R. Savtchenko, I. V. Baskakov, *J. Biol. Chem.* 284, 14386 (2009).
[26] I. V. Baskakov, *FEBS Lett.* 583, 2618 (2009).
[27] H. Wille, G.-F. Zhang, M. A. Baldwin, F. E. Cohen, S. B. Prusiner, *J. Mol. Biol.* 259, 608 (1996).
[28] L. Breydo *et al.*, *Biochemistry* 46, 852 (2007).
[29] D. W. Colby *et al.*, *Proc. Acad. Natl. Sci. U. S. A.* 104, 20914 (2007).
[30] R. Atarashi *et al.*, *Nature Methods* 4, 645 (2007).
[31] J. I. Kim *et al.*, *J. Biol. Chem.* 285, 14083 (2010).
[32] A. T. Petkova *et al.*, *Science* 307, 262 (2005).
[33] D. Eisenberg *et al.*, *Accounts Chem. Res.* 39, 568 (2006).
[34] N. Makarava, C. I. Lee, V. G. Ostapchenko, I. V. Baskakov, *J. Biol. Chem.* 282, 36704 (2007).
[35] V. G. Ostapchenko, N. Makarava, R. Savtchenko, I. V. Baskakov, *J. Mol. Biol.* 383, 1210 (2008).
[36] D. Peretz *et al.*, *Neuron* 34, 921 (2002).
[37] J. Castilla *et al.*, *Cell* 134, 757 (2008).
[38] K. M. Green *et al.*, *PLOS Pathog.* 4, e1000139 (2008).
[39] A. F. Hill, J. Collinge, *TRENDS in Microbiology* 11, 578 (2003).
[40] A. F. Hill *et al.*, *Proc. Natl. Acad. Sci. USA* 97, 10248 (2000).
[41] R. Race, A. Rainse, G. Raymond, B. Caughey, B. Chesebro, *J. Virology* 2001, 10106 (2001).
[42] K. Kimura, M. Kubo, T. Yokoyama, *J. Comp. Pathol.* 122, 123 (2000).
[43] R. Capobianco *et al.*, *PLOS Pathog.* 3, e31 (2007).
[44] G. Miller, *Science* 326, 1337 (2009).
[45] B. Frost, M. I. Diamond, *Nat Rev Neuroscience* 11, 155 (2010).
[46] A. Aguzzi, L. Rajendran, *Neuron* 64, 783 (2009).
[47] Y. S. Eisele *et al.*, *Science* 330, 980 (2010).
[48] L. Jean, B. Thomas, A. Tahiri-Alaoui, M. Shaw, D. J. Vaux, *Plos ONE* 2, e652 (2007).
[49] J. Yan *et al.*, *American Journal of Pathology* 171, 172 (2007).
[50] R. Morales *et al.*, *J. Neurosci.* 30, 4528 (2010).
[51] I. L. Derkatch, M. E. Bradley, P. Zhou, Y. O. Chernoff, S. W. Liebman, *Genetics* 147, 507 (1997).
[52] I. L. Derkatch, M. E. Bradley, J. Y. Hong, S. W. Liebman, *Cell* 106, 171 (2001).
[53] I. L. Derkatch *et al.*, *Proc. Acad. Natl. Sci. U. S. A.* 101, 12934 (2004).
[54] S. Haik *et al.*, *Acta Neuropath. (Berlin)* 103, 516 (2002).
[55] K. T. Adjou *et al.*, *J. Comp. Pathol.* 137, 78 (2007).
[56] M. Takahashi *et al.*, *Virchows Arch.* 429, 383 (1996).
[57] M. Miyazono, T. Kitamoto, K. Doh-ura, T. Iwaki, J. Tateishi, *Acta Neuropathol.* 84, 349 (1992).
[58] R. A. Galuske *et al.*, *Clin. Neuropathol.* 23, 113 (2004).

In: Prions and Prion Diseases: New Developments
Editor: Jean-Michel Verdier

ISBN: 978-1-62100-027-3
© 2012 Nova Science Publishers, Inc.

Chapter 4

SYNTHETIC PRIONS

Giuseppe Legname**, *Nhat Tran Thanh Le and Gabriele Giachin
Laboratory of Prion Biology, Scuola Internazionale Superiore di Studi Avanazati, Trieste, Italy

ABSTRACT

Prion diseases are invariably fatal neurodegenerative disorders affecting humans and many mammals. Here, we will discuss the current understanding of prion biology and the molecular biology of this group of illnesses. We introduce several aspects of prion biology, from the primary structure of the cellular form of the prion protein, PrP^C, to the conformational changes that occur during the conversion to the pathological form, PrP^{Sc}. In particular, we provide recent developments in our understanding of the molecular determinants of prion infectivity.

We present in detail the discovery of synthetic mammalian prions and the implications that such findings may have for the future of prion research.

1. INTRODUCTION

Prion diseases, also known as transmissible spongiform encephalopathies (TSEs), are fatal and incurable neurodegenerative disorders that occur in humans and several animal species. Prion diseases in animals include scrapie in sheep and goats, bovine spongiform encephalopathy in cattle and chronic wasting disease of deer, elk, and moose. In humans, prion diseases are rare neurological maladies such as Creutzfeldt-Jakob disease (CJD), Gerstmann-Sträussler-Scheinker (GSS) syndrome, Fatal Familial Insomnia (FFI) and kuru. Prion diseases are unique in medicine in that they can occur as spontaneous (sporadic or of unknown etiology), genetic (via point mutations in the coding region of the prion protein (PrP) gene (*PRNP*)), or infectious (through transmission from external contaminated sources)

* E-mail address: giuseppe.legname@sissa.it

[1]. In 1982, Stanley B. Prusiner hypothesized the existence of prions as infectious proteins able to adopt replicating conformations that would lead to neurodegenerative disease in an affected organism [2]. This postulate has been known ever since as the prion hypothesis. Prion diseases are now widely known to be caused by changes in the conformation of the endogenous normal cellular form of PrP, PrP^C, leading to an abnormally folded, disease-causing form denoted as PrP^{Sc} or prion. Structurally, PrP^C contains three α-helices and two short β-sheet structures in its C-terminal globular domain, and a largely unstructured N-terminal domain; whereas PrP^{Sc} has lower amount of α-helical content and mostly β-sheet structure [3,4]. The proteins PrP^C and PrP^{Sc} possess the same primary polypeptide sequence, but different secondary and tertiary structures. A nascent prion or PrP^{Sc} is produced by conversion of existing PrP^C into PrP^{Sc}. The molecular detail of the process by which PrP^{Sc} is made from PrP^C is still an area of intense research.

It is believed that this conversion occurs through PrP^C coming into contact with PrP^{Sc} and thereby PrP^C is induced to change into PrP^{Sc} [1]. Although it is clear that PrP^C is necessary for prion disease, there is still debate regarding whether other ancillary proteins or molecules are involved in the change of protein conformation *in vivo* [5,6]. The physiological cellular form PrP^C is a glysosylphosphatidylinositol (GPI) anchored polypeptide present on the outside leaflet of the cellular membrane of most cell types in mammals. The pre-pro-protein is composed of 253 amino acids in humans, which includes 22 amino acids of signal sequence at the N-terminus and 22 amino acids as GPI anchoring signal at the C-terminus. The N-terminal region of PrP^C encompasses five signature octarepeats that coordinate copper and, to a lesser extent, other metal ions. The physiological function of PrP^C has not been established with certainty and one additional and relevant focus of recent prion research indicates a possible role of the protein in neuronal differentiation and polarization [7].

Biochemical strategies for the identification of prions in biological samples have been relevant to support the pace of prion biology research. One assay that is still being used as standard for the identification of infectious prions is the proteinase digestion. In fact, limited proteolysis using, for example, proteinase K (PK) digestion is instrumental for detection of prions. The assay is typically followed by detection methods such as Western blotting or enzyme-linked immunosorbent assays. The read out is usually the partial resistance or sensitivity of prions to proteolitic digestion [8,9].

2. Strategies for De Novo Mammalian Prions Generation

One of the most important, recent advancement in prion biology has been the discovery of the *de novo* generation of prion infectivity from recombinant protein sources. Amyloid fibrils prepared *in vitro* from bacterially expressed PrP have confirmed that PrP^{Sc} is the principal, if not the sole, causative agent of TSEs, providing the definitive proof for the prion hypothesis. These PrP amyloid fibrils can be used as a synthetic surrogate of PrP^{Sc} to obtain a model for understanding the structural basis of prion conversion, for studying prion neurotoxicity, or for the development of drug leads able to halt the fibrillization process. In the past few years, considerable progress has been made in our understanding of prion diseases through the development of several protocols for producing amyloid fibrils from recombinant PrP (recPrP) (reviewed in [10,11]). This section recapitulates all relevant studies and experimental data that have led to the generation of synthetic prions (Table 1).

Table 1. Strategies used for *de novo* generation of prion *in vivo* and *in vitro*

Strategy	Methods	Results	Infectivity	Reference
Cell-free assay	Incubation of PrP^C with PrP^{Sc}	PK-resistant PrP^{Sc}	Negative on wild-type mice	[12-14]
Mouse transgenesis	Overexpression of PrP pathological mutants	*Bona fide* prion diseases	Negative on wild-type mice	[15-19]
	Knockin mice expressing FFI causing mutation	*Bona fide* FFI disease	Positive on WT mice carrying 3F4 epitope, and after passage in Tga20 mice	[20]
	Tg(1020) mice overexpressing mutations causing structural rigidity in the β_2-α_2 loop	*Bona fide* prion diseases	Positive in Tga20 mice; resistance to some prion strains.	[21,22]
PMCA	Amplification and conversion of Syrian hamster PrP^C in PrP^{Sc}	PK-resistant PrP^{Sc}	Positive in WT Syrian hamster	[23] [24,25]
	Generation of prions starting from normal brain homogenates in the absence of any PrP^{Sc} seed	PK-resistant PrP^{Sc}	Positive in Syrian hamster	[26]
	De novo prions starting from recombinant MoPrP, POPG and RNA	*Bona fide* prion disease	Positive in WT mice	[27,28]
ASA	Incubation in partially denaturing condition of recMoPrP(89-230)	*Bona fide* prion disease	Positive in Tg9949 and after passage in WT FVB mice and Tg4053	[29-33]
Annealing	Incubation of recPrP with normal brain homogenate at different heating/cooling cycles	*Bona fide* prion disease	Positive in WT Syrian hamsters	[34,35]
recPrP-PMCA	Similar to PMCA, but recPrP as substrate for the conversion instead of normal brain homogenate	PK-resistant PrP^{Sc}	Not determined	[36]
QuIC	recPrP as a substrate and automated tube shaking rather than sonication	PK-resistant PrP^{Sc}	Not determined	[37]
qPMCA	the PrP^{Sc} content is estimated by the number of PMCA rouds necessary for a positive response	PK-resistant PrP^{Sc}	Not determined	[38]
RT-Quic	Similar to ASA, but the PrP^{Sc} content is estimated by serial dilution of the seed	PK-resistant PrP^{Sc}	Not determined	[39-42]

2.1. Cell-Free Assay Using Mammalian Prions

The earliest efforts in defining the *in vitro* process of PrP^C conversion into PrP^{Sc} have been described in the 1990s by Caughey and collaborators. Radiolabelled, eucaryotically expressed, purified PrP^C was incubated with PrP^{Sc} derived from scrapie-diseased animals. The interaction with PrP^{Sc} resulted in the formation of a PK-resistant form of the radiolabelled progenitor [14].The same method has been used for inter and intraspecies transmission studies of prion diseases. The incubation of radiolabelled PrP^C with two different strains of PrP^{Sc}, the hyper (HY) and drowsy (DY) strains of hamster transmissible mink encephalopathy (TME), generated two distinct sets of PK-resistant progenitor forms [12]. Additionally, the mouse PrP MH2M variant (expressing a Syrian hamster (SHa) PrP sequence in the central region), extracted from cell culture, has been converted in a PK-resistant form after incubation with the SHa263K scrapie strain. However, no infectivity was detected when the converted material was inoculated into wild-type CD1 mice [13]. These pioneering studies recapitulate many features associated with prion transmission *in vitro*, demonstrating that the direct interaction between PrP^{Sc} and PrP^C is one of the key events during the conformational transition. Nevertheless, the PK-resistant PrP isoforms in the above mentioned studies could not be properly considered synthetic prions due to their lack of infectivity.

2.2. *De Novo* Generation of Prions by Mouse Transgenesis

A different approach that was largely explored for the purpose of generating *de novo* infectious material consisted in expressing PrP pathological mutants. These experiments were based on the hypothesis that PrP mutants should produce infectivity by increasing the likelihood of misfolding. This hypothesis is supported by evidences *in vitro* showing that some recPrP mutants (F198S and H187R) display an increased propensity to self-aggregate in amyloid PK-resistant fibrils reminiscent of natural prions [43,44]. Early efforts included the expression of two pathological mutants (six extra octapeptide insertions and the homologous human E200K) in stably transfected CHO cells, resulting in the formation of mutant proteins with biochemical properties similar to the scrapie isoform [45]. However, none of them were shown to be infectious.

Transgenic (Tg) mice expressing PrP containing pathological mutations develop a spectrum of neurological diseases that are reminiscent of TSEs [15-19]. However, none of the brain extracts from diseased Tg animals resulted able to reproduce the infectivity when inoculated in wild-type mice. Therefore, it has been argued that the identification of neurological symptoms similar to prion diseases observed in these Tg mice could be described as merely an acceleration of pre-existing diseases in the recipient mice, rather than *bona fide* transmission [18]. One possibility to explain the reason these experiments failed to develop *de novo* prions is that these models employed randomly integrated transgenes. In all these cases, mutant PrP trangene integrates in a random position, often with a variable copy number and without the control of the PrP promoter complex. The integration of multiple PrP copies causes an unusual high level of PrP expression, which would increase the likelihood of pathological conversion. Indeed, sometime an uncoupling of messenger RNA transcription levels and variable, usually lower proteins expression is described. The latter, may represent the complexity of protein expression regulation that often lacks in Tg mice.

New insights in the generation of *de novo* prions derived by experiments carried out in knockin mice expressing a PrP mutation (D179N-M129 with the 3F4 epitope tag) associated with a human prion disease FFI [20]. These mice developed biochemical, physiological, behavioral and neuropathological traits that were similar to FFI observed in humans. Interestingly, FFI knockin mice display protease sensitive PrP as well as human FFI cases [46-49], and other type of prion diseases [50]. Moreover, this spontaneous disease is infectious when transmitted to wild-type mice carrying the same 3F4 epitope, and to other Tg mice, namely Tga20 [51], expressing high level of wild-type PrP. These knockin mice were generated replacing the endogenous mouse *Prnp* gene with the construct carrying the FFI mutation, leaving the native regulatory elements unchanged. The implications of this work on the comprehension of prion diseases are remarkable. The presence of PK-sensitive PrP^{Sc} in FFI mice supports recent findings showing that novel synthetic prions become infectious yet the protein remains protease sensitive [29]. These results extend our notion about prions, which are not obligatory protease resistant [52,53]. The observation that only knockin mice developed *de novo* infectious materials suggest that PrP need to be expressed and regulated in particular cell types in order to generate TSE. Changes in the PrP regulatory elements or the overexpression of PrP may play a role by altering the physiological pathways in which PrP is involved. In any case, the observation that *de novo* prions were generated expressing a PrP mutant with endogenous expression level fulfills the prion hypothesis. Taken together, this work demonstrates that changing the PrP aminoacidic sequence is sufficient to generate *de novo* prions.

Recently, two papers reported the spontaneous appearance of infectivity from chimeric constructs of PrP inducing rigidity in the β_2-α_2 loop [21,22]. Sigurdson and coworkers [21] developed Tg mice (Tg1020), termed RL-PrP, overexpressing a PrP containing two artificial mutations, S170N and N174T, which confer a rigid structure to the β_2-α_2 loop in elk PrP [54]. These RL-PrP mice developed spontaneous and progressive clinico-pathological features similar to prion diseases, suggesting that these two aminoacidic substitutions are pathogenic for mice. These RL-PrP mice exhibited a very prolonged incubation time when infected with wild-type RML strain, arguing that the structural variation imposed by the artificial mutations creates transmission barrier to prion disease. Interestingly, sick animals are able to transmit disease to Tga20 mice (expressing wild-type PrP >2-fold higher levels than RL-PrP mice) causing similar symptoms after a long incubation time (481 ± 59 days post inoculation). However, when brain homogenates of RL-PrP mice were inoculated in Tga20 recipient mice, they caused similar neurological signs, but with shorter incubation periods. Both PK resistance and conformational stability increased after each passage. These data indicated the presence of a transmission barrier that was gradually overcome by repeated passaging. Finally, after serial passages in Tga20 mice the prion infected brain homogenates were transmissible to wild-type mice but not to PrP deficient mice. This work clearly confirms previous findings, demonstrating that *de novo* prions, could be generated by altering PrP sequence. Moreover, it underlies the role of β_2-α_2 loop region in modulating prion susceptibility and infectivity.

A further study by Aguzzi's group attempted to expand our knowledge about the significance of this epitope region on prion diseases development [22]. In this work, authors inoculated prions from five different species (mouse, deer, hamster, cattle and sheep) into RL-PrP mice and Tga20 mice in order to evaluate the effect of the "rigid loop" on the susceptibility on prion diseases. Interestingly, RL-PrP mice displayed strong transmission barriers against cattle and sheep prions, which efficiently infect Tga20 mice, and, conversely, were highly susceptible to SHa prions, for which wild-type mice are generally resistant [56,57]. These findings demonstrated that the single aminoacidic substitutions affecting the conformation of the β_2-α_2 loop significantly affect the susceptibility of a given species to prions. In particular, authors postulated that mammals carrying serine at codon 170 (responsible for the "*flexible loop*") could be easily infected by prions, whereas prions are poorly transmissible to animals carrying asparagine (responsible for the "*rigid loop*") at the same codon. In addition, several studies on species barriers support the model that the conformational flexibility of the β_2-α_2 loop represents a "*molecular switch*" for prion disease transmission.

These studies about *de novo* generation of prions by mouse transgenesis are a step ahead in showing that the infectivity is enciphered by PrP sequence. They provide invaluable insights for the comprehension on the effect of PrP pathological mutations, and on role of PrP epitopes involved in prion transmission and susceptibility. However, they do not address the issue about the infectivity generated *in vitro*, which represents the definitive proof of the prion hypothesis.

2.3. *In Vitro De Novo* Prions by PMCA

An invaluable contribution to the demonstration of the prion hypothesis is represented by an alternative conversion system, denoted as Protein Misfolding Cyclic Amplification or PMCA. It is based on the experience of the "*cell-free conversion*" developed by Caughey and collaborators, and it represents a widely used method to generate *de novo* prions *in vitro*. This approach developed by Soto's group [58,59] mimics the PrP^{Sc} autocatalytic amplification. It consists in the incubation of a large excess of PrP^{C} from healthy brain homogenate with an extremely low titer (usually 10^{-10} dilution factor) of PrP^{Sc} derived from TSE-infected animals. Basically, the mixture is then incubated to enlarge PrP^{Sc} conformers, and then subjected to multiple rounds of sonication in order to break down the aggregates and generate multiple smaller units of PrP^{Sc} conformers. The products are then diluted in new healthy brain homogenate for further amplification cycles allowing the elimination of the original PrP^{Sc} seed (10^{-20} dilution factor of the starting brain infectious material). The presence of newly generated PrP^{Sc} has been confirmed by different biochemical assays, such as the resistance to PK digestion, insolubility in non-ionic detergent or Fourier transform infrared spectroscopy [23]. Importantly, it has been shown that PMCA-generated PrP^{Sc} is infectious when intracerebrally injected into wild-type SHa, leading to a disease with biochemical and clinico-pathological features identical to the illness caused by the natural prion strain (for example the 263K scrapie strain). The only difference reported was the longer incubation time of the disease in the animal infected by PMCA-generate prion (177 ± 7.3 days) compared to the animals infected by 263K prion (106 ± 2.9 day), arguing a lower efficiency of infectivity [23]. Additionally, this method was used to amplify five different mouse strains, obtaining the same strain specific features (incubation time, biochemical and neuropathological characteristics) in wild-type mice infected by PMCA-generated PrP^{Sc} [60]. To rule out the possibility that other unknown agents in the TSE-infected brain homogenate may trigger in turn the conversion of PrP^{C} during the PMCA process, the same group demonstrated the *de novo* generation of prions starting from normal brain homogenates in the absence of any PrP^{Sc} seed [26]. Importantly, another group demonstrated the feasibility of the *de novo* prion generation by PMCA showing that PMCA of the DY and HY strains of TME recapitulate the strain specific properties of PrP^{Sc} when inoculated in wild-type SHa [24,25]. However, the presence of many unknown molecules in the brain homogenates used for the PMCA has brought on uncertainty about whether the infectivity is indeed derived from the prion agent only, or from other facilitating factors. The objective of inducing prion diseases in wild-type animals using only recPrP still represents a great challenge.

An important step forward defining the chemical composition of mammalian prions derived from studies showing that polyanions, particularly RNA [5,61-63], and lipids [64,65] facilitate the PrP conversion *in vitro*, and thus might promote the *de novo* prion formation. On the basis of these findings, Wang *et al.* recently applied PMCA to produce *de novo* prions starting from recPrP (murine full-length PrP) in the presence of both lipid (the synthetic phospholipid POPG) and RNA (total RNA isolated from mouse liver) [27,28]. To determine whether the newly PMCA generated PrP^{Sc} was capable to cause *bona fide* prion disease, authors infected wild-type CD1 mice. Animals developed classic neuropathological traits of prion diseases after about 150 days post infection. Moreover, infected brain homogenates were able to propagate the disease to recipient wild-type mice. These findings support the hypothesis that RNA and lipids are potentially important cofactors for the PrP conversions, and may represent a definitive answer to the question whether altered conformations of recPrP cause *bona fide* prion disease in wild-type mice. However, one of the major criticisms concerns the role of RNA for prion replication *in vivo*, since it is not clear whether nucleic acids are physiologically relevant or simply mimic other not well-characterized polyanionic molecules.

2.4. *De Novo* Prions by Amyloid Seeding Assay

Another largely explored strategy consisted of using several physico-chemical approaches to inducing misfolding of the recPrP into β-strand rich states. Such studies are relevant because they address the question whether PrP alone is sufficient for the spontaneous formation of prions without the presence of any exogenous agent or facilitator of the conversion. A plethora of studies have attempted to provide an answer to this question, but these experiments have largely failed in producing infectivity *in vivo* or the infectivity potential has not been tested so far (see, for instance, [66-73]). However, in 2004 the production of synthetic prions via the *in vitro* conversion of bacterially expressed recPrP was reported [31]. In a previous work [66], the same authors analyzed in detail the multiple misfolding pathways of recPrP (from residue 89 to 230) leading to β-sheet rich conformers. Depending on the reaction conditions, two misfolded forms were adopted: at acidic pH (3 to 5) and in the presence of partially denaturing urea concentration (4-5 M) a β-oligomer PrP^{Sc}-like is formed with no further aggregation; whereas under neutral or slightly acidic pH values and at low concentration of urea (1-2 M) recPrP aggregates in fibrillar structures which develop into amyloid. The polymerization process was monitored simply applying thioflavin T (ThT) in the reaction mixture. This dye shows strong increase of fluorescence upon binding to β-sheet rich structures like amyloid aggregates. Importantly, in this work authors discovered that the addition of a seed of pre-folded amyloid to the fresh reaction substantially reduces the time of the fibrillization (called lag phase) process, demonstrating that recPrP fibrils can be induced by seeding. Starting from these findings, Prusiner and collaborators [31] addressed the question to whether these synthetic fibrils were infectious when inoculated into mice. The pre-folded amyloid fibrils (denoted as "*unseeded*") and the seeded composed of recMoPrP(89-230) were intracerebrally injected into Tg9949 mice, which overexpress

MoPrP(89-230). Seeded amyloid fibrils exhibited shorter incubation time (382 days) and PK resistance than unseeded (473 days and PK sensitivity). Interestingly, also the neuropathological features associated with seeded and unseeded amyloids were different in terms, for instance, of vacuolation and gray matter PrP^{Sc} deposition. The authors argued that this result might be due to the creation of two new prion strains, denoted as MoSP1 (for Mouse **b**ynthetic Prion strain 1, obtained from seeded PrP amyloids) and as MoSP2 (from unseeded amyloid). Moreover, MoSP1 prion exhibited infectivity and shortened incubation periods upon serial passages to both wild-type FVB mice and different Tg mice lines [31-33]. The conformational stability of MoSP1, as measured by the GndHCl concentration required to denature half of the sample, was very high (~4.5 M) compared to other natural prion strains, confirming that a novel synthetic prion has been obtained [32]. Subsequent serial passages of this strain led to shorten incubation periods and a decreased conformational stability of the resulting prions. Combining these data with those available for naturally occurring prion strains, it was demonstrated that the length of the incubation time in mice is directly proportional to the conformational stability of the prion strain [30,33]. These results suggest that decreasing PrP^{Sc} stability increases the fragmentation of PrP^{Sc}. This in turn causes the generation of multiple seeds that can increase the rate of the conversion and shorten the incubation period. Consistent with this hypothesis, studies examining other fibrillogenic proteins (Sup35, Tau, synuclein and β-amyloid) demonstrate that less stable fibrils have a higher propensity to undergo breakage, creating new seeds for the conversion [74-80].

It has been reported that partially purified prion strains preparation may act as a seed for the polymerization of recPrP in amyloid fibrils. This conformational change can be monitored simply by a fluorescence shift in the dye ThT. When used in conjunction with multi-well plates and automated fluorescence plate readers, the ThT represents a feasible, highly sensitive, high-throughput approach for the detection of conformational changes of proteins. Authors denoted "*amyloid seeding assay*" (ASA), the method of amyloid fibrils formation seeded by preformed PrP^{Sc} and monitored by ThT fluorescence. The method of ASA is able to detect PrP^{Sc} (both PK sensitive or resistant) from different human or animal infected brain samples [29,30]. Another feature of ASA is the possibility to shake the sample in order to enhance the interaction between recPrP and the seed (included preformed amyloid from recPrP or partially purified PrP^{Sc} from infected sample) and promote the generation of multiple seeds. Additionally, the partial unfolding of recPrP is enhanced by the presence of low denaturant concentration (usually GndHCl).

The same group recently reported the generation of protease-sensitive, synthetic prions *in vitro* during the polymerization of recPrP into amyloid fibers [29]. The inoculation of this amyloid preparation to Tg9949 mice resulted in novel, protease-sensitive, synthetic prions, which caused severe neuropathology and were transmissible both in Tg9949 mice and in Tg4053 mice, which moderately overexpress the full-length MoPrP. These results demonstrate that also PK-sensitive synthetic prions are able to transmit prion disease and change our notion that the protease resistance is not an obligatory feature of PrP^{Sc}, as it has been reported in some sporadic [50] and genetic [46-49] cases of prion disease.

The findings that different synthetic prions are able to generate TSE *de novo* provided the strongest evidence that PrP^{Sc} is the only element needed for infectivity. The main criticism about these findings is the observation that transgenic animals overexpressing PrP develop prion-like disease spontaneously [81-83]. Therefore, it could not be ruled out that the effects observed might be just an acceleration of a disease process. However, it is important to note that the authors clearly answered to these criticisms demonstrating by means of different assays (ASA, PK digestion and histopathology) that the spontaneous neurological dysfunctions observed in Tg9949 control mice are not related to spontaneous generation of prions, but rather to aging of the animals [29].

2.5. *De Novo* Prions by Annealing Technique

Additional evidence has been shown that synthetic prions can be generated when amyloid fibrils from full length SHaPrP are intracerebrally inoculated in wild-type hamster [35]. Authors converted recPrP into cross-β-sheet amyloids and subjected to "*annealing*". Basically, this procedure consisted in the incubation of recPrP with normal brain homogenate, and then in subjecting the mixture to different heating and cooling cycles [34]. The result was then verified by PK-treatment. No disease was produced in the first passage although PrP^{Sc} was detected in the brain. However, serial transmission gave rise to a TSE disease phenotype with highly unique clinical and neuropathological features and a very long incubation time.

2.6. Concluding Remarks and New Emerging Techniques for Prion Detection and Generation

The previous sections have recapitulated all relevant studies and experimental data on the generation of synthetic prions. It has been shown that PMCA and ASA are largely used methods to generate *de novo* prions *in vitro*. Moreover, they have many applications for effective prion disease diagnosis due to their high sensitivity. Indeed, the minimal PrP^{Sc} quantity that can be detected and propagated by PMCA and ASA is 1.3 ag (corresponding to about 26 PrP^{Sc} molecules) and about 1 fg (1.8×10^4 molecules detected), respectively [30,58]. However, the limits of the PMCA detection include the long experimental time (about 3 weeks), a read-out of the assay based only on PK-resistant prions visualized by immunoblotting, the impossibility to detect protease sensitive prions and the use of sonication, which is inherently difficult to control. Conversely, ASA is a higher-throughput approach for prions detection in short experimental time (usually 3-4 days), but a potentially confounding aspect is the frequent spontaneous formation of recPrP fibrils (without seeding by prions) before prion-seeded reactions [30,58].

To improve the speed and practicality of prion detection assays, new techniques have been developed. The recPrP-PMCA [36] represents an improvement of the classical PMCA because it employs recPrP as substrate for the conversion reaction instead of normal brain homogenate. This method still uses periodic sonication and serial reaction rounds but is faster (2-3 days) and highly sensitive. To circumvent problems associated with sonications, a new assay has been developed, denoted QuIC for quaking-induced conversion [37]. QuiC uses recPrP as a substrate and automated tube shaking rather than sonication. This assay can detect about one lethal prion dose within a day and it is faster and simpler than previous described techniques. The technique QuIC has several advantages over conventional PMCA: it is faster, highly sensitive, simple and easy to duplicate. It is able to seed prions even without GndHCl, which it is thought to increase the spontaneous fibril formation [39]. However, a major limitation of all these methods is the lack of prion quantification. Very recently, a method has been developed called quantitative PMCA (qPMCA), in which the PrP^{Sc} content is estimated by the number of PMCA rounds necessary for a positive response [38]. This last new *in vitro* amplification technology for PrP^{Sc} is called real-time QuiC or RT-QuiC [42]. The method combines several aspects of ASA, such as intermittent shaking, recPrP as a substrate, sample preparation, the fluorescence ThT readout and sensitivity. Indeed, RT-QuIC can rapidly determine the relative prion concentration on the basis of serial dilutions of the infected samples and of statistically estimation of the seeding dilution at which 50% of the reaction becomes ThT positive. Moreover, RT-QuiC might represent a valuable new means for the early, rapid, *ante mortem* diagnosis for TSEs. In particular, its ability to detect PrP^{Sc} not only from infected brain samples but also from nasal lavages [42], cerebrospinal fluid [39] and blood, has been shown [41].

The new emerging techniques here described represents a step forward defining the methods for effective diagnoses of prion disease, but the newly generated prions have not been tested *in vivo* for infectivity. So far, the only *in vitro* high-throughput technique for prion detection and generation remains the ASA developed in the Prusiner's laboratory.

3. Structural Biology of Natural and Synthetic Prions

One of the most important challenges in prion biology is determining the structural traits of prions. Detailed information about PrP^{Sc} structure is crucial not only for understanding the molecular basis of conversion and transmission, but also for effective pharmacological intervention.

Several spectroscopic studies revealed that the amyloid form of PrP is β-sheet enriched [84-89]. However, all the structural studies on prions are limited by the disorder and insolubility of PrP^{Sc}, or PrP27-30, and are still lacking to demonstrate its structure at atomic level. In absence of direct experimental evidences, two models have attempted to describe the putative PrP^{Sc} structure: the "***β**-helical*" and the "*spiral*" models. The first originates from cryo-electron microscopy data and structural modeling and proposes that PrP^{Sc} forms β-sheets in the region from 89 to 171, which are rearranged in left-handed β-helices [90]. In the spiral model the proposed PrP^{Sc} structure derives from an all-atom explicit solvent molecular dynamic simulation [91,92]. According to this model, during prion conversion the two native β-sheets elongate in a longer single β-strand, which forms intermolecular β-sheets with other PrP molecules leading to polymerization. The basic subunit of the oligomers was also modeled according to a trimer.

From the experimental point of view, several research groups investigated the molecular mechanism of the conversion process by means of different methods. Table 2 summarizes all the relevant studies, which have tried to elucidate the mechanism of conversion from PrP^{C} to PrP^{Sc} using biochemical, biophysical and structural approaches. In this section we focus our analysis on the most relevant studies regarding the structural biology of natural prions and synthetic prions.

3.1. Structural Studies on Natural and Synthetic Prions

In the previous section we underlined that the sole component of mammalian prion is PrP^{Sc}. Limited proteolysis on PrP^{Sc} usually generates a smaller C-terminal PK-resistant molecule composed by approximately 142 residues starting from residue ~90. Historically, PrP^{Sc} is denoted also as PrP27-30 because of its electrophoretic mobility, which encompasses a molecular weight from 27 to 30 kDa [1]. In the presence of detergent PrP27-30 polymerizes into rod-shaped particles, which exhibit morphological and tinctorial features of amyloids [93]. According to the modern biophysical definition, amyloids are fibers composed by assemblies of misfolded proteins whose repeating structural unit consists of cross-β–sheet. This motif results from hydrogen bonded β–sheets running perpendicularly to the filament axis [94]. By means of electron microscopy, amyloids are identified as long, non-branched filaments with diameters of around 6-12 nm [95]. The repeating cross-β–sheet motif gives rise to a distinctive X-ray fiber diffraction pattern, including a strong meridional intensity at about 4.75 Å resolution (corresponding to the inter-β strand spacing), and an equatorial reflection at about 10 Å resolution (corresponding to the distance between stacked β–sheets) [96].

The distinctive cross-β fiber diffraction pattern has been recently observed also from natural infectious prions [97]. Authors obtained X-ray diffraction data from both natural and synthetic prions, including the SHa Sc237 PrP27-30 strain (SHaSc237), the mouse RML prion (MoRML), the mouse adapted MoSP1 synthetic prion [31-33,98], the mouse recPrP(89-230) [recMoPrP(89-230)] and recSHa(90-231) amyloids. Interestingly, fiber diffraction patterns of SHaSc237, MoRML and MoSP1 exhibited a marked intensity maximum at 4.8 Å resolutions, confirming the presence of β-strands running at right angles to the filament axis and typical for amyloid structures. Diffraction patterns exhibited a series of equatorial maxima, which diminished in intensity with increasing resolution. Equatorial diffraction from brain isolated natural and synthetic prions also included an intense, moderately sharp, low-angle reflection (63.3 Å). The presence of reflection at low-angle is characteristic of fibers with poorly ordered para-crystalline packing. Conversely, diffraction patterns from both recMoPrP(89-230) and recSHa(90-231) amyloids resulted different from brain-extracted prions. Recombinant amyloids showed a well-defined 4.8 Å meridional layer line, but with an equatorial broad maximum at 10.5 Å. This diffraction pattern is consistent with a stacked β-sheet structure for the major component of recPrP amyloids. These differences imply that recPrP fibrils do not have the same amyloid structure as brain adapted prions. This structural information might also explain the substantial differences in their infectivity.

The implications of the studies reported by Wille *et al.* are remarkable. The X-ray diffraction patterns of brain-extracted prions demonstrate that PrP^{Sc} fibrils present a cross-β structure consistent with the "*β-helical*" model, confirming that prion can form amyloid. On the contrary, *in vitro* generated synthetic prions do not display the cross-β structure, suggesting that their lower infectivity may be due to an undetectable contribution of fibers with a structure similar to brain-derived prions. This work represents the only available study carried out on synthetic prions, including both MoSP1 and the infectious recMoPrP(89-230) amyloid. All the other structural studies on recPrP fibrils summarized in Table 2 cannot be properly considered synthetic prions due to the lack of infectivity.

Recently, Surewicz and collaborators examined by hydrogen-deuterium exchange the structural organization of PrP^{Sc} extracted from Tg mice expressing unglycosilated PrP^{C} lacking GPI anchor (ΔGPI) [99]. In contrast to the β-helical model, these data indicate that the PrP^{Sc} structure might include a continuum of short β-strands from residue ~90 to the entire C-terminal region.

Table 2. Proposed region involved in the conversion from PrP^{C} and PrP^{Sc}.

Methods	Fibril core region	Substrate	Refs.
Limited proteolisis	78/82/97-231	Type 1 Human PrP27-30	[100,101]
	92/97/103-231	Type 2 Human PrP27-30	[102,103]
	154/156/162/167-231	Sporadic CJD	[102]
	74/80-231; 146/153-231	GSS	[102]
	86/90/92/98/101/117/119/ 135/139/142/154-231	Drowsy (DY) Syrian hamster strain	[104,105]
Chemical cross-linking	From G90-231	PrP27-30 purified from scrapie-infected SHa	[106]
Antibody labeling	90-120	PrP27-30 purified from scrapie-infected SHa	[107,108]
Solution-state NMR	145-223	RecHuPrP(90-231)	[109]
Cryo-EM (β-helix model)	89-174	PrP27-30 purified from scrapie-infected SHa	[90,97,110]
Hydrogen-deuterium exchange	~80/90-231	ΔGPI 22L PrP^{Sc} extracted from Tg mice	[99]
	~163-223	recSHa(90-231), recSHa(23-231)	[111]
	~178-213	PMCA generated recSHa(90-231), recSHa(23-231)	[111]
	~160-220	recHuPrP(90-231, D178N)	[112]
	~169-213	recHuPrP(90-231)	[113]
Solid State NMR	112-141	recHuPrP23-144	[114] [115]
	175-225	recSHa(23-231)	[116]
high-pressure NMR	~175-231	recSHa(90-231)	[117,118]
In silico studies	~175-231	HuPrP(124-228)	[119,120]
	116-119; 129-132; 160-164 (spiral model)	HuPrP(23-231)	[91,92]

While the X-ray diffraction data demonstrate the presence of cross-β structure in brain-extracted prions consistent with the β-helical model, the last work of Surewicz clearly indicates that other structural models cannot be ruled out.

3.2. Lesson from Human Prion Protein Pathological Mutants

In section 2.2, we reported different studies in which Tg mice carrying pathological PrP mutations develop a spectrum of neurological diseases sharing some features with TSEs. Moreover, mutants are able to generate *de novo* prions only by altering the PrP coding sequence. It has been proposed that disease-linked mutations increase the likelihood of misfolding by the thermodynamic destabilization of PrP^C [121-123]. However, this cannot be taken as a general mechanism because individual mutations differently affect PrP^C stability. Besides influencing the stability of PrP^C, mutations may also alter its surface properties triggering in turn an abnormal interaction with other, not yet identified cofactors [6,124], or causing an aberrant trafficking and accumulation inside the cell [125]. Most point mutations linked to inherited prion diseases are clustered in the structural region between helices 2 and 3. Interestingly, this region has been suggested to be involved in structural reorganization during the conversion process to PrP^{Sc} by different experimental and *in silico* data (Table 2). Therefore, solution NMR studies on PrP carrying mutations localized in the globular domain might help in the identification of "hot spots" in PrP^C involved in the pathogenic conversion. Recently, we determined the NMR structures of two mutations causing familial prion diseases: Q212P [126] and V210I [127] linked to GSS syndrome and familial CJD, respectively [128]. The comparison with the structure of the wild-type human (Hu) PrP revealed that, although the structures share similar globular architecture, mutations introduce novel local structural differences (Figure 1). The observed variations are mostly clustered in the β_2-α_2 loop region and in α_2-α_3 inter-helical interface. The β_2-α_2 loop is poorly defined and highly disordered in the mutants due to the interruption of aromatic and hydrophobic interactions between Tyr163, Met166, Tyr169, Phe175 and Tyr218, which stabilize the overall fold in the wild-type (Figure 1b). Consequently, this affects the exposition to the solvent of the aforementioned residues, and the distance between this loop and the C-terminal part of α_3 increases upon mutation, as illustrated in Figure 1a and 1b. In support, similar findings have been reported also in the NMR structure of the E200K mutant [129], in the F198S and D178N X-ray crystal structures [130], and in several independent molecular dynamic studies [131-135]. Moreover, various studies on species barriers support the model that the conformational flexibility of the β_2-α_2 loop represents a "*molecular switch*" for prion disease transmission [21,22].

In conclusion, our findings on Q212P and V210I mutants provide new clues about the possible early events of PrP^C misfolding. The structural disorder of the β_2–α_2 loop together with the increased distance between this loop and α_3 helix observed in different mutants leads to exposure of hydrophobic residues to solvent. This might have an effect on the long-range interactions that govern the correct folding of α_2 and α_3 helices and promotes the protein conformational changes and intermolecular interactions.

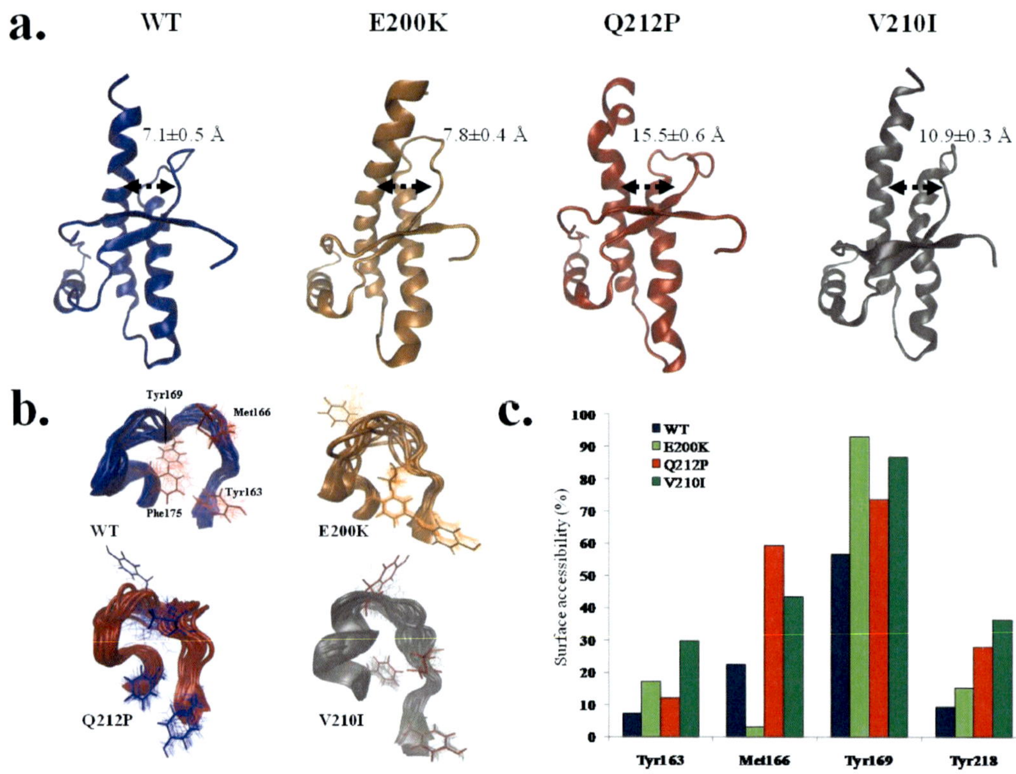

Figure 1. Effects of pathological mutations on the HuPrP structure. (a.) Ribbon representation of different HuPrP NMR structures: wild-type, WT (1QM1), E200K (1FO7), Q212P (2KUN) and V210I (2LEJ). Distances between C_{α}-Met166 and C_{α}-Glu221 are highlighted. (b.) Structural details of the β_2-α_2 loop region. (c.) Average values of solvent accessibility (%) of selected residues calculated from the structures using GETAREA.

Conclusion

The generation of synthetic prions demonstrated that PrP^{Sc} is the principal, if not the sole, causative agent of TSEs, providing important information about the structural basis of prion conversion and the understanding of prion susceptibility and infectivity. However, one of the most significant challenges in prion biology is the identification of the structural determinants of prion conversion. At present, only low-resolution techniques attempted sheding light on the PrP^{Sc} structure often with contrasting results. The fact that in mammals more than a dozen of different prion strains are documented can explain the multitude of PrP^{Sc} structural organizations [136]. The different structural organizations of amyloid prions are the basis for understanding the nature of strain-specific species barriers in mammals. The phenomena of prion adaptation observed after serial transmission experiments might be explained as a new conformation adopted by PrP^{Sc}, which enables itself to replicate in the host. Many combinations of assemblies, the presence of polymorphism/mutations and other chemical modifications (such as distinct physiological environments or the glycosylation patterns) may give rise to a plethora of amyloid states, which present virtually indefinite structural features and physiological activities. Therefore, it is reasonable to argue that the identification of a common structural motif for amyloids composed by PrP^{Sc} is still hard to be detected.

An alternative scenario for the comprehension of prion diseases may arise from studies aimed at clarifying which are the PrP epitopes involved in the conversion. In particular, the use of pathological mutants represents an invaluable strategy for this purpose since mutations seem to share a common mechanism of misfolding. Moreover, new insights may derive from studies focused on the structural and biochemical characterization of the PrP^{C} intermediate state, denoted as PrP* [118,137]. Such studies are relevant in the pursuit of isolating PrP isoforms, including the *bona fide* monomeric PrP^{Sc} β-sheet rich state, and may provide the ultimate information regarding the "*hot spots*" of prion conversion.

REFERENCES

[1] Prusiner SB (1998) Prions. Proc Natl Acad Sci U S A 95: 13363-13383.

[2] Prusiner SB (1982) Novel proteinaceous infectious particles cause scrapie. Science 216: 136-144.

[3] Prusiner SB (1998) The prion diseases. Brain Pathol 8: 499-513.

[4] Prusiner SB (2001) Shattuck lecture--neurodegenerative diseases and prions. N Engl J Med 344: 1516-1526.

[5] Deleault NR, Lucassen RW, Supattapone S (2003) RNA molecules stimulate prion protein conversion. Nature 425: 717-720.

[6] Telling GC, Scott M, Mastrianni J, Gabizon R, Torchia M, et al. (1995) Prion propagation in mice expressing human and chimeric PrP transgenes implicates the interaction of cellular PrP with another protein. Cell 83: 79-90.

[7] Kanaani J, Prusiner SB, Diacovo J, Baekkeskov S, Legname G (2005) Recombinant prion protein induces rapid polarization and development of synapses in embryonic rat hippocampal neurons in vitro. J Neurochem 95: 1373-1386.

[8] Bolton DC, McKinley MP, Prusiner SB (1982) Identification of a protein that purifies with the scrapie prion. Science 218: 1309-1311.

[9] Safar JG, Scott M, Monaghan J, Deering C, Didorenko S, et al. (2002) Measuring prions causing bovine spongiform encephalopathy or chronic wasting disease by immunoassays and transgenic mice. Nat Biotechnol 20: 1147-1150.

[10] Benetti F, Legname G (2009) De novo mammalian prion synthesis. Prion 3: 213-219.

[11] Legname G, Giachin G, F B (in press) Structural studies of prion proteins and prions. Pre-fibrillar amyloidogenic protein assemblies-common cytotoxins underlying degenerative diseases: Springer Publishing.

[12] Bessen RA, Kocisko DA, Raymond GJ, Nandan S, Lansbury PT, et al. (1995) Non-genetic propagation of strain-specific properties of scrapie prion protein. Nature 375: 698-700.

[13] Hill AF, Antoniou M, Collinge J (1999) Protease-resistant prion protein produced in vitro lacks detectable infectivity. J Gen Virol 80 (Pt 1): 11-14.

[14] Kocisko DA, Come JH, Priola SA, Chesebro B, Raymond GJ, et al. (1994) Cell-free formation of protease-resistant prion protein. Nature 370: 471-474.

[15] Chiesa R, Piccardo P, Ghetti B, Harris DA (1998) Neurological illness in transgenic mice expressing a prion protein with an insertional mutation. Neuron 21: 1339-1351.
[16] Dossena S, Imeri L, Mangieri M, Garofoli A, Ferrari L, et al. (2008) Mutant prion protein expression causes motor and memory deficits and abnormal sleep patterns in a transgenic mouse model. Neuron 60: 598-609.
[17] Hsiao KK, Scott M, Foster D, Groth DF, DeArmond SJ, et al. (1990) Spontaneous neurodegeneration in transgenic mice with mutant prion protein. Science 250: 1587-1590.
[18] Nazor KE, Kuhn F, Seward T, Green M, Zwald D, et al. (2005) Immunodetection of disease-associated mutant PrP, which accelerates disease in GSS transgenic mice. EMBO J 24: 2472-2480.
[19] Shmerling D, Hegyi I, Fischer M, Blattler T, Brandner S, et al. (1998) Expression of amino-terminally truncated PrP in the mouse leading to ataxia and specific cerebellar lesions. Cell 93: 203-214.
[20] Jackson WS, Borkowski AW, Faas H, Steele AD, King OD, et al. (2009) Spontaneous generation of prion infectivity in fatal familial insomnia knockin mice. Neuron 63: 438-450.
[21] Sigurdson CJ, Nilsson KP, Hornemann S, Heikenwalder M, Manco G, et al. (2009) De novo generation of a transmissible spongiform encephalopathy by mouse transgenesis. Proc Natl Acad Sci U S A 106: 304-309.
[22] Sigurdson CJ, Nilsson KP, Hornemann S, Manco G, Fernandez-Borges N, et al. (2010) A molecular switch controls interspecies prion disease transmission in mice. J Clin Invest 120: 2590-2599.
[23] Castilla J, Saa P, Hetz C, Soto C (2005) In vitro generation of infectious scrapie prions. Cell 121: 195-206.
[24] Ayers JI, Schutt CR, Shikiya RA, Aguzzi A, Kincaid AE, et al. (2011) The strain-encoded relationship between PrP replication, stability and processing in neurons is predictive of the incubation period of disease. PLoS Pathog 7: e1001317.
[25] Shikiya RA, Ayers JI, Schutt CR, Kincaid AE, Bartz JC (2010) Coinfecting prion strains compete for a limiting cellular resource. J Virol 84: 5706-5714.
[26] Barria MA, Mukherjee A, Gonzalez-Romero D, Morales R, Soto C (2009) De novo generation of infectious prions in vitro produces a new disease phenotype. PLoS Pathog 5: e1000421.
[27] Wang F, Wang X, Ma J (2011) Conversion of bacterially expressed recombinant prion protein. Methods 53: 208-213.
[28] Wang F, Wang X, Yuan CG, Ma J (2010) Generating a prion with bacterially expressed recombinant prion protein. Science 327: 1132-1135.
[29] Colby DW, Wain R, Baskakov IV, Legname G, Palmer CG, et al. (2010) Protease-sensitive synthetic prions. PLoS Pathog 6: e1000736.
[30] Colby DW, Zhang Q, Wang S, Groth D, Legname G, et al. (2007) Prion detection by an amyloid seeding assay. Proc Natl Acad Sci U S A 104: 20914-20919.
[31] Legname G, Baskakov IV, Nguyen HO, Riesner D, Cohen FE, et al. (2004) Synthetic mammalian prions. Science 305: 673-676.
[32] Legname G, Nguyen HO, Baskakov IV, Cohen FE, DeArmond SJ, et al. (2005) Strain-specified characteristics of mouse synthetic prions. Proc Natl Acad Sci U S A 102: 2168-2173.

[33] Legname G, Nguyen HO, Peretz D, Cohen FE, DeArmond SJ, et al. (2006) Continuum of prion protein structures enciphers a multitude of prion isolate-specified phenotypes. Proc Natl Acad Sci U S A 103: 19105-19110.

[34] Bocharova OV, Makarava N, Breydo L, Anderson M, Salnikov VV, et al. (2006) Annealing prion protein amyloid fibrils at high temperature results in extension of a proteinase K-resistant core. J Biol Chem 281: 2373-2379.

[35] Makarava N, Kovacs GG, Bocharova O, Savtchenko R, Alexeeva I, et al. (2010) Recombinant prion protein induces a new transmissible prion disease in wild-type animals. Acta Neuropathol 119: 177-187.

[36] Atarashi R, Moore RA, Sim VL, Hughson AG, Dorward DW, et al. (2007) Ultrasensitive detection of scrapie prion protein using seeded conversion of recombinant prion protein. Nat Methods 4: 645-650.

[37] Atarashi R, Wilham JM, Christensen L, Hughson AG, Moore RA, et al. (2008) Simplified ultrasensitive prion detection by recombinant PrP conversion with shaking. Nat Methods 5: 211-212.

[38] Chen B, Morales R, Barria MA, Soto C (2010) Estimating prion concentration in fluids and tissues by quantitative PMCA. Nat Methods 7: 519-520.

[39] Atarashi R, Satoh K, Sano K, Fuse T, Yamaguchi N, et al. (2011) Ultrasensitive human prion detection in cerebrospinal fluid by real-time quaking-induced conversion. Nat Med 17: 175-178.

[40] Orru CD, Caughey B (2011) Prion Seeded Conversion and Amplification Assays. Top Curr Chem.

[41] Orru CD, Wilham JM, Raymond LD, Kuhn F, Schroeder B, et al. (2011) Prion disease blood test using immunoprecipitation and improved quaking-induced conversion. MBio 2.

[42] Wilham JM, Orru CD, Bessen RA, Atarashi R, Sano K, et al. (2010) Rapid end-point quantitation of prion seeding activity with sensitivity comparable to bioassays. PLoS Pathog 6: e1001217.

[43] Hosszu LL, Tattum MH, Jones S, Trevitt CR, Wells MA, et al. (2010) The H187R mutation of the human prion protein induces conversion of recombinant prion protein to the PrP(Sc)-like form. Biochemistry 49: 8729-8738.

[44] Vanik DL, Surewicz WK (2002) Disease-associated F198S mutation increases the propensity of the recombinant prion protein for conformational conversion to scrapie-like form. J Biol Chem 277: 49065-49070.

[45] Lehmann S, Harris DA (1996) Two mutant prion proteins expressed in cultured cells acquire biochemical properties reminiscent of the scrapie isoform. Proc Natl Acad Sci U S A 93: 5610-5614.

[46] Brown P, Kenney K, Little B, Ironside J, Will R, et al. (1995) Intracerebral distribution of infectious amyloid protein in spongiform encephalopathy. Ann Neurol 38: 245-253.

[47] 47. Little BW, Brown PW, Rodgers-Johnson P, Perl DP, Gajdusek DC (1986) Familial myoclonic dementia masquerading as Creutzfeldt-Jakob disease. Ann Neurol 20: 231-239.

[48] Medori R, Montagna P, Tritschler HJ, LeBlanc A, Cortelli P, et al. (1992) Fatal familial insomnia: a second kindred with mutation of prion protein gene at codon 178. Neurology 42: 669-670.

[49] Zarranz JJ, Digon A, Atares B, Rodriguez-Martinez AB, Arce A, et al. (2005) Phenotypic variability in familial prion diseases due to the D178N mutation. J Neurol Neurosurg Psychiatry 76: 1491-1496.
[50] Gambetti P, Puoti G, Zou WQ (2011) Variably Protease-Sensitive Prionopathy: a Novel Disease of the Prion Protein. J Mol Neurosci.
[51] Fischer M, Rulicke T, Raeber A, Sailer A, Moser M, et al. (1996) Prion protein (PrP) with amino-proximal deletions restoring susceptibility of PrP knockout mice to scrapie. EMBO J 15: 1255-1264.
[52] McKinley MP, Bolton DC, Prusiner SB (1983) A protease-resistant protein is a structural component of the scrapie prion. Cell 35: 57-62.
[53] Tremblay P, Ball HL, Kaneko K, Groth D, Hegde RS, et al. (2004) Mutant PrPSc conformers induced by a synthetic peptide and several prion strains. J Virol 78: 2088-2099.
[54] Gossert AD, Bonjour S, Lysek DA, Fiorito F, Wuthrich K (2005) Prion protein NMR structures of elk and of mouse/elk hybrids. Proc Natl Acad Sci U S A 102: 646-650.
[55] 55. Perez DR, Damberger FF, Wuthrich K (2010) Horse prion protein NMR structure and comparisons with related variants of the mouse prion protein. J Mol Biol 400: 121-128.
[56] Kimberlin RH, Walker CA (1978) Evidence that the transmission of one source of scrapie agent to hamsters involves separation of agent strains from a mixture. J Gen Virol 39: 487-496.
[57] Race R, Meade-White K, Raines A, Raymond GJ, Caughey B, et al. (2002) Subclinical scrapie infection in a resistant species: persistence, replication, and adaptation of infectivity during four passages. J Infect Dis 186 Suppl 2: S166-170.
[58] Saa P, Castilla J, Soto C (2005) Cyclic amplification of protein misfolding and aggregation. Methods Mol Biol 299: 53-65.
[59] Saborio GP, Permanne B, Soto C (2001) Sensitive detection of pathological prion protein by cyclic amplification of protein misfolding. Nature 411: 810-813.
[60] Castilla J, Morales R, Saa P, Barria M, Gambetti P, et al. (2008) Cell-free propagation of prion strains. EMBO J 27: 2557-2566.
[61] Deleault NR, Geoghegan JC, Nishina K, Kascsak R, Williamson RA, et al. (2005) Protease-resistant prion protein amplification reconstituted with partially purified substrates and synthetic polyanions. J Biol Chem 280: 26873-26879.
[62] Deleault NR, Harris BT, Rees JR, Supattapone S (2007) Formation of native prions from minimal components in vitro. Proc Natl Acad Sci U S A 104: 9741-9746.
[63] Geoghegan JC, Valdes PA, Orem NR, Deleault NR, Williamson RA, et al. (2007) Selective incorporation of polyanionic molecules into hamster prions. J Biol Chem 282: 36341-36353.
[64] Wang F, Yang F, Hu Y, Wang X, Jin C, et al. (2007) Lipid interaction converts prion protein to a PrPSc-like proteinase K-resistant conformation under physiological conditions. Biochemistry 46: 7045-7053.
[65] White SH, Ladokhin AS, Jayasinghe S, Hristova K (2001) How membranes shape protein structure. J Biol Chem 276: 32395-32398.
[66] Baskakov IV, Legname G, Baldwin MA, Prusiner SB, Cohen FE (2002) Pathway complexity of prion protein assembly into amyloid. J Biol Chem 277: 21140-21148.

[67] Bjorndahl TC, Zhou GP, Liu X, Perez-Pineiro R, Semenchenko V, et al. (2011) Detailed biophysical characterization of the acid-induced PrP(c) to PrP(beta) conversion process. Biochemistry 50: 1162-1173.

[68] Bocharova OV, Breydo L, Parfenov AS, Salnikov VV, Baskakov IV (2005) In vitro conversion of full-length mammalian prion protein produces amyloid form with physical properties of PrP(Sc). J Mol Biol 346: 645-659.

[69] Cobb NJ, Apetri AC, Surewicz WK (2008) Prion protein amyloid formation under native-like conditions involves refolding of the C-terminal alpha-helical domain. J Biol Chem 283: 34704-34711.

[70] Jackson GS, Hosszu LL, Power A, Hill AF, Kenney J, et al. (1999) Reversible conversion of monomeric human prion protein between native and fibrilogenic conformations. Science 283: 1935-1937.

[71] Jones EM, Surewicz WK (2005) Fibril conformation as the basis of species- and strain-dependent seeding specificity of mammalian prion amyloids. Cell 121: 63-72.

[72] Lee S, Eisenberg D (2003) Seeded conversion of recombinant prion protein to a disulfide-bonded oligomer by a reduction-oxidation process. Nat Struct Biol 10: 725-730.

[73] Polano M, Bek A, Benetti F, Lazzarino M, Legname G (2009) Structural insights into alternate aggregated prion protein forms. J Mol Biol 393: 1033-1042.

[74] Kryndushkin DS, Alexandrov IM, Ter-Avanesyan MD, Kushnirov VV (2003) Yeast [PSI+] prion aggregates are formed by small Sup35 polymers fragmented by Hsp104. J Biol Chem 278: 49636-49643.

[75] Lee S, Fernandez EJ, Good TA (2007) Role of aggregation conditions in structure, stability, and toxicity of intermediates in the Abeta fibril formation pathway. Protein Sci 16: 723-732.

[76] Sun Y, Makarava N, Lee CI, Laksanalamai P, Robb FT, et al. (2008) Conformational stability of PrP amyloid fibrils controls their smallest possible fragment size. J Mol Biol 376: 1155-1167.

[77] Tanaka M, Collins SR, Toyama BH, Weissman JS (2006) The physical basis of how prion conformations determine strain phenotypes. Nature 442: 585-589.

[78] Li X, Xue X, Li PC (2009) Real-time detection of the early event of cytotoxicity of herbal ingredients on single leukemia cells studied in a microfluidic biochip. Integr Biol (Camb) 1: 90-98.

[79] Yonetani M, Nonaka T, Masuda M, Inukai Y, Oikawa T, et al. (2009) Conversion of wild-type alpha-synuclein into mutant-type fibrils and its propagation in the presence of A30P mutant. J Biol Chem 284: 7940-7950.

[80] Zhou Z, Fan JB, Zhu HL, Shewmaker F, Yan X, et al. (2009) Crowded cell-like environment accelerates the nucleation step of amyloidogenic protein misfolding. J Biol Chem 284: 30148-30158.

[81] Castilla J, Gutierrez-Adan A, Brun A, Pintado B, Parra B, et al. (2004) Different behavior toward bovine spongiform encephalopathy infection of bovine prion protein transgenic mice with one extra repeat octapeptide insert mutation. J Neurosci 24: 2156-2164.

[82] Chiesa R, Drisaldi B, Quaglio E, Migheli A, Piccardo P, et al. (2000) Accumulation of protease-resistant prion protein (PrP) and apoptosis of cerebellar granule cells in

transgenic mice expressing a PrP insertional mutation. Proc Natl Acad Sci U S A 97: 5574-5579.
[83] Westaway D, DeArmond SJ, Cayetano-Canlas J, Groth D, Foster D, et al. (1994) Degeneration of skeletal muscle, peripheral nerves, and the central nervous system in transgenic mice overexpressing wild-type prion proteins. Cell 76: 117-129.
[84] Caughey B, Raymond GJ, Bessen RA (1998) Strain-dependent differences in beta-sheet conformations of abnormal prion protein. J Biol Chem 273: 32230-32235.
[85] Caughey BW, Dong A, Bhat KS, Ernst D, Hayes SF, et al. (1991) Secondary structure analysis of the scrapie-associated protein PrP 27-30 in water by infrared spectroscopy. Biochemistry 30: 7672-7680.
[86] Gasset M, Baldwin MA, Fletterick RJ, Prusiner SB (1993) Perturbation of the secondary structure of the scrapie prion protein under conditions that alter infectivity. Proc Natl Acad Sci U S A 90: 1-5.
[87] Goormaghtigh E, Cabiaux V, Ruysschaert JM (1990) Secondary structure and dosage of soluble and membrane proteins by attenuated total reflection Fourier-transform infrared spectroscopy on hydrated films. Eur J Biochem 193: 409-420.
[88] Pan KM, Baldwin M, Nguyen J, Gasset M, Serban A, et al. (1993) Conversion of alpha-helices into beta-sheets features in the formation of the scrapie prion proteins. Proc Natl Acad Sci U S A 90: 10962-10966.
[89] Spassov S, Beekes M, Naumann D (2006) Structural differences between TSEs strains investigated by FT-IR spectroscopy. Biochim Biophys Acta 1760: 1138-1149.
[90] 90. Govaerts C, Wille H, Prusiner SB, Cohen FE (2004) Evidence for assembly of prions with left-handed beta-helices into trimers. Proc Natl Acad Sci U S A 101: 8342-8347.
[91] DeMarco ML, Silveira J, Caughey B, Daggett V (2006) Structural properties of prion protein protofibrils and fibrils: an experimental assessment of atomic models. Biochemistry 45: 15573-15582.
[92] DeMarco ML, Daggett V (2004) From conversion to aggregation: protofibril formation of the prion protein. Proc Natl Acad Sci U S A 101: 2293-2298.
[93] McKinley MP, Meyer RK, Kenaga L, Rahbar F, Cotter R, et al. (1991) Scrapie prion rod formation in vitro requires both detergent extraction and limited proteolysis. J Virol 65: 1340-1351.
[94] Tycko R (2011) Solid-state NMR studies of amyloid fibril structure. Annu Rev Phys Chem 62: 279-299.
[95] Sunde M, Blake C (1997) The structure of amyloid fibrils by electron microscopy and X-ray diffraction. Adv Protein Chem 50: 123-159.
[96] Sunde M, Serpell LC, Bartlam M, Fraser PE, Pepys MB, et al. (1997) Common core structure of amyloid fibrils by synchrotron X-ray diffraction. J Mol Biol 273: 729-739.
[97] Wille H, Bian W, McDonald M, Kendall A, Colby DW, et al. (2009) Natural and synthetic prion structure from X-ray fiber diffraction. Proc Natl Acad Sci U S A 106: 16990-16995.
[98] Colby DW, Giles K, Legname G, Wille H, Baskakov IV, et al. (2009) Design and construction of diverse mammalian prion strains. Proc Natl Acad Sci U S A 106: 20417-20422.

[99] Smirnovas V, Baron GS, Offerdahl DK, Raymond GJ, Caughey B, et al. (2011) Structural organization of brain-derived mammalian prions examined by hydrogen-deuterium exchange. Nat Struct Mol Biol 18: 504-506.

[100] Worrall BB, Herman ST, Capellari S, Lynch T, Chin S, et al. (1999) Type 1 protease resistant prion protein and valine homozygosity at codon 129 of PRNP identify a subtype of sporadic Creutzfeldt-Jakob disease. J Neurol Neurosurg Psychiatry 67: 671-674.

[101] Zanusso G, Farinazzo A, Prelli F, Fiorini M, Gelati M, et al. (2004) Identification of distinct N-terminal truncated forms of prion protein in different Creutzfeldt-Jakob disease subtypes. J Biol Chem 279: 38936-38942.

[102] Zou WQ, Capellari S, Parchi P, Sy MS, Gambetti P, et al. (2003) Identification of novel proteinase K-resistant C-terminal fragments of PrP in Creutzfeldt-Jakob disease. J Biol Chem 278: 40429-40436.

[103] Parchi P, Zou W, Wang W, Brown P, Capellari S, et al. (2000) Genetic influence on the structural variations of the abnormal prion protein. Proc Natl Acad Sci U S A 97: 10168-10172.

[104] Bessen RA, Marsh RF (1994) Distinct PrP properties suggest the molecular basis of strain variation in transmissible mink encephalopathy. J Virol 68: 7859-7868.

[105] Sajnani G, Pastrana MA, Dynin I, Onisko B, Requena JR (2008) Scrapie prion protein structural constraints obtained by limited proteolysis and mass spectrometry. J Mol Biol 382: 88-98.

[106] Onisko B, Fernandez EG, Freire ML, Schwarz A, Baier M, et al. (2005) Probing PrPSc structure using chemical cross-linking and mass spectrometry: evidence of the proximity of Gly90 amino termini in the PrP 27-30 aggregate. Biochemistry 44: 10100-10109.

[107] Peretz D, Williamson RA, Matsunaga Y, Serban H, Pinilla C, et al. (1997) A conformational transition at the N terminus of the prion protein features in formation of the scrapie isoform. J Mol Biol 273: 614-622.

[108] Williamson RA, Peretz D, Pinilla C, Ball H, Bastidas RB, et al. (1998) Mapping the prion protein using recombinant antibodies. J Virol 72: 9413-9418.

[109] Kumar J, Sreeramulu S, Schmidt TL, Richter C, Vonck J, et al. (2010) Prion protein amyloid formation involves structural rearrangements in the C-terminal domain. Chembiochem 11: 1208-1213.

[110] Wille H, Michelitsch MD, Guenebaut V, Supattapone S, Serban A, et al. (2002) Structural studies of the scrapie prion protein by electron crystallography. Proc Natl Acad Sci U S A 99: 3563-3568.

[111] Smirnovas V, Kim JI, Lu X, Atarashi R, Caughey B, et al. (2009) Distinct structures of scrapie prion protein (PrPSc)-seeded versus spontaneous recombinant prion protein fibrils revealed by hydrogen/deuterium exchange. J Biol Chem 284: 24233-24241.

[112] Cobb NJ, Sonnichsen FD, McHaourab H, Surewicz WK (2007) Molecular architecture of human prion protein amyloid: a parallel, in-register beta-structure. Proc Natl Acad Sci U S A 104: 18946-18951.

[113] Lu X, Wintrode PL, Surewicz WK (2007) Beta-sheet core of human prion protein amyloid fibrils as determined by hydrogen/deuterium exchange. Proc Natl Acad Sci U S A 104: 1510-1515.

[114] Helmus JJ, Surewicz K, Nadaud PS, Surewicz WK, Jaroniec CP (2008) Molecular conformation and dynamics of the Y145Stop variant of human prion protein in amyloid fibrils. Proc Natl Acad Sci U S A 105: 6284-6289.

[115] Helmus JJ, Surewicz K, Surewicz WK, Jaroniec CP (2010) Conformational flexibility of Y145Stop human prion protein amyloid fibrils probed by solid-state nuclear magnetic resonance spectroscopy. J Am Chem Soc 132: 2393-2403.

[116] Tycko R, Savtchenko R, Ostapchenko VG, Makarava N, Baskakov IV (2010) The alpha-helical C-terminal domain of full-length recombinant PrP converts to an in-register parallel beta-sheet structure in PrP fibrils: evidence from solid state nuclear magnetic resonance. Biochemistry 49: 9488-9497.

[117] Kuwata K, Kamatari YO, Akasaka K, James TL (2004) Slow conformational dynamics in the hamster prion protein. Biochemistry 43: 4439-4446.

[118] Kuwata K, Li H, Yamada H, Legname G, Prusiner SB, et al. (2002) Locally disordered conformer of the hamster prion protein: a crucial intermediate to PrPSc? Biochemistry 41: 12277-12283.

[119] Dima RI, Thirumalai D (2002) Exploring the propensities of helices in PrP(C) to form beta sheet using NMR structures and sequence alignments. Biophys J 83: 1268-1280.

[120] Dima RI, Thirumalai D (2004) Probing the instabilities in the dynamics of helical fragments from mouse PrPC. Proc Natl Acad Sci U S A 101: 15335-15340.

[121] Swietnicki W, Petersen RB, Gambetti P, Surewicz WK (1998) Familial mutations and the thermodynamic stability of the recombinant human prion protein. J Biol Chem 273: 31048-31052.

[122] Liemann S, Glockshuber R (1999) Influence of amino acid substitutions related to inherited human prion diseases on the thermodynamic stability of the cellular prion protein. Biochemistry 38: 3258-3267.

[123] Apetri AC, Surewicz K, Surewicz WK (2004) The effect of disease-associated mutations on the folding pathway of human prion protein. J Biol Chem 279: 18008-18014.

[124] Kaneko K, Zulianello L, Scott M, Cooper CM, Wallace AC, et al. (1997) Evidence for protein X binding to a discontinuous epitope on the cellular prion protein during scrapie prion propagation. Proc Natl Acad Sci U S A 94: 10069-10074.

[125] Ashok A, Hegde RS (2009) Selective processing and metabolism of disease-causing mutant prion proteins. PLoS Pathog 5: e1000479.

[126] Ilc G, Giachin G, Jaremko M, Jaremko L, Benetti F, et al. (2010) NMR structure of the human prion protein with the pathological Q212P mutation reveals unique structural features. PLoS One 5: e11715.

[127] Biljan I, Ilc G, Giachin G, Raspadori A, Zhukov I, et al. (2011) Toward the molecular basis of inherited prion diseases: NMR structure of the human prion protein with V210I mutation. J Mol Biol 412: 660-673.

[128] Kovacs GG, Trabattoni G, Hainfellner JA, Ironside JW, Knight RS, et al. (2002) Mutations of the prion protein gene phenotypic spectrum. J Neurol 249: 1567-1582.

[129] Zhang Y, Swietnicki W, Zagorski MG, Surewicz WK, Sonnichsen FD (2000) Solution structure of the E200K variant of human prion protein. Implications for the mechanism of pathogenesis in familial prion diseases. J Biol Chem 275: 33650-33654.

[130] Lee S, Antony L, Hartmann R, Knaus KJ, Surewicz K, et al. (2010) Conformational diversity in prion protein variants influences intermolecular beta-sheet formation. EMBO J 29: 251-262.

[131] van der Kamp MW, Daggett V (2010) Pathogenic mutations in the hydrophobic core of the human prion protein can promote structural instability and misfolding. J Mol Biol 404: 732-748.

[132] van der Kamp MW, Daggett V (2011) Molecular Dynamics as an Approach to Study Prion Protein Misfolding and the Effect of Pathogenic Mutations. Top Curr Chem.

[133] Meli M, Gasset M, Colombo G (2011) Dynamic diagnosis of familial prion diseases supports the beta2-alpha2 loop as a universal interference target. PLoS One 6: e19093.

[134] Rossetti G, Cong X, Caliandro R, Legname G, Carloni P (2011) Common Structural Traits across Pathogenic Mutants of the Human Prion Protein and Their Implications for Familial Prion Diseases. J Mol Biol.

[135] Rossetti G, Giachin G, Legname G, Carloni P (2010) Structural facets of disease-linked human prion protein mutants: a molecular dynamic study. Proteins 78: 3270-3280.

[136] Weissmann C (2005) Birth of a prion: spontaneous generation revisited. Cell 122: 165-168.

[137] Khan MQ, Sweeting B, Mulligan VK, Arslan PE, Cashman NR, et al. (2010) Prion disease susceptibility is affected by beta-structure folding propensity and local side-chain interactions in PrP. Proc Natl Acad Sci U S A 107: 19808-19813.

In: Prions and Prion Diseases: New Developments
Editor: Jean-Michel Verdier
ISBN: 978-1-62100-027-3
© 2012 Nova Science Publishers, Inc.

Chapter 5

RECENT DEVELOPMENTS IN CELL BIOLOGY: ROLE OF GLYCOSYLATION IN PRION DISEASES

Hanin Abdel-Haq*
Department of Cell Biology and Neurosciences, Istituto Superiore di Sanità, Rome, Italy

ABSTRACT

It is thought that efficiency of the conversion of PrP^C to the abnormal partially protease-resistant form (PrP^{Sc}), which is the characteristic event of prion diseases or transmissible spongiform encephalopathies (TSEs), may be strongly dependent on alteration in the PrP^C glycosylation state. However, the mechanism of glycosylation alteration is still unknown. To elucidate some dynamics of the glycosylation alteration, using a panel of biotinylated lectins and two capturing anti PrP monoclonal antibodies in enzyme-linked immunosorbent and immunoblotting assays, in the first part of this chapter; I investigated effect of the infection *in vivo* with the prion strain 263K of scrapie on the glycosylation of hamster brain total glycoproteins and PrP^C, and then I compared it with the effect of treatment *in vitro* with proteinase-K (PK) and guanidine hydrochloride (GdnHCl). I found that both scrapie infection and PK and GdnHCl cause marked alterations in the lectin binding profiles of PrP^C and other proteins of hamster brain. Comparison between the *in vivo* and *in vitro* effects revealed a similar lectin binding alteration profiles of determined sugars. In the second part of this chapter, I subjected hamster plasma, collected at increasing time-point from scrapie infection, to lectin staining to determine whether the glycosylation alteration concerns also blood glycoproteins especially in the preclinical phase of the disease. I found that glycosylation pattern of plasma glycoproteins begins to show alteration at a time as early as 10 days after the infection.

Taken together, proteolytic agents and denaturants might constitute potential candidates as inducers of the glycosylation alteration observed in prion diseases, while, detection of glycosylation alterations of plasma total glycoproteins at distance of few days from the infection when the animals are still asymptomatic and apparently healthy, may constitute the basis for a promising early-stage diagnostic test for TSEs and for disease progression monitoring.

---

* Department of Cell Biology and Neurosciences, Istituto Superiore di Sanità, Rome, Italy. Viale Regina Elena, 299, 00161-Rome, Italy, E-mail address: hanin.abdelhaq@iss.it

INTRODUCTION

Glycosylation consists in the introduction of sugar chains of different length onto specific sites which confer proteins new biochemical properties and functions. Glycosylated proteins called glycoproteins are involved in the regulation of various systems including the nervous system [1 - 3], and they play an important role in pathological and physiological conditions. The oligosaccharide moiety is responsible for many of glycoproteins functions such as synthesis, stability, recognition and regulation of the proteins themselves and many of their diverse interactions. Therefore, its alteration is often accompanied by serious functional disorders [4, 5] such as autoimmune diseases, tumors and neurodegenerative diseases [6, 7]. In this regard, in a recent work it has been revealed that cleavage *in vivo* by reactive oxygen species (ROS) of oligosaccharides of serum glycoproteins may participate into the development of acute hepatitis [8].

Regarding neurodegenerative diseases, prion diseases such as scrapie in sheep [9], bovine spongiform encephalopathy (BSE) in cattle [10] or new variant Creutzfeldt-Jakob disease (vCJD) in humans [11], are a group of transmissible spongiform encephalopathies (TSEs) that cause neurodegenerative disorders characterized by behavioral changes, gradual loss of motor skills and mental impairment with dementia.

TSEs are transmissible from one individual or species to another by different infection routs. Although, the oral rout which is on the basis of the transmission of kuru [12], transmissible mink encephalopathy (TME) [13], BSE and vCJD which occurred in humans following the consumption of BSE-contaminated meat products [14], is the ascertained rout of infection [15], the natural route/ s of transmission have not yet been determined.

Blood has demonstrated to constitute not only a consistent risk for the transmission of prion diseases; whereas TSE transmission by blood either experimentally from animal-to-animal [16 - 22] or naturally from human-to-human [23 - 26] has been occurred, but also in reference to a recent evidence on a significant role of the haematogenous route in TSE neuroinvasion in sheep [27], it may have a role in the propagation of TSE infectivity. Moreover, prion infections by blood have been occurred in recipients following transfusions with blood from vCJD-asymptomatic and apparently healthy donors who later died of vCJD [23, 24] or even from subclinically vCJD-infected donors who later never develop disease as it was hypothesized by Chohan and colleagues [28] indicating that some blood donors could be potentially infectious remaining, permanently, clinically asymptomatic. This increased alarming evidence on the risk of blood which is essential for transfusions and constitutes the unique starting material for various life saving plasma-derived products, highlights the need for enhancing the level of blood safety. A screening blood test for detecting TSE agent in human blood as well as an early diagnosis of prion diseases are still unavailable [29, 30] because a reliable diagnostic marker of the early-stage of the disease has not yet been found.

The unique reliable marker of prion diseases is the protease-resistant form (PrP^{Sc} or PrPres) of the cellular prion protein (PrP^{C}) [31 - 33] which accumulates mainly in the central nervous system [10] and significantly detectable at a time close to the symptomatic stage of the disease [33]. PrP^{Sc} has been sought in blood by several researchers using different kinds of *in vitro* protocols and methods [some of them: 34 - 43]. However, only few of them were able to detect it because level of TSE infectivity of blood was found to be many orders of magnitude lower than that of brain tissue from the same animals [16, 17, 29, 44], and since

TSE infectivity has been generally associated with PrP^{Sc} presence after digestion with proteinase-K (PK) [33, 45 - 47]; consequently, its theoretical concentration in blood should be very small to be detected by methods none sufficiently sensitive.

Additionally, in the past decade, it has been largely demonstrated the presence of high amounts (approximately 80%) of PK-sensitive but disease related abnormal isoforms of PrP [48 - 53]. And in the light of this evidence, it was reasoned that PK-digestion step used to digest PrP^{C} present in mixture with PrP^{Sc}, might digest also the PK-sensitive portion of the total amount of PrP^{Sc} reducing, further, its extremely low concentration in blood and therefore decreasing the sensitivity of blood-based tests [54, 55]. It is thought that the PK-sensitive PrP^{Sc} is involved in the determination of the duration of the incubation period of each single TSE strain and plays an important role in prion disease pathogenesis [48, 49].

Among all PrP^{Sc} detection methods, of particular importance are the protein misfolding cyclic amplification (PMCA) [38], the enhanced QuIC (eQuIC) [42] and the solid-state capture matrix coupled with direct immunodetection of the surface-bound material [41]. They are methods of recent development which succeeded in detecting PrP^{Sc} in blood, improving the expectance for a diagnostic test for prion diseases. The PMCA technique was developed by Saborio and colleagues [56] and has been proposed by Saà and colleagues [38] as a promising blood test for the early-stage of prion diseases since it is able to detect small amounts of PrP^{Sc} from hamster blood of the preclinical phase of the disease by its amplification to a level detectable by conventional methods by application numerous cycles of incubation and sonication. PMCA is a technique that does not seem of easy application in a routine diagnostic test, besides the high risk of the spontaneous generation of protease resistant PrP de novo [57, 58]. The eQuIC method [42] is a combined assay between the quaking-induced conversion (QuIC) which can be as sensitive as an *in vivo* bioassay where prions induce the polymerization of recombinant PrP^{C} ($rPrP^{C}$) into amyloid fibrils by applying cycles of shaking and rest [59, 60], and a specific immunoprecipitation of PrP^{Sc} using 15B3 antibody [61 - 63]. This assay is able to detect PrP^{Sc} from human plasma spiked with high dilutions of either hamster scrapie or human vCJD brain homogenate, and from hamster plasma of the preclinical phase of the disease. However, this promising blood test is relatively long and does not yet seem ready for a routine diagnostic test. Finally, the solid-state capture matrix-ELISA method developed by Edgeworth and colleagues [41] consists in capturing vCJD PrP^{Sc} from human whole blood on stainless steel beads and their subsequent immunodetection in ELISA. The assay was able to detect PrP^{Sc} from human whole blood spiked with high dilutions of vCJD-infected brain homogenate, and from whole blood of 15 symptomatic patients with vCJD. This assay may allow the development of large-scale screening tests for asymptomatic vCJD prion infection. However, it is complex and not yet enough sensitive for routine use [30].

Nature of the infectious agent causing TSEs is now undefined. According to the protein-only or prion hypothesis the infectious agent is devoid of nucleic acid and represented by PrP^{Sc} [10, 64].

Although a huge mole of studies, treating various aspects of prions, have been done, many doubts and uncertainty are still characterizing prion diseases pathogenesis [29, 65]. This issue is of fundamental importance not only for the comprehension of the reason of disease onset, but also it is helpful in determining the factors involved in its early and late dynamic. In fact, many factors identified and characterized through studying disease pathogenesis have demonstrated in many cases to constitute a specific markers of diseases of different nature and origin, and to be useful in monitoring disease progression. Studying disease pathogenesis is also of great help in the determination of specific targets of the early and late phase of a disease having the possibility to apply specific and effective therapeutic approaches or strategies [66, 67]. In this regard, many therapeutic approaches for the treatment of prion diseases, have been suggested [65, 67], but although some of these proposed therapies have shown very promising prospects [68 - 73], to present date no effective treatment has been found [65 - 67] properly because still lacking the knowledge of the key target/ s tightly related to the pathogenesis on which acting therapeutically.

It is thought that the fundamental event in prion diseases pathogenesis is the conversion of PrP^C to PrP^{Sc} [45, 46, 64, 74], whereas the mechanism by which it occurs is still unknown. Glycosylation, also, is likely to play a crucial role in the pathogenesis of TSEs. In fact, the acetylcholinesterase enzyme and the insulin receptor are two glycoproteins whose glycosylation have been found substantially altered in patients with Creutzfeldt-Jakob disease and in scrapie-infected neuroblastoma cells respectively [75, 76]. Upon alteration, the acetylcholinesterase glycoprotein has shown a reduction in its enzymatic activity followed by progressive reduction in the cholinergic system function until dementia [75], while; the insulin receptor glycoprotein has shown alteration in its correct processing and trafficking [76].

These findings besides emphasizing the role of glycosylation alteration of some glycoproteins in the pathogenesis of prion diseases, they may also suggest that clinical symptoms of prion diseases could be the reflex of the dysfunction of systems regulated by specific glycoproteins. Thereby, identification and characterization of the altered glycoproteins may provide a new target for the therapy of prion diseases and for disease progression monitoring.

PrP^C is an ubiquitous glycoprotein that when converts into PrP^{Sc} acquires detergent insolubility [77], resistance to proteases [46,78], higher content of beta-sheet structure [79 - 81], capability to form amyloid fibrils deposits into the brain [82] and especially shows an altered glycosylation pattern [4, 83, 84]. PrP has two glycosylation sites, and typically both PrP^C and PrP^{Sc} are composed of a mixture of un- mono- and diglycosylated isoforms [85]. The proportion of each of these forms varies among brain regions or animal species [86, 87]. PrP^{Sc} is specific for each prion strain [88] and for that it has been exploited by several researchers for the glycotyping of various prion strains [89 - 91] as a method to distinguish among them.

Based on the revelation that glycosylation pattern of PrP^{Sc} changes by changing the region of brain in which a TSE strain replicates and the fact that PrP^C glycosylation in different regions of the brain of Syrian hamsters and mice is different, it has been postulated that TSE strains action depends on the host PrP^C glycosylation; since, they select regions of the brain where the neurons express a compatible PrP^C glycosylation pattern [92]. Accordingly, a recent pharmacokinetic study in mice using highly purified radioactively labelled PrP^{Sc} demonstrated that glycosylation of PrP^{Sc} does not affect its kinetic of distribution [93]. Moreover, a possible link between the glycosylation alterations on aging PrP^C and the PrP^C that converts to PrP^{Sc} upon prion infection was suggested by Goh and colleagues [94]; who found that glycosylation of mouse brain PrP^C is subjected to alteration during the normal aging process whereas some of the glycosylation changes are similar to those observed on PrP^{Sc} [94].

Thus, involvement of PrP^C glycosylation in the pathogenesis of prion diseases is clear. However, little is known about the precise role of the N-linked glycosylation in the neurodegenerative process.

It was reported that mutations at the first N-linked glycosylation site of human PrP causes genetic CJD [95, 96], and amino acid substitution at one of the N-linked glycosylation sites of mouse PrP expressed in transgenic mice caused prion disease when mice had been inoculated with scrapie prions [97, 98]. While, studies on short synthetic PrP peptides have shown that glycosylation can alter the kinetic equilibrium between monomeric PrP^C and an aggregated form [92]. And, accumulated evidence, suggests that loss or inhibition of PrP^C glycosylation enhances the production of PrP^{Sc} in prion-infected cell lines [99 - 103].

Literature data clearly indicate that efficiency of the conversion event may be strongly dependent on alteration in the PrP^C glycosylation state. However, the mechanism of glycosylation alteration is still unknown.

With the aim to elucidate some dynamics of the glycosylation alteration, in the first part of this chapter; using a panel of biotinylated lectins and two capturing monoclonal antibodies raised against different epitopes of PrP in enzyme-linked immunosorbent and immunoblotting assays, I investigated effect of the infection *in vivo* with the prion strain 263K of scrapie on the glycosylation of hamster brain total glycoproteins and PrP^C, and then I compared it with the effect of treatment *in vitro* with PK and guanidine hydrochloride (GdnHCl). In the second part of this chapter, seeking for an early-stage diagnostic marker for prion diseases, I subjected hamster plasma, collected at increasing time-point from scrapie infection, to lectin staining in order to determine whether the glycosylation alteration concerns also blood glycoproteins especially in the preclinical phase of the disease.

Lectins are a group of proteins which specifically bind or crosslink carbohydrates in glycoproteins making possible either the quantification or the identification of different sugar types. Changes in lectins binding property to glycoproteins from the infected sample with respect to glycoproteins from the normal sample was used as indicator of alteration in the glycosylation.

In the first part of this chapter, I focused my efforts on studying the mechanism of glycosylation alteration where through a set of experiments on hamster brain homogenate I tried to elucidate some aspects of this issue and to answer the question of how glycosylation is involved in the pathogenesis of prion diseases.

To achieve this goal, the first step of the investigation was determination of the glycosylation alterations and their extent in total glycoproteins and PrP^{Sc} of scrapie-infected hamster brain.

Therefore, binding of seven biotinylated lectins to glycoproteins from normal and 263K-infected brain homogenate, under native conditions, was adopted as tool to determine in ELISA the sugars of hamster brain total glycoproteins greatly subjected to alteration by the infection with 263K strain of scrapie. I found that glycosylation of the total proteins was differentially affected by the 263K strain (Fig. 1A). While, ConA, WGA, PNA and UEA-I did not change binding activity to the specific sugars, the binding of RCA and SBA was considerably increased (31.3 and 29.4% respectively) and that of DBA was instead significantly reduced (36.3%, P= 0.015). This result demonstrates that a discrete percent of hamster total glycoproteins carries sugars that had been selectively and markedly altered by the 263K infection, whereas galactose residues seem to be the most affected.

On the other hand, determination of the sugars on PrP^C subjected to alteration by the 263K strain was performed by capturing PrP with 3F4 (directed against an epitope between aa 109 - 112) or 6H4 (directed against an epitope between aa 144 - 152) monoclonal antibodies and the subsequent identification by the lectins. I found that under native conditions, glycosylation of PrP^{Sc} was generally reduced with respect to that of PrP^C: all the lectins except RCA, have shown lower binding activity to the sugars on PrP^{Sc} either captured by 3F4 or 6H4; whereas this latter has shown capturing properties similar to those of 3F4 but allowing better exposure for mannose and N-acetylgalactosamine recognized by ConA and RCA respectively (Fig. 2A, B). This result indicates that glycosylation of hamster PrP^C is subjected to substantial alterations when challenged with scrapie confirming an earlier study on glycosylation differences between PrP^C and PrP^{Sc} from hamsters [4].

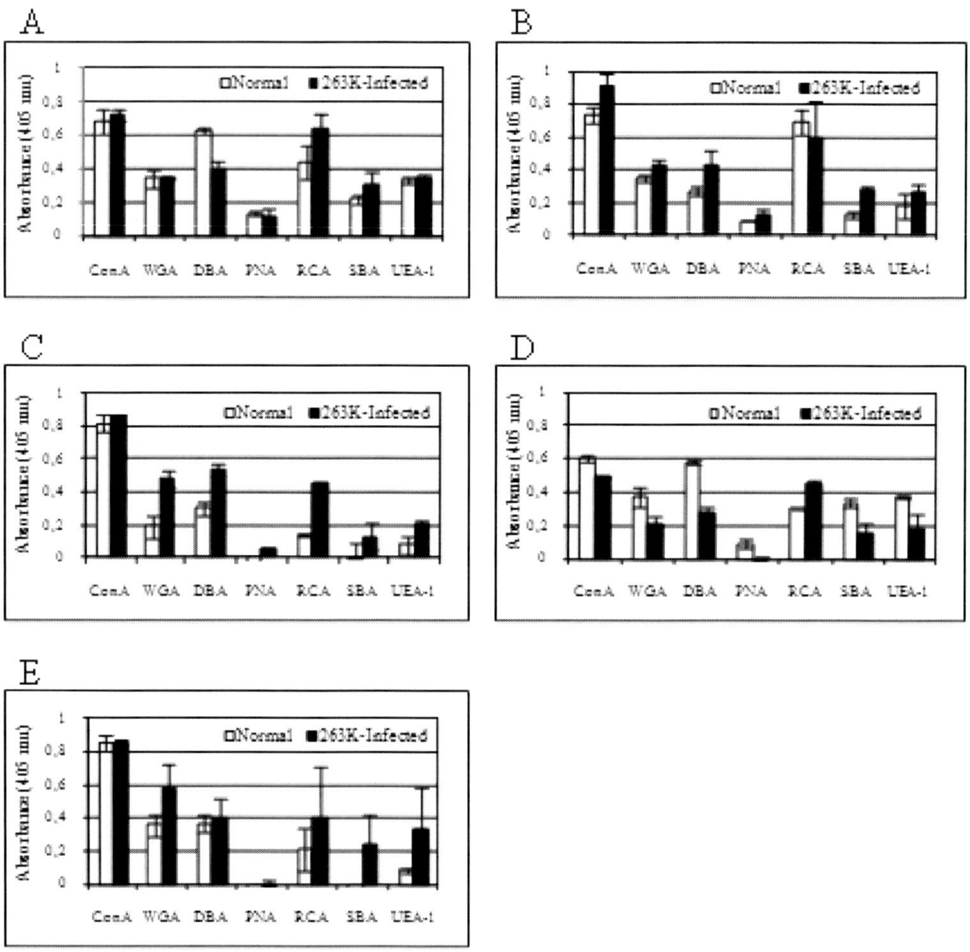

Figure 1. Lectins binding profile to total glycoproteins from normal and scrapie-infected hamster brain. Equal amounts of total proteins of normal and 263K-infected brain homogenate were loaded on 96-well ELISA plates, and lectins binding profile was determined by staining with a panel of seven biotinylated lectins. (A) native conditions, (B) after treatment with PK, (C) after treatment with GdnHCl before loading, (D) after treatment with GdnHCl after loading and (E) after treatment with PK and GdnHCl added before loading. Results are average ± standard deviation (SD) of duplicates.

The second step of the investigation was comparing the glycosylation alterations occurred *in vivo* and carried out in the first result with glycosylation alterations induced *in vitro* by treatment with PK and GdnHCl.

Effect of PK treatment on hamster brain total glycoproteins and PrP N-linked sugars was investigated by treating normal and 263K-infected brain homogenate with 50 μg/ml of PK for 1 h at 37 °C. Treatment caused reduction in the binding activity of UEA-I, SBA and PNA, and enhancement in that of ConA and RCA to glycoproteins from both normal and infected samples (Fig. 1B *vs* 1A). Instead, WGA and DBA binding activity was opposite between normal and infected samples indicating that the specific sugars recognized by these two lectins have been altered on glycoproteins of the infected sample (Fig. 1B). This result indicates that proteolytic enzymes are able to produce alterations in the glycosylation of hamster brain total proteins.

When PrP^C and PrP^{Sc} were captured by 3F4, PK treatment produced substantial reduction in the binding activity of all the lectins except RCA, to both PrP^C and PrP^{Sc} (Fig. 2C *vs* 2A). While when proteins were captured by 6H4, treatment produced an effect similar to that of 3F4 but with improved exposure of the sugars recognized by ConA and WGA (Fig. 2D *vs* 2B). Glycosylation of PrP^C was markedly decreased by the PK but not completely abolished suggesting presence of PrP^C with some PK-resistance. Moreover, after PrP^C treatment with PK, particular is the profile of N-acetylgalactosamine recognized by RCA: on one side; it reflects the occurrence *in vitro* of an alteration in the glycosylation of PrP^C because although the PK digestion with consequent substantial reduction of the quantity of PrP^C that binds to the 3F4 antibody, binding activity of RCA instead of reducing it increased, and on the other side; it shows a profile similar to that obtained with native PrP^{Sc} (Fig. 2C *vs* 2A) suggesting that proteolytic enzymes may be involved in the PrP^C glycosylation alterations occurred *in vivo*.

Effect of GdnHCl treatment on hamster brain total glycoproteins and PrP N-linked sugars was investigated treating normal and 263K-infected brain homogenate with GdnHCl either before or after loading on ELISA plate. Treatment with GdnHCl before loading decreased the binding activity of all the lectins except ConA to glycoproteins from normal sample, while toward glycoproteins from infected sample it decreased the binding activity of PNA, RCA, SBA and UEA-I, and increased that of ConA, WGA and DBA (Fig. 1C *vs* 1A). Binding activity of ConA, PNA, RCA, SBA and UEA-I to glycoproteins from both normal and infected samples was proportionally increased or reduced, while that of WGA and DBA was opposite between normal and infected samples indicating that the specific sugars have been altered on glycoproteins of the infected sample. The result besides indicating that glycosylation is also affected by denaturing agents; it suggests that the effect of PK and GdnHCl on N-acetylglucosamine and α-N-acetylgalactosamine recognized by WGA and DBA respectively is unspecific. Treatment after loading produced reduction in the binding activity of all the lectins to glycoproteins from the infected sample with respect to glycoproteins from the normal sample where in these latter, lectins binding to the sugars was differentially affected by GdnHCl; in fact, ConA, PNA and RCA have shown reduced binding activity, SBA has shown increased binding activity and WGA, DBA and UEA-I did not change their binding activity (Fig. 1D *vs* 1A). This result indicates that these latter four sugars have been altered on glycoproteins of the infected sample and suggests that alteration of sugars exposure by denaturing agents may occur at different levels and could be observed at the native state or only upon treatment with GdnHCl. Comparison between effect of PK and GdnHCl treatments, added before loading, on lectins binding profile to glycoproteins from normal and infected samples revealed a similar binding profile with both treatments except for RCA, ConA and PNA. This revelation on one side; indicates that PK and GdnHCl may act at the same site of a glycoprotein, and on the other side, taking into account the previous data I obtained in the current chapter; it indicates that PK may affect specifically the two sugars recognized by ConA and RCA since upon treatment with PK but not GdnHCl of glycoproteins from normal samples, these two lectins produced a binding profile similar to that observed with native-infected glycoproteins (Fig. 3). PNA binding profile, instead, may suggest absence of action by both PK and GdnHCl on the specific sugar, and finally; binding profile of SBA and UEA-I may reflect a specific interaction of GdnHCl, added after loading, with the sugars recognized by these two lectins because only upon such treatment, normal glycoproteins regenerated the profile observed with native-infected glycoproteins (Fig. 3).

Treatment of PrP with GdnHCl before loading, increased lectins binding to PrP^{Sc} either captured by 3F4 or 6H4 antibody (Fig. 2E and F *vs* 2A and B). Interestingly, the same treatment decreased the binding of all the lectins to PrP^{C} when it was captured by 3F4 and decreased the binding of 3 lectins only leaving unchanged or increased the binding of the others when PrP^{C} was captured by 6H4 (Fig. 2E and F *vs* 2A and B). I noticed that, while binding of UEA-I was opposite between PrP^{C} and PrP^{Sc} when they were captured by both 3F4 and 6H4, binding of PNA was opposite between PrP^{C} and PrP^{Sc} when they were captured by 6H4 only, and binding of DBA and WGA was opposite between PrP^{C} and PrP^{Sc} when they were captured by 3F4 only. This result suggests that the exposure of some sugars was altered on PrP^{Sc} and that the identification of such alterations seems to be antibody dependent.

Treatment with GdnHCl after loading, produced a proportional reduction of ConA and RCA binding activity and a proportional increasing in the binding of the other lectins, when PrP^{C} and PrP^{Sc} were captured by 3F4 (Fig. 2G *vs* 2A). While, when PrP^{C} and PrP^{Sc} were captured by 6H4, treatment increased binding activity of WGA, DBA and UEA-I and reduced that of ConA, RCA and SBA, to both proteins (Fig. 2H *vs* 2B). PNA binding was opposite between PrP^{C} and PrP^{Sc} indicating that the exposure of the specific sugar was altered on PrP^{Sc} (Fig. 2H *vs* 2B). This result supports the idea on the dependency of the identification of sugar-exposure alterations on the capturing antibody.

Collectively, this result indicates that PrP^{C} glycosylation is subjected to exposure alterations of some sugars whereas singular sugars may not be influenced similarly. Moreover, it demonstrates that exposure of the epitope of PrP^{C} recognized by 3F4 antibody is influenced by the glycosylation alterations since lectins binding activity toward the treated PrP^{C} (before loading only) was reduced with respect to that toward both the native PrP^{C} and the treated PrP^{Sc} indicating that the exposure of the same epitope was greater before PrP^{C} treatment and increased in PrP^{Sc} after treatment. It is largely known that this epitope is buried in PrP^{Sc} compared to PrP^{C} and treating with GdnHCl greatly improves its exposure in PrP^{Sc} [48], here surprisingly, such treatment changed the exposure of this epitope also in PrP^{C} reducing it, making believe that following prion infection this epitope may become buried in PrP^{C} rather than in PrP^{Sc}.

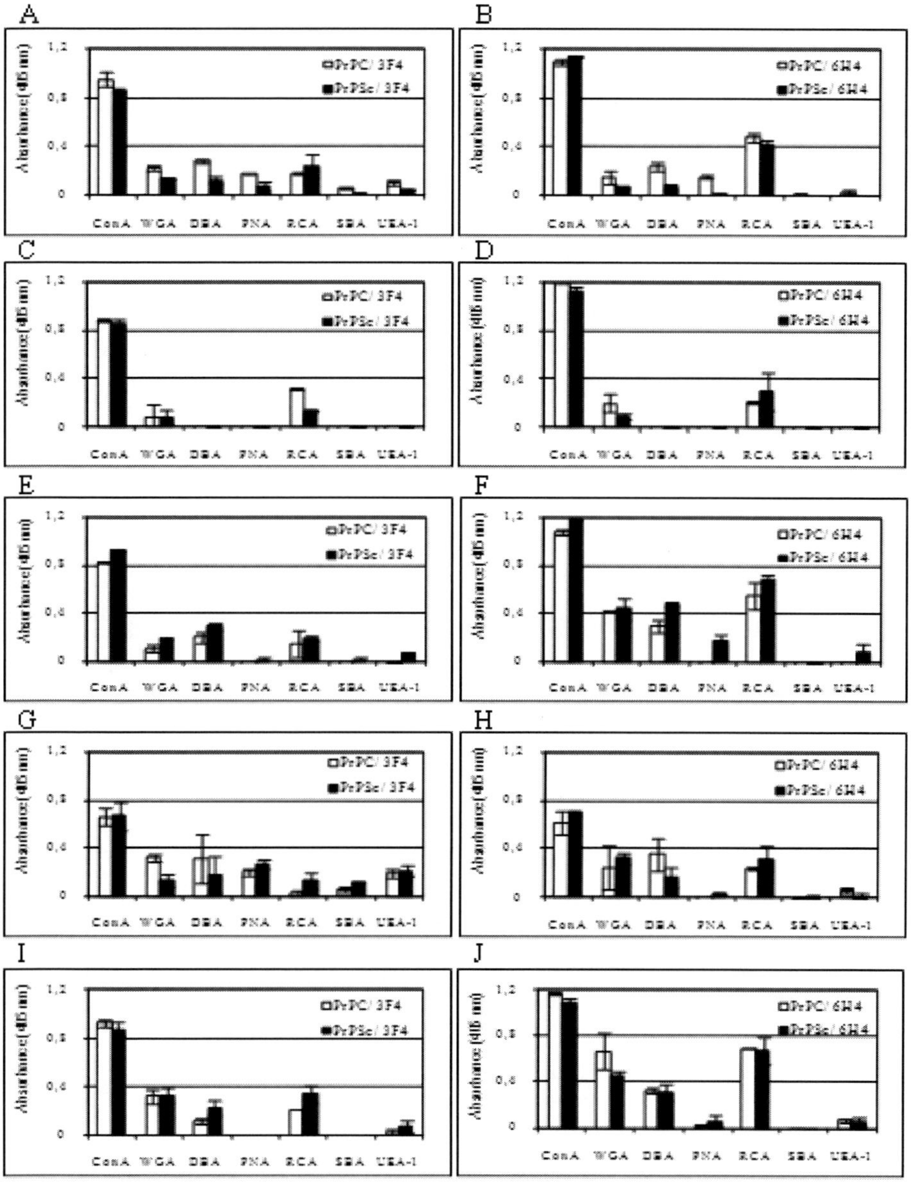

Figure 2. Lectins binding profile to hamster brain PrP^C and PrP^{Sc}. Equal amounts of total proteins of normal and 263K-infected brain homogenate were loaded on 96-well ELISA plates precoated with capturing anti-PrP monoclonal antibodies 3F4 or 6H4, and lectins binding profile was determined by staining with a panel of seven biotinylated lectins. (A and B) native conditions, (C and D) after treatment with PK, (E and F) after treatment with GdnHCl before loading, (G and H) after treatment with GdnHCl after loading and (I and J) after treatment with PK and GdnHCl added before loading. Results are average ± standard deviation (SD) of duplicates.

Taken together, results attribute a certain specificity of action to both PK and GdnHCl; to ascertain this issue, I treated normal and infected brain homogenate before loading at the same time with PK and GdnHCl because if the action is specific, binding profile of a lectin to a sugar on native-infected glycoprotein and on treated-normal glycoprotein should be similar only following a single treatment and not a combined one. Treatment caused reduction in the binding activity of all the lectins except ConA, WGA and DBA, to glycoproteins from normal and infected samples (Fig. 1E *vs* 1A). ConA binding was proportionally increased while that of WGA and DBA was opposite between normal and infected samples indicating presence of alterations. Under this condition of treatment only WGA and DBA produced on glycoproteins from normal sample a binding profile similar to that revealed under native conditions for infected glycoproteins confirming the none specificity of PK and GdnHCl action toward N-acetylglucosamine and α-N-acetylgalactosamine recognized by WGA and DBA respectively, and the specificity of PK action toward mannose and N-acetylgalactosamine recognized by ConA and RCA respectively, and the specificity of GdnHCl action toward α-D-N-acetylgalactosamine and fucose recognized by SBA and UEA-I respectively, and the absence of action toward galactosyl (β-1,3) GalNAc recognized by PNA. As seen, sugars are differentially affected by these two agents indicating that the interaction occurs with a certain degree of specificity.

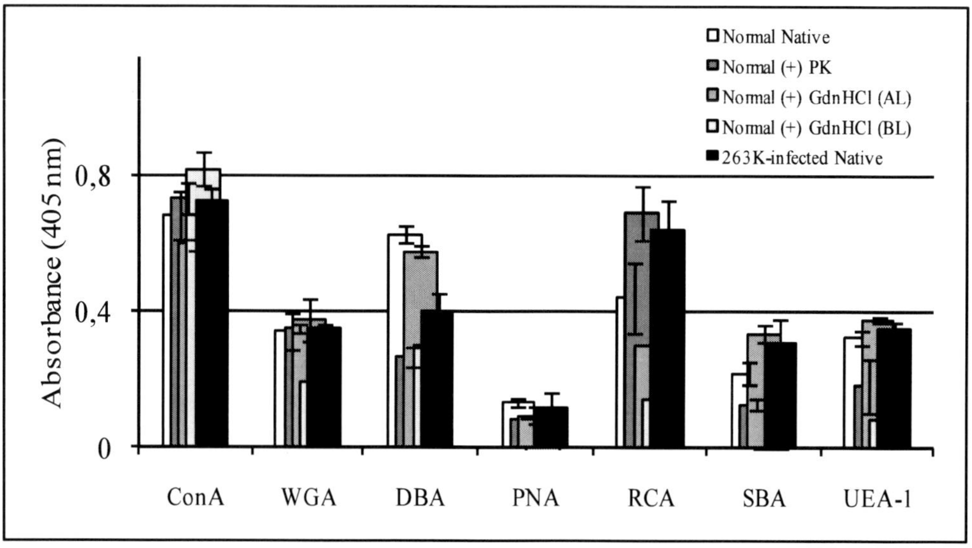

Figure 3. Comparison between lectins binding profile to native scrapie-infected and treated normal hamster brain homogenate. It is clearly shown that lectins binding profile is similar between infected-native and normal-treated glycoproteins but, only for distinct sugars sensitive to the action of determined agents. AL and BL indicate after and before loading of proteins on ELISA plate, respectively.

The combined treatment with PK and GdnHCl unchanged, increased or reduced lectins binding to PrP^C and PrPres when they were captured by both 3F4 and 6H4. Whereas, DBA and UEA-I have shown altered binding activity with 3F4 (Fig. 2 I *vs* 2A) and PNA instead with 6H4 (Fig. 2 J *vs* 2B). Also in this case, the specificity of PK for N-acetylgalactosamine recognized by RCA has been confirmed.

Table 1 reports the lectins that have altered their binding activity to the specific sugars, present on PrP^{Sc} and glycoproteins from 263K-infected brain homogenate with respect to PrP^C and normal glycoproteins, under native, proteolytic and denaturing conditions.

These results provided evidence on the occurrence of alterations in the glycosylation of the total proteins and on possible potential candidates' factors that might be involved in the glycosylation alteration dynamic. Results provided also a characterization of the glycosylation alteration of scrapie-infected hamster brain total glycoproteins using the lectin ELISA method which although its numerous advantages is unable to identify specifically and singularly glycoproteins that carry substantial glycosylation alterations for a future consideration as disease biomarkers. Therefore, characterization of the glycosylation alteration of scrapie-infected hamster brain total glycoproteins by the lectin blotting method was the third and last step of this investigation. Equal amounts of normal and infected brain homogenate subjected to lectin staining by the seven biotinylated lectins revealed that glycosylation of four glycoproteins at approximately 29, 18, 15 and 12 kDa was strongly increased in the infected sample compared to the normal one, whereas; fucose was markedly increased in the first, galactose residues recognized by PNA and SBA in the second, all the sugars in the third and galactose residues recognized by DBA and PNA in the fourth (Fig. 4A). This result complete and support the previous results confirming galactose as the most affected although fucose seems to be considerably involved. Interestingly, when I compared equal amounts of three different preparations of normal brain homogenate with three different preparations of infected brain homogenate on a single blot I observed that for some glycoproteins there were no differences in the intensity of the bands either were from normal or infected samples (Fig. 4B) suggesting that these glycoproteins were not absolutely subjected to glycosylation alterations. Instead, when glycoproteins were subject to glycosylation alterations there were substantial differences between normal and infected glycoproteins bands intensity but; while the intensity of the bands for the same glycoprotein was similar among the three normal preparations it was different among the three infected preparations although equal amounts of total proteins were loaded (Fig. 4B). This, was observed with all the seven lectins indicating on one hand, that the alteration of the glycosylation is selective concerning only distinct glycoproteins and on the other hand, that the degree and extent of the alteration is variable among the infected animals. Since the scrapie-infected hamsters used in this study were genetically identical and had received the same prion agent at the moment of the infection, I suppose that the variability in the degree of glycosylation alteration might be due to cellular or metabolic differences among the animals, whose interaction with the infectious agent affect differentially the glycosylation. This supposition is consistent with the affirmation that the cellular environment can contribute into glycosylation alterations [101] and it is also in line with the conclusive results I obtained in the current chapter because the physiological levels of proteolytic agents, denaturants and other factors such as clearance can be different from animal to animal and consequently they may cause a heterogeneous alteration of the glycosylation. Finally, immunoreactivity of the seven biotinylated lectins to glycoproteins from both normal and infected brain homogenate was proportional to increasing amounts of the total proteins loaded onto polyacrylamide gels (Fig. 4C) as a further proof that the glycosylation alterations discussed in this chapter were true and not due to quantitative differences.

In the second part of this chapter, I focused the study on the impact of the scrapie infection on the glycosylation of hamster blood glycoproteins with the aim to set up the basis of a blood test for the early-stage of prion diseases exploiting any significant glycosylation alteration between glycoproeins from infectious and normal plasma.

Table 1. Summary of the alteration of lectins immunoreactivity to sugars on native and treated glycoproteins from hamster brain

Lectin	Abbreviation	Sugar specificity	Lectin immunoreactivity											
			Total glycoproteins				PrP^{Sc}							
							3F4				6H4			
			Native	PK	GdnHCl	PK+ GdnHCl	Native	PK	GdnHCl	PK+ GdnHCl	Native	PK	GdnHCl	PK+ GdnHCl
Concanavalin A	ConA	α–linked mannose	-	-	-	-	Δ	-	-	-	-	-	-	-
Peanut Agglutinin	PNA	galactosyl (β-1,3) (GalNAc)	-	-	-	-	Δ*	-	-	-	Δ***	-	Δ*	Δ
Ricinus communis agglutinin-I	RCA	N-acetylgalactosamine	Δ	-	-	-	Δ	Δ***	-	-	-	-	-	-
Soybean agglutinin	SBA	α-D-N-acetylgalactosamine	Δ	-	-	-	Δ***	-	-	-	Δ***	-	-	-
Ulex europaeus agglutinin I	UEA-I	(α-1, 2) linked fucose	-	-	-	-	Δ*	-	Δ**	Δ	Δ**	-	Δ*	-
Wheat Germ Agglutin	WGA	N-acetylglucosamine (GlcNAc)	-	Δ*	Δ*	Δ	Δ*	-	Δ**	-	Δ	-	-	-
Dolichos biflorus Agglutinin	DBA	α-N-acetylgalactosamine	Δ*	Δ	Δ**	Δ	Δ**	-	Δ	Δ	Δ***	-	-	-

All PK and GdnHCl treatments reported in the table were done before loading on ELISA plate. (Δ) indicates alteration in the immunoreactivity of the lectins to sugars on glycoproteins from scrapie-infected hamster brain. (-) indicates absence of alterations. (*) indicates a statistically significant alteration whereas; * $P < 0.05$, ** $P \leq 0.01$, *** $P \leq 0.001$ as evaluated by student's t-test.

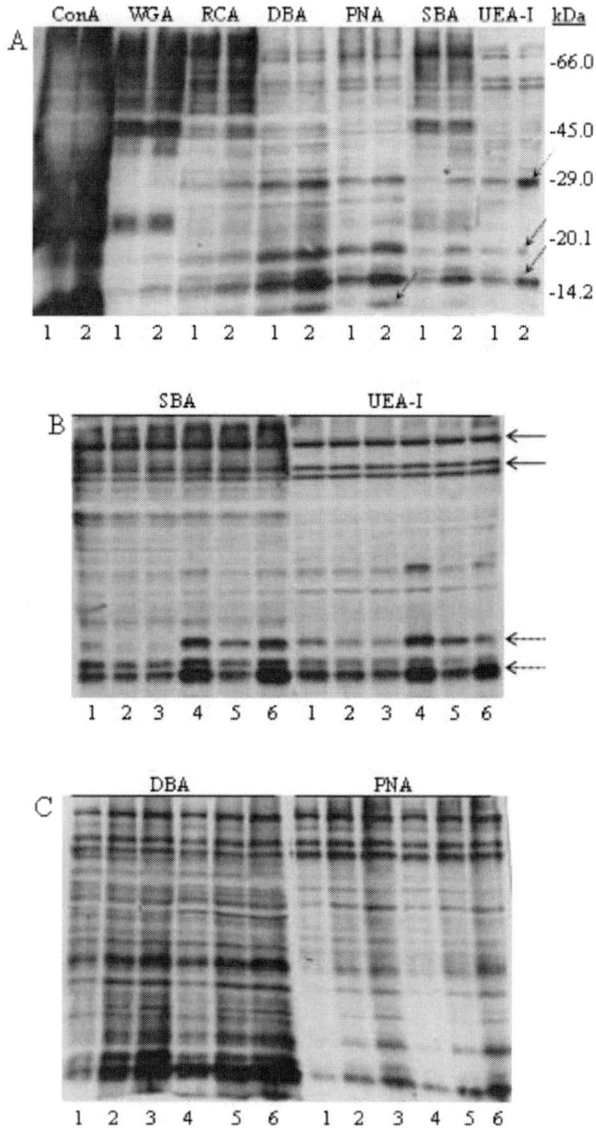

Figure 4. Characterization by lectin blotting of the glycosylation alteration of scrapie-infected hamster brain total glycoproteins. Brain homogenates were electrophoresed on 12% polyacrylamide gels, blotted onto nitrocellulose membrane and then stained with the seven biotinylated lectins. (A) Immunoreactivity of the lectins to equal amounts of normal (lane 1) and infected (lane 2) brain homogenate, arrows indicate glycoproteins whose glycosylation is greatly altered in the infected sample with respect to the normal. (B) Representative blot of lectins immunoreactivity to equal amounts of brain homogenate from three different normal (lanes 1, 2, 3) and infected (lanes 4, 5, 6) brains, solid arrows indicate glycoproteins whose glycosylation is not absolutely affected by the prion infection while dotted arrows indicate glycoproteins whose glycosylation is similar among the normal samples and of different extent besides being altered; among the infected samples. (C) Representative blot of lectins immunoreactivity to increasing amounts (12.5, 25 and 50 μg/ml total proteins) of normal (lanes 1, 2, 3) and infected (lanes 4, 5, 6) brain homogenate. Molecular mass markers are indicated in kilodaltons on the right.

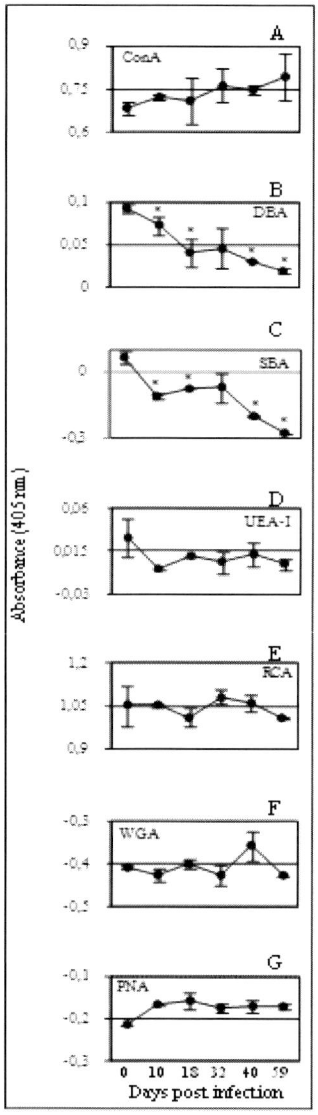

Figure 5. Lectins binding profile to total glycoproteins from normal and endogenously scrapie-infected hamster plasma. Equal amounts of total proteins of normal and 263K-infected plasma were loaded on 96-well ELISA plates, and lectins binding profile was determined, under native conditions, by staining with (A) ConA, (B) DBA, (C) SBA, (D) UEA-1, (E) RCA, (F) WGA and (G) PNA. Results are average ± standard deviation (SD) of duplicates. * $P \leq 0.05$.

To achieve this objective I subjected hamster plasma collected before scrapie infection and then at 10, 18, 32, 40 and 59 days after the infection to lectins analysis in ELISA. I observed a differential alteration of binding reactivity of the lectins to the specific sugars present on glycoproteins of the infected samples compared to the normal: ConA and DBA have shown a linear relationship between incubation period (days post infection) and binding alteration (R^2 = 0.842 and 0.906, respectively) but, while ConA binding reactivity was increased (Fig. 5A), that of DBA was decreased in significant manner ($P \leq 0.05$) immediately at 10 days (21.2%) and through the whole incubation period reaching more than 50% reduction already at 18 days and 78.8% at the terminal stage (59 days) (Fig. 5B). SBA binding reactivity has shown a significant ($P \leq 0.05$) and marked reduction already at 10 days post infection reaching more than 50% reduction which was maintained almost unchanged till 32 days post infection when it started again to show further significant reductions (Fig. 5C). UEA-I binding reactivity was reduced to almost the maximum already at 10 days post infection maintaining invariable this trend through the whole incubation period (Fig. 5D). RCA has shown a similar binding reactivity before and after scrapie infection (Fig. 5E), while WGA and PNA at this tested quantity of total proteins have shown negative measures (Fig. 5F and G).

Results indicates that plasma glycoproteins are subjected to substantial glycosylation alteration as soon as possible after exposure to the prion agent regardless of the infection rout which here was the intracerebral. With this result I demonstrated that a diagnostic blood test, based on the revelation of glycosylation alteration of the total plasma glycoproteins, is possible and may be useful also in monitoring disease progression through measuring percentage of alteration of lectins binding reactivity. And also, determination of the kind of the sugar mostly involved in the alteration, may provide information on the disease progression. Of all the tested lectins, DBA binding activity demonstrated to be the most altered, either in blood or brain, as suggested from some parameters of analysis such as significance, linearity and reduction percentages, and for that, detecting alteration in its binding activity may be considered as a reliable marker of the disease.

To further characterize glycosylation alteration of scrapie-infected hamster blood total glycoproteins, I studied plasma glycoproteins by the lectin blotting method through separation by gel electrophoresis and subsequent staining with lectins of equal amounts of normal and infected plasma. Lectin blot confirmed the occurrence of glycosylation alteration showing clearly marked alterations of the glycosylation of some proteins (Fig. 6). Moreover, it showed that proteins glycosylation alteration may concern even a single sugar only (Fig. 6). Among the glycoproteins with high molecular mass, glycosylation of three glycoproteins at approximately 150, 116 and 60 kDa was consistently altered in the infected plasma with respect to the normal (Fig. 6). Particularly, the 60 kDa glycoprotein which is composed of a double band has shown increased glycosylation of the upper band and disappearance of that lower in the infected plasma with respect to the normal. This latter particular change was observed obviously with WGA and less with RCA, only. Glycosylation alteration of the glycoprotein at almost 150 kDa concerned galactose residues recognized by DBA, PNA and SBA, while that of the glycoprotein at almost 116 kDa concerned fucose recognized by UEA-I and α-N-acetylgalactosamine recognized by DBA. Among the glycoproteins with middle molecular mass, glycosylation of two glycoproteins at approximately 50 and 40 kDa was altered in the infected plasma with respect to the normal. Whereas, the glycoprotein at almost 50 kDa has shown alteration of all the sugars although in different measures and the glycoprotein at almost 40 kDa which may be the most altered has shown alteration of N-acetylglucosamine (GlcNAc) and N-acetylgalactosamine recognized by WGA and RCA respectively. Among the glycoproteins with low molecular mass, glycosylation of a glycoprotein at almost 24 kDa was altered concerning, apparently, only mannose recognized by ConA.

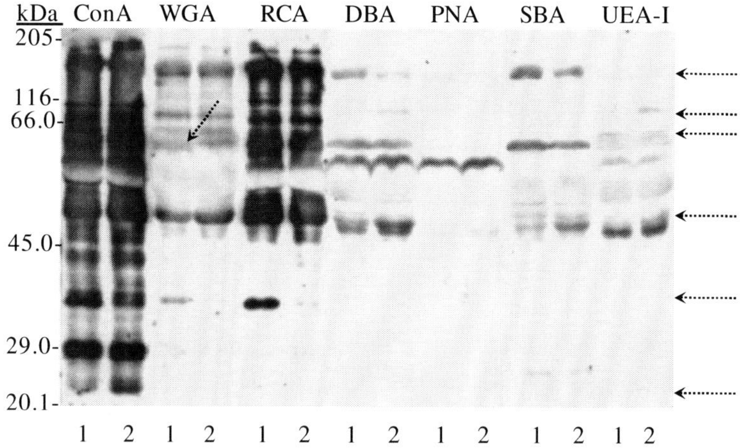

Figure 6. Characterization by lectin blotting of the glycosylation alteration of endogenously scrapie-infected hamster plasma total glycoproteins. Equal amounts of normal and endogenously infected plasma were electrophoresed on 10% polyacrylamide gels, blotted onto nitrocellulose membrane and then stained with the seven biotinylated lectins. Lane 1 (normal), lane 2 (infected). Arrows indicate glycoproteins whose glycosylation is greatly altered in the infected sample with respect to the normal. Molecular mass markers are indicated in kilodaltons on the left.

As seen, sugars were increased, decreased or unchanged in the infected plasma with respect to the normal. Also in the case of the blood, glycosylation alteration seems to be selective not only to some glycoproteins but also to some sugars of a single glycoprotein.

Lectin blot provided elements for a promising diagnostic blood test especially with respect to the glycoprotein at approximately 40 kDa. Further immunological analysis able to identify with precision this protein may be necessary to validate it as a specific biomarker for the diagnosis of scrapie and perhaps of other prion diseases.

The main objective of this part of the chapter was finding a biomarker for prion diseases different from PrP^{Sc} since it was largely demonstrated that levels of this protein in blood are too much low to be detected by the classic diagnostic methods [16, 17, 44]. However; since PrP^{Sc} has been already characterized and easily recognized by various monoclonal antibodies either in its full length or as fragments, I tried to detect it directly from endogenously infected hamster plasma by lectin ELISA. Thus, using 3F4 monoclonal antibody, PrP^{C} or PrP^{Sc} from equal amounts of normal and infected plasma respectively, were captured on ELISA plates and then detected by lectin staining. I was able to record an altered binding reactivity to PrP^{Sc} with respect to PrP^{C} of all the tested lectins (DBA, UEA-I, SBA and PNA) except SBA which showed negative readings at the used quantity of plasma total proteins (Fig. 7A, B, C and D). DBA binding reactivity was markedly and significantly ($P \leq 0.01$) decreased not only at 40 days post infection (46.0%) but even at a time as early as 18 days post infection reaching a 72.6% reduction (Fig. 7A). UEA-I binding reactivity has shown a significant increase at 40 days post infection ($P = 0.04$) (Fig. 7B) and finally, PNA binding reactivity was curious because it was substantially decreased (63.8%) although with a $P = 0.06$ at 18 days post infection, and instead was increased drastically and significantly (66.2 %, $P = 0.014$) at 40 days post infection (Fig. 7C).

α-N-acetylgalactosamine recognized by DBA is the most altered sugar either in the total glycoproteins or in the PrP^{Sc} at both levels central and peripheral showing coherently a signal that results always significantly reduced in the infected samples compared to the normal. Therefore, alteration of the proportions of this sugar could be considered as a marker of scrapie and may be also for other prion diseases.

The differences found between PrP^{C} and PrP^{Sc} are due to different glycosylation and not to quantitative differences. Because, first of all, as above mentioned, equal amounts of normal and infected plasma were loaded. Second, an excess of PrP (1100 μg total proteins) was captured by a small but similar quantity of 3F4 antibody in order to bind always the same quantity of PrP regardless of its total quantity in the samples and, therefore, the differences in lectins binding reactivity between PrP^{C} and PrP^{Sc} should be due to glycosylation alterations and not to quantitative differences. A similar consideration for a similar evaluation has been reported by Goh and colleagues [94]. Third, both 3F4 antibody and the lectins are specific for the relative antigen.

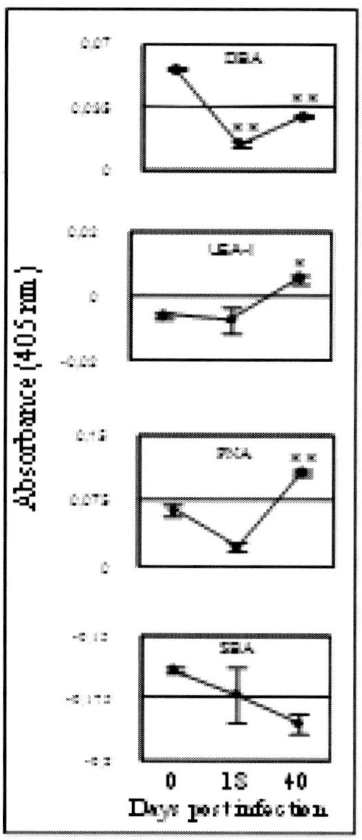

Figure 7. Lectins binding profile to hamster plasma PrP^{C} and PrP^{Sc}. Equal amounts of total proteins of normal and endogenously infected plasma were loaded on 96-well ELISA plates precoated with 3F4 antibody, and lectins binding profile was determined, under native conditions, by staining with (A) DBA, (B) UEA-1, (C) PNA and (D) SBA. Results are average ± standard deviation (SD) of duplicates. * $P \leq 0.05$, ** $P \leq 0.01$.

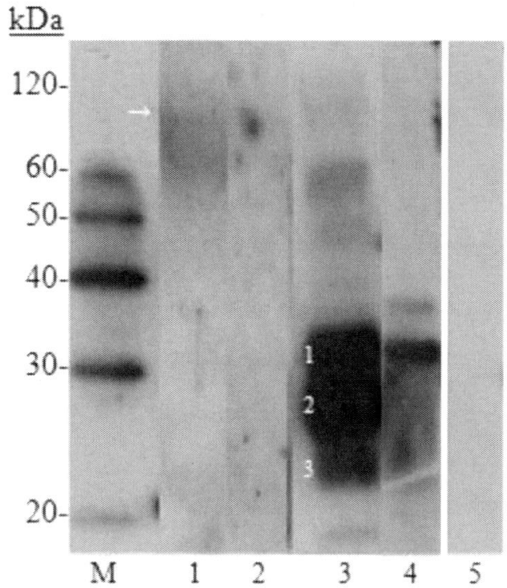

Figure 8. Electrophoretic profile of hamster plasma PrP. Plasma PrP released from ELISA plates was electrophoresed on a 12% polyacrylamide gel and then detected by immuno blotting. Lanes 1, 2, and 3 were probed with 3F4 antibody: M (Molecular mass markers), lane 1 (blank control), lane 2 (plasma PrP), lane 3 (brain homogenate not released from ELISA plate but added as positive control). Lanes 4 and 5 were probed with PNA lectin: lane 4 (plasma PrP) and lane 5 (blank control). Control lanes (lane 1 and 5) were included to show that the signal detected by 3F4 and PNA was specific and due to an interaction with the PrP. Numbers 1, 2 and 3 on lane 3, indicate the di-, mono- and non-glycosylated bands of PrP, respectively. Arrow indicates 3F4 antibody IgG bands from lanes 1 and 2. Molecular mass markers are indicated in kilodaltons on the left. Image has been cropped to remove lanes that are not relevant to this data.

Electrophoretic profile of plasma PrP species captured in ELISA by 3F4 antibody was determined by releasing PrP from ELISA plate and its subsequent analysis by lectins and 3F4 on an immunoblot. Plasma PrP was identified by the lectins showing a major band with an apparent molecular mass of approximately 32 kDa (Fig 8, lane 4). Figure 8 shows two bands (lane 4), detected with PNA, of which the upper one is faint and the lower one is strong and they seem corresponding to the di and monoglycosylated glycoforms of PrP respectively, although they are slightly higher as compared with the banding of PrP^{Sc} from brain homogenate (lane 3), detected with 3F4. The reason of this small difference in the apparent molecular mass of PrP^{Sc} between the antibody and lectins detection is not clear but it may be attributed to the different structures involved in the immunoreaction. A similar result has been reported by Xanthopoulos and colleagues [104] who found that the apparent molecular mass of monoglycosylated PrP^{Sc} is slightly higher when blotted with Datura stramonium lectin (DSL) than with 6H4 monoclonal antibody. Author's interpretation was that lectins bind a subpopulation of the PrP^{Sc} molecules presenting the suitable sugar moiety for recognition, while the antibody binds all the PrP^{Sc} molecules present.

This result confirms that the carbohydrate portion detected in ELISA is belonging to PrP species and, in addition, it indicates that the antibody is much less sensitive than biotynilated lectins since it was not able to detect plasma PrP, released from ELISA plate, at its actual loaded quantities (Fig. 8, lane 2).

Conclusion

In this chapter, I confirmed that not only glycosylation of PrP^C but also that of other glycoproteins is profoundly altered by scrapie prions. Instead, with difference to earlier studies [4, 105] which described alterations in the quantity of bi-, tri- and tetraantennary glycans present on PrP^{Sc}; with respect to PrP^C, and hypothesized that alterations in the levels of glycans processing enzymes (GlcNAc transferases) in prion-infected cells, has to be responsible for these alterations, I carried out exposure alterations of the glycosylation.

Since the two results (earlier and current) concerned in both cases the carbohydrate portion of PrP from normal and scrapie-infected Syrian hamster, I reasoned that the exposure alteration is that which might be involved in the pathogenesis and the quantitative alteration is only a consequence. An exposure alteration of the glycosylation may consequently cause alteration of the proportion of some sugars on functional glycoproteins, and as a compensatory mechanism, glycans processing enzymes are evoked to readjust glycans proportions producing consequently further alteration of the protein glycosylation. Obviously, also levels of the glycans processing enzymes involved in the reaction are subjected to alteration.

Based on this rational, the earlier results are in good agreement with my conclusion that proteolytic agents and denaturants could constitute potential candidates as inducers of the *in vivo* glycosylation alterations. This conclusion is based on the similar lectins-binding profile to native-pathological glycoproteins and PK or GdnHCl-treated-normal glycoproteins reflecting similarities between the relative N-linked glycans and suggesting that the *in vitro* treatment caused glycosylation alterations apparently similar to those induced by the *in vivo* prion infection. A potential involvement of such agents in glycosylation alterations does not sound so new, a protective role of the glycosylation against proteolytic agents by rendering vulnerable cleavage sites of PrP and other proteins inaccessible to their action has always been known [100, 105 - 108]. It was also found that the N-linked glycans play a role in protecting proteins from the action of proteases during T cell engagement in a process which may take several hours [109]. On the other hand, glycosylation has shown to have a protective role also against denaturing conditions [110] whose effect on the *in vivo* conversion of PrP^C into PrP^{Sc} was reported and found to be responsible for the conformational changes that facilitate amyloid and prion self-assembly [111]. In fact, it is known that denaturants (such as heat, variation of the pH; of the urea concentration; of inorganic salts concentrations; of heavy metals, and many other factors) are able to cause conformational alterations conferring proteins new physical-biochemical characteristics ranging from loss of solubility to increased aggregation. Such characteristics besides being typical of PrP^{Sc} [112] they are also observed when glycosylation state is subjected to alteration [92, 105, 107,113 - 115] especially in denaturing environment [110]. Thus, since a relationship between PrP^C conversion process and its glycosylation state alteration exists (see introduction section), and since both events confer it identical physical-biochemical properties it is plausible that the two events would occur in a similar denaturing environment, if not in the same.

On these basis, glycosylation alteration of a protein may be consequence of an its tentative to hide the sites greatly susceptible to proteolysis and denaturation, as a further mechanism of protection when the challenge persists. In line with this supposition my demonstration that alteration in the PrP^C glycosylation is strongly correlated with alteration in the exposure of an its epitope (aa 109 - 112) recognized by 3F4 antibody which is a specific feature of the PrP^C-to-PrP^{Sc} conversion process in prion diseases [48, 116 - 118].

This correlation led the current results to support the idea that following prion infection; alteration of the PrP^C glycosylation and the exposure of its epitope 109 - 112 would occur before its conversion into PrP^{Sc}. Accordingly, other authors sustained such affirmation [104]. Thereby, an irreversible alteration of the PrP^C glycosylation might be the promoter of the conversion process and PrP^{Sc} seems to be only the final result of alterations occurred to PrP^C. Consistent with this my supposition the finding that subtle changes in the PrP^C glycosylation and the cellular environment in which the conversion occurs *in vivo* can influence the final glycosylation pattern of PrP^{Sc} [101].

By providing evidence on glycosylation alteration of hamster plasma total glycoproteins at a time as early as 10 days post infection, I together with other researchers previously mentioned in the current chapter, may open a true prospective for a promising diagnostic blood test for prion diseases but, with the difference that the blood test proposed by me being extremely rapid, very simple, sensitive, does not require pre-treatment of plasma samples, need small volumes of blood, not invasive and reliable, it may be more suitable as a routine diagnostic test. Furthermore, this test presents several advantages represented firstly by the possibility to provide an early diagnosis of the disease before the development of symptoms allowing a more favorable prognosis since treatment at this point is more effective than treatment initiated at a later stage of the disease [65, 119]. Secondly, it may be useful for the prediction of the potential infectivity of blood by a simple screening making possible its exclusion before being employed in the plasma-derived manufacturing or transfusions, enhancing, so, blood safety. Thirdly, this diagnostic test may own the advantage of being able to monitor disease progression and a therapeutic treatment predicting its efficacy.

Detection, here, of PrP^{Sc} in endogenously infected blood through its carbohydrate portion which resulted different from that of PrP^C, allowed the discrimination between them at the native state without using the classic digestion with PK or any other treatment that could be source of artifact results or/ and underestimation of PrP^{Sc} effective amounts due to the digestion of the PK-sensitive portion of PrP^{Sc} [48 - 53].

Finally, demonstration that prion infection affects selectively glycosylation of some proteins at both central and peripheral levels at few distance from the infection, suggests that this biochemical process might be effectively involved in the pathogenesis of prion diseases since its early onset. And, its impact on the pathogenesis of prion diseases might be represented by participating at molecular level into the PrP^C-to-PrP^{Sc} conversion process (subsequent alteration of the glycosylation of PrP^C), and at clinical level causing systematic dysfunctions (subsequent alteration of the glycosylation of different functional glycoproteins).

In this chapter, I explored and discussed some new concepts regarding glycosylation alteration of hamster glycoproteins providing not only novel insights on the role of glycosylation in prion diseases pathogenesis but also identifying new candidates targets for the early and late therapy of the disease and proposing an innovative diagnostic approach for the early-stage of illness. Therefore, these studies should be extended to other animal species and TSE strains with particular regard to that of the human vCJD.

EXPERIMENTAL PROCEDURES

Preparation of Brain Homogenate

10% brain homogenate was prepared from brains of normal or terminally ill Syrian hamsters infected with the 263K strain of scrapie, by homogenization in ice-cold phosphate-buffered saline (PBS; pH 7.4). After centrifugation of the brain homogenate at 2000 x g for 10 minutes at 4 °C, supernatants were collected, divided into single aliquots and stored at - 80 °C until use. Total proteins amount was measured by the bicinchoninic acid (BCA) protein assay (performed as the manufacture instructions, Sigma Chemical Co.).

Digestion with Proteinase-K (PK)

Aliquots of normal and 263K-infected brain homogenate were incubated with 50 μg/ml of proteinase-K (PK, Sigma Chemical Co.) for 1 h with shaking at 37 °C. After PK inactivation by adding phenylmethylsulfonil fluoride (Sigma Chemical Co.) and measuring total proteins amount, samples were subjected to detection by lectins.

Treatment with Guanidine Hydrochloride (GdnHCL)

Some aliquots of brain homogenate were treated with guanidine hydrochloride 4 M (GdnHCl, Sigma Chemical Co.) before loading on a 96-well plate: GdnHCl was added to the brain homogenate at a ratio 1:1 (v/v) and after heating at 100 °C for 10 minutes with shaking, the denatured samples were brought to the requested dilution with PBS. And, other aliquots were treated after loading on a 96-well plate: samples before saturation with PBS containing 0.1% Tween-20 (PBS-T) were incubated with 100 μl of GdnHCl for 1-2 h with shaking at 37 °C.

Plasma Preparation

Blood was collected, in tubes containing sodium citrate (3.8%) as anti-coagulant at time 0 and at 10, 18, 32, 40 and 59 days after infection with the 263K strain of scrapie, from Syrian hamsters. Blood was, then, separated into components by centrifugation at 2000 x g for 15 minutes at room temperature (RT). Supernatants (plasma) were collected into 0.5 ml aliquots, immediately frozen on dry ice and then stored at - 80 °C until analysis.

Lectin-ELISA

96-well ELISA plates (Nunc, Nunclon delta Surface) were loaded and incubated overnight at 4 °C with equal amounts of total proteins of normal and 263K-infected brain homogenate (70 μg total proteins) or plasma (290 μg total proteins) diluted in carbonate buffer pH 9.6 containing protease inhibitors cocktail (Complete, Roche Diagnostics, Mannheim, Germany). For sandwich-lectin ELISA, plates were precoated overnight at 4 °C with 100 µl of capturing anti-PrP monoclonal antibodies 3F4 (aa 109 – 112) or 6H4 (aa 144 – 152) diluted in carbonate buffer pH 9.6 containing protease inhibitors cocktail.

Samples, after blocking unspecific sites of binding with 200 µl of PBS-T at room temperature for 1h, were incubated at room temperature for 2 h with 100 µl of different biotinylated lectins (Vector Laboratories) diluted in PBS-T at a final concentration of 10 µg/ml. The lectins used are reported in table 1 and include: Concanavalin A (ConA), specific for α–linked mannose; Ricinus communis agglutinin I (RCA I), specific for N-acetylgalactosamine; Ulex europaeus agglutinin I (UEA I), specific for (α-1, 2) linked fucose; Peanut agglutinin (PNA), specific for galactosyl (β-1, 3) GalNAc; Wheat germ agglutinin (WGA), specific for N-acetylglucosamine (GlcNAc); Soybean agglutinin (SBA), specific for α-D-N-acetylgalactosamine and Dolichos biflorus agglutinin (DBA), specific for α-N-acetylgalactosamine. At the end of the incubation, wells were washed 3 times with PBS-T and incubated at room temperature for 1h with 100 µl of a streptavidin-coniugated horseradish peroxidase (Vector Laboratories) diluted in PBS-T at a final concentration of 2.5 µg/ml. Finally, after washing 5 times with PBS-T and incubation in the dark at room temperature for 30 minutes with 100 µl of the ABTS Substrate (Vector Laboratories); optical density of the developed colour was measured at 405 nm by a microplate reader (Bio-Rad). Blank wells, in which no brain homogenate or plasma was added, were also included. The results presented, are average of duplicates and all the experiments were repeated 3 times.

Lectin Blotting

Equal or increasing amounts of total proteins of normal and 263K-infected brain homogenate or plasma were diluted in sample buffer, boiled for 10 minutes at 100 °C and electrophoresed on (12% for brain homogenate and 10% for plasma) polyacrylamide gels. At the end of the run, separated proteins were blotted onto nitrocellulose membrane (Amersham Biosciences) using a semi-dry transfer apparatus at 125 mA for 1h. Membranes were blocked for 1 h at room temperature in Tris-buffered saline containing 0.1% Tween-20 (TBS-T, pH 7.5) and then incubated for 2 h at room temperature with the different biotinylated lectins diluted in TBS-T at a final concentration of 1 µg/ml. After washing six times with TBS-T, blots were incubated for 1 h at room temperature with a streptavidin-conjugated horseradish peroxidase and then developed using an ECL detection system (Santa Cruz).

Releasing of PrP from ELISA Plates

Plasma PrP was removed from ELISA plates, which were used in the lectin ELISA assay, by incubation with sample buffer for one hour at 37 °C under constant agitation.

ACKNOWLEDGMENTS

I am very grateful to Maria Grazia Mancini for the help offered during reading ELISA plates and for using the microplate reader.

REFERENCES

[138] S. C. Fu and J. W. Gurd, Developmental changes in the oligosaccharide composition of synaptic junctional glycoproteins, *J. Neurochem.* 41, 1726-34 (1983).

[139] R. Kleene and M. Schachner, Glycans and neural cell interactions, *Nat. Rev. Neurosci.* 5, 195-208 (2004).

[140] Y. Sato and T. Endo, Alteration of brain glycoproteins during aging, *Geriatr. Gerontol. Int.* 10, S32-40 (2010).

[141] P. M. Rudd, T. Endo, C. Colominas, D. Groth, S. F. Wheeler, D. J. Harvey, M. R. Wormald, H. Serban, S. B. Prusiner, A. Kobata and R. A. Dwek, Glycosylation differences between the normal and pathogenic prion protein isoforms, *Proc. Natl. Acad. Sci.* U S A 96, 13044-9 (1999).

[142] A. Kobata, A journey to the world of glycobiology, *Glycoconj. J.* 17, 443-64 (2000).

[143] F. Liu, T. Zaidi, K. Iqbal, I. Grundke-Iqbal, R. K. Merkle, C. X. Gong, Role of glycosylation in hyperphosphorylation of tau in Alzheimer's disease, *FEBS Lett.* 512, 101-6 (2002).

[144] J. Sáez-Valero, L. R. Fodero, M. Sjögren, N. Andreasen, S. Amici, V. Gallai, H. Vanderstichele, E. Vanmechelen, L. Parnetti, K. Blennow and D. H. Small, Glycosylation of acetylcholinesterase and butyrylcholinesterase changes as a function of the duration of Alzheimer's disease, *J. Neurosci. Res.*72, 520-6 (2003).

[145] J. Yasuda, H. Eguchi, N. Fujiwara, T. Ookawara, S. Kojima, Y. Yamaguchi, M. Nishimura, J. Fujimoto and K. Suzuki, Reactive oxygen species modify oligosaccharides of glycoproteins in vivo: a study of a spontaneous acute hepatitis model rat (LEC rat), *Biochem. Biophys. Res. Commun.* 342, 127-34 (2006).

[146] I. Batxelli-Molina, N. Salvetat, O. Andréoletti, L. Guerrier, G. Vicat, F. Molina and C. Mourton-Gilles, Ovine serum biomarkers of early and late phase scrapie, *BMC Vet. Res.* 6, 49 (2010).

[147] S. B. Prusiner, Prions, *Proc. Natl. Acad. Sci.* U S A 95, 13363-83 (1998).

[148] R. G. Will, J. W. Ironside, M. Zeidler, S. N. Cousens, K. Estibeiro, A. Alperovitch, S. Poser, M. Pocchiari, A. Hofman and P. G. Smith, A new variant of Creutzfeldt-Jakob disease in the UK, *Lancet* 347, 921-5 (1996).

[149] J. Collinge, J. Whitfield, E. McKintosh, J. Beck, S. Mead, D. J. Thomas and M. P. Alpers, Kuru in the 21st century--an acquired human prion disease with very long incubation periods, *Lancet* 367, 2068-74 (2006).

[150] R. A. Bessen and R. F. Marsh, Distinct PrP properties suggest the molecular basis of strain variation in transmissible mink encephalopathy, *J. Virol.* 68, 7859-68 (1994).

[151] H. J. Ward, D. Everington, S. N. Cousens, B. Smith-Bathgate, M. Leitch, S. Cooper, C. Heath, R. S. Knight, P. G. Smith and R. G. Will, Risk factors for variant Creutzfeldt-Jakob disease: a case–control study, *Ann. Neurol.* 59, 111–20 (2006).

[152] A. M. Thackray, M. A. Klein and R. Bujdoso, Subclinical prion disease induced by oral inoculation, *J. Virol.* 77, 7991-8 (2003).

[153] P. Brown, R. G. Rohwer, B. C. Dunstan, C. MacAuley, D. C. Gajdusek and W. N. Drohan, The distribution of infectivity in blood components and plasma derivatives in experimental models of transmissible spongiform encephalopathy, *Transfusion* 38, 810-6 (1998).

[154] P. Brown, L. Cervenáková, L. M. McShane, P. Barber, R. Rubenstein and W. N. Drohan, Further studies of blood infectivity in an experimental model of transmissible spongiform encephalopathy, with an explanation of why blood components do not transmit Creutzfeldt-Jakob disease in humans, *Transfusion* 39, 1169-78 (1999).

[155] F. Houston, J. D. Foster, A. Chong, N. Hunter and C. J. Bostock, Transmission of BSE by blood transfusion in sheep, *Lancet* 356, 999-1000 (2000).

[156] K. Holada, J. G. Vostal, P. W. Theisen, C. MacAuley, L. Gregori and R. G. Rohwer, Scrapie infectivity in hamster blood is not associated with platelets, *J. Virol.* 76, 4649-50 (2002).

[157] N. Hunter, J. Foster, A. Chong, S. McCutcheon, D. Parnham, S. Eaton, C. MacKenzie and F. Houston, Transmission of prion diseases by blood transfusion, *J. Gen. Virol.* 83, 2897-905 (2002).

[158] L. Cervenakova, O. Yakovleva, C. McKenzie, S. Kolchinsky, L. McShane, W. N. Drohan and P. Brown, Similar levels of infectivity in the blood of mice infected with human-derived vCJD and GSS strains of transmissible spongiform encephalopathy, *Transfusion* 43, 1687-94 (2003).

[159] R. G. Rohwer, Titer, distribution, and transmissibility of blood-borne TSE infectivity. Presented at the Cambridge Healthtech Institute 6th Annual Meeting, "Blood Product Safety: TSE, Perception versus Reality", Feb 13-15; Maclean, VA (2000).

[160] C. A. Llewelyn, P. E. Hewitt, R. S. Knight, K. Amar, S. Cousens, J. Mackenzie and R. G. Will, Possible transmission of variant Creutzfeldt-Jakob disease by blood transfusion, *Lancet* 363, 417-21 (2004).

[161] A. H. Peden, M. W. Head, D. L. Ritchie, J. E. Bell and J. W. Ironside, Preclinical vCJD after blood transfusion in a PRNP codon 129 heterozygous patient, *Lancet* 364, 527-9 (2004).

[162] S. J. Wroe, S. Pal, D. Siddique, H. Hyare, R. Macfarlane, S. Joiner, J. M. Linehan, S. Brandner, J. D. Wadsworth, P. Hewitt and J. Collinge, Clinical presentation and pre-mortem diagnosis of variant Creutzfeldt-Jakob disease associated with blood transfusion: a case report, *Lancet* 368, 2061-7 (2006).

[163] Health Protection Agency, Fourth case of transfusion associated variant-CJD, *Health Prot. Rep.* 1, (2007).

[164] S. Sisó, M. Jeffrey and L. González, Neuroinvasion in sheep transmissible spongiform encephalopathies: the role of the haematogenous route, *Neuropathol. Appl. Neurobiol.* 35, 232-46 (2009).

[165] G. Chohan, C. Llewelyn, J. Mackenzie, S. Cousens, A. Kennedy, R. Will and P. Hewitt, Variant Creutzfeldt-Jakob disease in a transfusion recipient: coincidence or cause?, *Transfusion* 50, 1003-6 (2010).

[166] R. Knight, The risk of transmitting prion disease by blood or plasma products, *Transfus. Apher. Sci.* 43, 387-91(2010).

[167] L. Gregori, A prototype assay to detect vCJD-infected blood, *Lancet* 377, 444-6 (2011).

[168] A. Aguzzi, Neuro-immune connection in spread of prions in the body?, *Lancet* 349, 742-3 (1997).

[169] A. Aguzzi, Understanding the diversity of prions, *Nat. Cell. Biol.* 6, 290-2 (2004).

[170] C. Soto, Diagnosing prion diseases: needs, challenges and hopes, *Nat. Rev. Microbiol.* 2, 809-19 (2004).

[171] Y. Murayama, M. Yoshioka, H. Okada, M. Takata, T. Yokoyama and S. Mohri, Urinary excretion and blood level of prions in scrapie-infected hamsters, *J. Gen. Virol.* 88, 2890-8 (2007).

[172] L. Trieschmann, A. Navarrete Santos, K. Kaschig, S. Torkler, E. Maas, H. Schätzl and G. Böhm, Ultra-sensitive detection of prion protein fibrils by flow cytometry in blood from cattle affected with bovine spongiform encephalopathy, *BMC Biotechnol.* 5, 26 (2005).

[173] B. Chang, X. Cheng, S. Yin, T. Pan, H. Zhang, P. Wong, S. C. Kang, F. Xiao, H. Yan, C. Li, L. L. Wolfe, M. W. Miller, T. Wisniewski, M. I. Greene and M. S. Sy, Test for detection of disease-associated prion aggregate in the blood of infected but asymptomatic animals, *Clin. Vaccine Immunol.* 14, 36-43 (2007).

[174] K. Tsukui, M. Takata and K. Tadokoro, A potential blood test for transmissible spongiform encephalopathies by detecting carbohydrate-dependent aggregates of PrPres-like proteins in scrapie-Infected hamster plasma, *Microbiol. Immunol.* 51, 1221-31 (2007).

[175] P. Saá, J. Castilla and C. Soto, Presymptomatic detection of prions in blood, *Science* 313, 92-4 (2006).

[176] S. S. An, K. T. Lim, H. J. Oh, B. S. Lee, E. Zukic, Y. R. Ju, T. Yokoyama, S. Y. Kim, E. Welker, Differentiating blood samples from scrapie infected and non-infected hamsters by detecting disease-associated prion proteins using Multimer Detection System, *Biochem. Biophys. Res. Commun.* 392, 505-9 (2010).

[177] L. A. Terry, L. Howells, J. Hawthorn, J. C. Edwards, S. J. Moore, S. J. Bellworthy, H. Simmons, S. Lizano, L. Estey, V. Leathers and S. J. Everest, Detection of PrPsc in blood from sheep infected with the scrapie and bovine spongiform encephalopathy agents, *J. Virol.* 83, 12552-8 (2009).

[178] J. A. Edgeworth, M. Farmer, A. Sicilia, P. Tavares, J. Beck, T. Campbell, J. Lowe, S. Mead, P. Rudge, J. Collinge and G. S. Jackson, Detection of prion infection in variant Creutzfeldt-Jakob disease: a blood-based assay, Lancet 377, 487-93 (2011).

[179] C. D. Orrú, J. M. Wilham, L. D. Raymond, F. Kuhn, B. Schroeder, A. J. Raeber and B. Caughey, Prion disease blood test using immunoprecipitation and improved quaking-induced conversion, *MBio* 2, e00078-11 (2011).

[180] M. H. Tattum, S. Jones, S. Pal, J. Collinge and G. S. Jackson, Discrimination between prion-infected and normal blood samples by protein misfolding cyclic amplification, *Transfusion* 50, 996-1002 (2010).

[181] L. Gregori, N. McCombie, D. Palmer, P. Birch, S. O. Sowemimo-Coker, A. Giulivi and R. G. Rohwer, Effectiveness of leucoreduction for removal of infectivity of transmissible spongiform encephalopathies from blood, *Lancet* 364, 529-31 (2004).

[182] S. B. Prusiner, S. P. Cochran, D. F. Groth, D. E. Downey, K. A. Bowman and H. M. Martinez, Measurement of the scrapie agent using an incubation time interval assay, *Ann. Neurol.* 11, 353-8 (1982).

[183] D. C. Bolton, M. P. McKinley and S. B. Prusiner, Identification of a protein that purifies with the scrapie prion, *Science* 218, 1309-11 (1982).
[184] J. D. Wadsworth, S. Joiner, K. Fox, J. M. Linehan, M. Desbruslais, S. Brandner, E. A. Asante and J. Collinge, Prion infectivity in variant Creutzfeldt-Jakob disease rectum, *Gut* 56, 90-4 (2007).
[185] J. Safar, H. Wille, V. Itri, D. Groth, H. Serban, M. Torchia, F. E. Cohen, S. B. Prusiner, Eight prion strains have PrP(Sc) molecules with different conformations, *Nat. Med.* 4, 1157-65 (1998).
[186] J. Safar, F. E. Cohen and S. B. Prusiner, Quantitative traits of prion strains are enciphered in the conformation of the prion protein, *Arch. Virol. Suppl.* 16, 227-35 (2000).
[187] A. M. Thackray, L. Hopkins and R. Bujdoso, Proteinase K-sensitive disease-associated ovine prion protein revealed by conformation-dependent immunoassay, *Biochem. J.* 401, 475-83 (2007).
[188] P. Tremblay, H. L. Ball, K. Kaneko, D. Groth, R. S. Hegde, F. E. Cohen, S. J. DeArmond, S. B. Prusiner and J. G. Safar, Mutant PrPSc conformers induced by a synthetic peptide and several prion strains, *J. Virol.* 78, 2088-99 (2004).
[189] S. Tzaban, G. Friedlander, O. Schonberger, L. Horonchik, Y. Yedidia, G. Shaked, R. Gabizon and A. Taraboulos, Protease-sensitive scrapie prion protein in aggregates of heterogeneous sizes, *Biochemistry* 41, 12868-75 (2002).
[190] M. A. Pastrana, G. Sajnani, B. Onisko, J. Castilla, R. Morales, C. Soto and J. R. Requena, Isolation and characterization of a proteinase K-sensitive PrPSc fraction, *Biochemistry* 45, 15710-7 (2006).
[191] O. Yakovleva, A. Janiak, C. McKenzie, L. McShane, P. Brown and L. Cervenakova, Effect of protease treatment on plasma infectivity in variant Creutzfeldt-Jakob disease mice, *Transfusion* 44, 1700-5 (2004).
[192] P. Brown, Creutzfeldt-Jakob disease: blood infectivity and screening tests, *Semin. Hematol.* 38, 2-6 (2001).
[193] G. P. Saborio, B. Permanne and C. Soto, Sensitive detection of pathological prion protein by cyclic amplification of protein misfolding, *Nature* 411, 810-3 (2001).
[194] L. Thorne and L. A. Terry, In vitro amplification of PrPSc derived from the brain and blood of sheep infected with scrapie, *J. Gen. Virol.* 89, 3177-84 (2008).
[195] N. R. Deleault, B. T. Harris, J. R. Rees and S. Supattapone, Formation of native prions from minimal components in vitro, *Proc. Natl. Acad. Sci.* U S A. 104, 9741-6 (2007).
[196] R. Atarashi, J. M. Wilham, L. Christensen, A. G. Hughson, R. A. Moore, L. M. Johnson, H. A. Onwubiko, S. A. Priola and B. Caughey, Simplified ultrasensitive prion detection by recombinant PrP conversion with shaking, *Nat. Methods* 5, 211-2 (2008).
[197] C. D. Orrú, J. M. Wilham, A. G. Hughson, L. D. Raymond, K. L. McNally, A. Bossers, C. Ligios and B. Caughey, Human variant Creutzfeldt-Jakob disease and sheep scrapie PrP(res) detection using seeded conversion of recombinant prion protein, *Protein Eng. Des. Sel.* 22, 515-21 (2009).
[198] C. Korth, B. Stierli, P. Streit, M. Moser, O. Schaller, R. Fischer, W. Schulz-Schaeffer, H. Kretzschmar, A. Raeber, U. Braun, F. Ehrensperger, S. Hornemann, R. Glockshuber, R. Riek, M. Billeter, K. Wüthrich and B. Oesch, Prion (PrPSc)-specific epitope defined by a monoclonal antibody, *Nature* 390, 74-7 (1997).

[199] E. Biasini, M. E. Seegulam, B. N. Patti, L. Solforosi, A. Z. Medrano, H. M. Christensen, A. Senatore, R. Chiesa, R. A. Williamson and D. A. Harris, Non-infectious aggregates of the prion protein react with several PrPSc-directed antibodies, *J. Neurochem.* 105, 2190-204 (2008).

[200] E. Biasini, L. Tapella, S. Mantovani, M. Stravalaci, M. Gobbi, D. A. Harris and R. Chiesa, Immunopurification of pathological prion protein aggregates, *PLoS One* 4, e7816 (2009).

[201] S. B. Prusiner, Novel proteinaceous infectious particles cause scrapie, *Science* 216, 136-44 (1982).

[202] A. Rigter, J. P. Langeveld, F. G. van Zijderveld and A. Bossers, Prion protein self-interactions: a gateway to novel therapeutic strategies?, *Vaccine* 28, 7810-23 (2010).

[203] C. Soto and N. Satani, The intricate mechanisms of neurodegeneration in prion diseases, *Trends in Molecular Medicine* 17, 14-24 (2011).

[204] B. S. Appleby and C. G. Lyketsos, Rapidly progressive dementias and the treatment of human prion diseases, *Expert. Opin. Pharmacother.* 12, 1-12 (2011).

[205] N. V. Todd, J. Morrow, K. Doh-ura, S. Dealler, S. O'Hare, P. Farling, M. Duddy and N. G. Rainov, Cerebroventricular infusion of pentosan polysulphate in human variant Creutzfeldt-Jakob disease, *J. Infect.* 50, 394-6 (2005).

[206] I. Bone, L. Belton, A. S. Walker and J. Darbyshire, Intraventricular pentosan polysulphate in human prion diseases: an observational study in the UK, *Eur. J. Neurol.* 15, 458-64 (2008).

[207] H. Abdel-Haq, M. Lu, F. Cardone, Q. G. Liu, M. Puopolo and M. Pocchiari, Efficacy of phthalocyanine tetrasulfonate against mouse-adapted human prion strains, *Arch. Virol.* 154, 1005-7 (2009).

[208] C. Riemer, M. Burwinkel, A. Schwarz, S. Gültner, S. W. Mok, I. Heise, N. Holtkamp and M. Baier, Evaluation of drugs for treatment of prion infections of the central nervous system, *J. Gen. Virol.* 89, 594-7 (2008).

[209] G. Forloni, M. Salmona, G. Marcon and F. Tagliavini, Tetracyclines and prion infectivity, *Infect. Disord. Drug Targets* 9, 23-30 (2009).

[210] M. D. White, M. Farmer, I. Mirabile, S. Brandner, J. Collinge and G. R. Mallucci, Single treatment with RNAi against prion protein rescues early neuronal dysfunction and prolongs survival in mice with prion disease, *Proc. Natl. Acad. Sci.* U S A 105, 10238-43 (2008).

[211] D. A. Kocisko, P. T. Lansbury Jr, and B. Caughey, Partial unfolding and refolding of scrapie-associated prion protein: evidence for a critical 16-kDa C-terminal domain, *Biochemistry* 35, 13434-42 (1996).

[212] M. X. Silveyra, N. Cuadrado-Corrales, A. Marcos, M. S. Barquero, A. Rábano, M. Calero and J. Sáez-Valero, Altered glycosylation of acetylcholinesterase in Creutzfeldt-Jakob disease, *J. Neurochem.* 96, 97-104 (2006).

[213] D. Nielsen, H. Gyllberg, P. Ostlund, T. Bergman and K. Bedecs, Increased levels of insulin and insulin-like growth factor-1 hybrid receptors and decreased glycosylation of the insulin receptor alpha- and beta-subunits in scrapie-infected neuroblastoma N2a cells, *Biochem. J.* 380, 571-9 (2004).

[214] R. Gabizon, M. P. McKinley and S. B. Prusiner, Purified prion proteins and scrapie infectivity copartition into liposomes, *Proc. Natl. Acad. Sci.* U S A 84, 4017-21 (1987).

[215] B. Oesch, D. Westaway, M. Wälchli, M. P. McKinley, S. B. Kent, R. Aebersold, R. A. Barry, P. Tempst, D. B. Teplow, L. E. Hood, et al., A cellular gene encodes scrapie PrP 27-30 protein, *Cell* 40, 735-46 (1985).
[216] B. W. Caughey, A. Dong, K. S. Bhat, D. Ernst, S. F. Hayes and W. S. Caughey, Secondary structure analysis of the scrapie-associated protein PrP 27-30 in water by infrared spectroscopy, *Biochemistry* 30, 7672-80 (1991).
[217] M. Gasset, M. A. Baldwin, R. J. Fletterick and S. B. Prusiner, Perturbation of the secondary structure of the scrapie prion protein under conditions that alter infectivity, *Proc. Natl. Acad. Sci.* U S A 90, 1-5 (1993).
[218] K. M. Pan, M. Baldwin, J. Nguyen, M. Gasset, A. Serban, D. Groth, I. Mehlhorn, Z. Huang, R. J. Fletterick, F. E. Cohen, et al., Conversion of alpha-helices into beta-sheets features in the formation of the scrapie prion proteins, *Proc. Natl. Acad. Sci.* U S A 90, 10962-6 (1993).
[219] C. L. Masters and E. P. Richardson Jr, Subacute spongiform encephalopathy (Creutzfeldt-Jakob disease), The nature and progression of spongiform change, *Brain* 101, 333-44 (1978).
[220] T. Pan, R. Li, B. S. Wong, S. C. Kang, J. Ironside and M. S. Sy, Novel antibody-lectin enzyme-linked immunosorbent assay that distinguishes prion proteins in sporadic and variant cases of Creutzfeldt-Jakob disease, *J. Clin. Microbiol.* 43, 1118-26 (2005).
[221] I. E. Triantaphyllidou, T. Sklaviadis and D. H. Vynios, Detection, quantification, and glycotyping of prion protein in specifically activated enzyme-linked immunosorbent assay plates, *Anal. Biochem.* 359, 176-82 (2006).
[222] B. Caughey, R. E. Race, D. Ernst, M. J. Buchmeier and B. Chesebro, Prion protein biosynthesis in scrapie-infected and uninfected neuroblastoma cells, *J. Virol.* 63, 175-81 (1989).
[223] R. A. Somerville, Host and transmissible spongiform encephalopathy agent strain control glycosylation of PrP, *J. Gen. Virol.* 80, 1865-72 (1999).
[224] S. J. DeArmond, Y. Qiu, H. Sànchez, P. R. Spilman, A. Ninchak-Casey, D. Alonso and V. Daggett, PrPc glycoform heterogeneity as a function of brain region: implications for selective targeting of neurons by prion strains, *J. Neuropathol. Exp. Neurol.* 58, 1000-9 (1999).
[225] P. Parchi, R. Castellani, S. Capellari, B. Ghetti, K. Young, S. G. Chen, M. Farlow, D. W. Dickson, A. A. Sima, J. Q. Trojanowski, R. B. Petersen and P. Gambetti, Molecular basis of phenotypic variability in sporadic Creutzfeldt-Jakob disease, *Ann. Neurol.* 39, 767-78 (1996).
[226] J. Collinge, K. C. Sidle, J. Meads, J. Ironside and A. F. Hill, Molecular analysis of prion strain variation and the aetiology of 'new variant' CJD, *Nature* 383, 685-90 (1996).
[227] P. Parchi, A. Giese, S. Capellari, P. Brown and W. Schulz-Schaeffer, Classification of sporadic Creutzfeldt-Jakob disease based on molecular and phenotypic analysis of 300 subjects, *Ann. Neurol.* 46, 224-33 (1999).
[228] A. F. Hill, S. Joiner, J. D. Wadsworth, K. C. Sidle, J. E. Bell, H. Budka, J. W. Ironside and J. Collinge, Molecular classification of sporadic Creutzfeldt-Jakob disease, *Brain* 126, 1333-46 (2003).
[229] V. A. Lawson, S. J. Collins, C. L. Masters and A. F. Hill, Prion protein glycosylation, *J. Neurochem.* 93, 793-801 (2005).

[230] A. Urayama, R. Morales, M. L. Niehoff, W. A. Banks and C. Soto, Initial fate of prions upon peripheral infection: half-life, distribution, clearance, and tissue uptake, *FASEB J.* 25, 2792-2803 (2011).

[231] A. X. Goh, C. Li, M. S. Sy and B. S. Wong, Altered prion protein glycosylation in the aging mouse brain, *J. Neurochem.* 100, 841-54 (2007).

[232] R. Nitrini, S. Rosemberg, M. R. Passos-Bueno, L. S. da Silva, P. Iughetti, M. Papadopoulos, P. M. Carrilho, P. Caramelli, S. Albrecht, M. Zatz and A. LeBlanc, Familial spongiform encephalopathy associated with a novel prion protein gene mutation, *Ann. Neurol.* 42, 138-46 (1997).

[233] E. Grasbon-Frodl, H. Lorenz, U. Mann, R. M. Nitsch, O. Windl and H. A. Kretzschmar, Loss of glycosylation associated with the T183A mutation in human prion disease, *Acta. Neuropathol.* 108, 476-84 (2004).

[234] F. Wiseman, E. Cancellotti and J. Manson, Glycosylation and misfolding of PrP, *Biochem. Soc. Trans.* 33, 1094-5 (2005).

[235] E. Neuendorf, A. Weber, A. Saalmueller, H. Schatzl, K. Reifenberg, E. Pfaff and M. H. Groschup, Glycosylation deficiency at either one of the two glycan attachment sites of cellular prion protein preserves susceptibility to bovine spongiform encephalopathy and scrapie infections, *J. Biol. Chem.* 279, 53306-16 (2004).

[236] A. Taraboulos, M. Rogers, D. R. Borchelt, M. P. McKinley, M. Scott, D. Serban and S. B. Prusiner, Acquisition of protease resistance by prion proteins in scrapie-infected cells does not require asparagine-linked glycosylation, *Proc. Natl. Acad. Sci.* U S A 87, 8262-6 (1990).

[237] S. Lehmann and D. A. Harris, Blockade of glycosylation promotes acquisition of scrapie-like properties by the prion protein in cultured cells, *J. Biol. Chem.* 272, 21479-87 (1997). Erratum in, *J. Biol. Chem.* 273, 5988 (1998).

[238] I. Vorberg and S. A. Priola, Molecular basis of scrapie strain glycoform variation, *J. Biol. Chem.* 277, 36775-81 (2002).

[239] K. F. Winklhofer, U. Heller, A. Reintjes and J. Tatzelt, Inhibition of complex glycosylation increases the formation of PrPsc, *Traffic* 4, 313-22 (2003).

[240] C. Korth, K. Kaneko and S. B. Prusiner, Expression of unglycosylated mutated prion protein facilitates PrP(Sc) formation in neuroblastoma cells infected with different prion strains, *J. Gen. Virol.* 81, 2555-63 (2000).

[241] K. Xanthopoulos, M. Polymenidou, S. J. Bellworthy, S. L. Benestad, T. Sklaviadis, Species and strain glycosylation patterns of PrPSc, *PLoS One* 4, e5633 (2009).

[242] P. M. Rudd, M. R. Wormald, D. R. Wing, S. B. Prusiner and R. A. Dwek, Prion glycoprotein: structure, dynamics, and roles for the sugars, *Biochemistry* 40, 3759-66 (2001).

[243] J. Zuegg and J. E. Gready, Molecular dynamics simulation of human prion protein including both N-linked oligosaccharides and the GPI anchor, *Glycobiology* 10, 959-74 (2000).

[244] M. Ermonval, S. Mouillet-Richard, P. Codogno, O. Kellermann and J. Botti, Evolving views in prion glycosylation: functional and pathological implications, *Biochimie* 85, 33-45 (2003).

[245] C. R. Carter, K. M. Whitmore and R. Thorpe, The significance of carbohydrates on G-CSF: differential sensitivity of G-CSFs to human neutrophil elastase degradation, *J. Leukoc. Biol.* 75, 515-22 (2004).

[246] P. M. Rudd, T. Elliott, P. Cresswell, I. A. Wilson and R. A. Dwek, Glycosylation and the immune system, *Science* 291, 2370-6 (2001).

[247] M. Oh-eda, M. Hasegawa, K. Hattori, H. Kuboniwa, T. Kojima, T. Orita, K. Tomonou, T. Yamazaki and N. Ochi, O-linked sugar chain of human granulocyte colony-stimulating factor protects it against polymerization and denaturation allowing it to retain its biological activity, *J. Biol. Chem.* 265, 11432-5 (1990).

[248] J. W. Kelly, The environmental dependency of protein folding best explains prion and amyloid diseases, *Proc. Natl. Acad. Sci.* U S A 95, 930-2 (1998).

[249] D. Riesner, Biochemistry and structure of PrP(C) and PrP(Sc), *Br. Med. Bull.* 66, 21-33 (2003).

[250] B. Imperiali and K. W. Rickert, Conformational implications of asparagine-linked glycosylation, *Proc. Natl. Acad. Sci.* U S A 92, 97-101 (1995).

[251] D. H. Live, R. A. Kumar, X. Beebe and S. J. Danishefsky, Conformational influences of glycosylation of a peptide: a possible model for the effect of glycosylation on the rate of protein folding, *Proc. Natl. Acad. Sci.* U S A 93, 12759-61 (1996).

[252] K. Nieznanski, M. Rutkowski, M. Dominik and D. Stepkowski, Proteolytic processing and glycosylation influence formation of porcine prion protein complexes, *Biochem. J.* 387, 93-100 (2005).

[253] Z. Huang, S. B. Prusiner and F. E. Cohen, Scrapie prions: a three-dimensional model of an infectious fragment, *Fold Des.* 1, 13-9 (1995).

[254] D. Peretz, R. A. Williamson, Y. Matsunaga, H. Serban, C. Pinilla, R. B. Bastidas, R. Rozenshteyn, T. L. James, R. A. Houghten, F. E. Cohen, S. B. Prusiner and D. R. Burton, A conformational transition at the N terminus of the prion protein features in formation of the scrapie isoform, *J. Mol. Biol.* 273, 614-22 (1997).

[255] S. Yin, N. Pham, S. Yu, C. Li, P. Wong, B. Chang, S. C. Kang, E. Biasini, P. Tien, D. A. Harris and M. S. Sy, Human prion proteins with pathogenic mutations share common conformational changes resulting in enhanced binding to glycosaminoglycans, *Proc. Natl. Acad. Sci.* U S A 104, 7546-51 (2007).

[256] C. R. Herman, H. K. Gill, J. Eng and L. L. Fajardo, Screening for preclinical disease: test and disease characteristics, *AJR. Am. J. Roentgenol.* 179, 825-31 (2002).

In: Prions and Prion Diseases: New Developments
Editor: Jean-Michel Verdier
ISBN: 978-1-62100-027-3
© 2012 Nova Science Publishers, Inc.

Chapter 6

TRANSMISSIBILITY OF PRION DISEASES IN RODENT MODELS: ATYPICAL STRAINS

T. Baron
Anses, Laboratoire de Lyon, Unité Maladies Neurodégénératives,
Lyon, France

ABSTRACT

Transmission experiments in rodents have been widely used to study transmissible spongiform encephalopathies (TSEs) following the demonstration that some of them could transmit a disease in mice or hamsters. These studies first highlighted the diversity of the transmissible agents involved and then strengthened the hypothesis of a link between the disease-associated prion protein (PrPd) and the biological diversity of these transmissible agents. However, the spectrum of these diseases has been considerably enlarged in the recent past, especially in ruminants. Two "atypical" forms of atypical BSE were identified in cattle (H and L-type), whereas "atypical" or "Nor98" scrapie was found in sheep and goats. This was a result of the greatly increased surveillance in cattle and small ruminants in Europe, following the discovery that BSE was transmissible from cattle to other species, including humans. The recent availability of diagnosis tests, based on the possible identification of PrPd in the brain of animals, has been an essential factor in this improved surveillance. Attempts to transmit them in rodent models revealed the variable behaviour of these diseases and confirmed that they were previously unknown forms of TSE. However, TSEs often fail to transmit a disease when inoculated in wild-type rodents, so the recent availability of a large panel of transgenic mouse models that express the bovine or ovine prion proteins has been essential for their characterization. In this review, recent data from transmission studies of the recently identified forms of TSEs in ruminants, in wild-type and transgenic mouse models, are compared with background knowledge about classical scrapie in small ruminants and classical BSE in cattle, established in the past. It is clear that a number of crucial questions remain unanswered, notably regarding the possible relationship between some of these diseases and their potential transmissibility across species.

Introduction

Transmissibility in rodents was recognized as an invaluable tool for studying transmissible spongiform encephalopathies (TSEs) following initial discoveries that scrapie from small ruminants could be experimentally transmitted to wild-type mice, voles or hamsters [1, 2]. These findings motivated vast amounts of work, from which emerged one of the most intriguing characteristics of these neurodegenerative diseases. The disease features were observed to vary in a given experimental model, especially with regard to disease incubation periods and the localization of neurodegenerative lesions, and could be stably reproduced during serial passages in the same experimental model. This was demonstrated particularly from scrapie in sheep and goats after transmission studies in wild-type mice [3, 4], but also from transmissible mink encephalopathy (TME) that occurred in ranch-raised minks, after transmission studies in hamsters [5]. These unexpected findings led to the notion that such diseases could involve different "strains" of transmissible agents, as in infectious diseases caused by exogenous pathogens, at a time when the origin of the TSEs remained entirely elusive. So far, the search for conventional pathogens specifically associated with these diseases in natural conditions has failed and the existence of "strains" appeared even more challenging when the theory was proposed that these diseases could be caused by post-translational modification of a protein [6], the prion protein (PrP), that later, according to studies in an experimental model of scrapie transmitted to hamsters, appeared to be encoded by the host genome [7]. However, experimental studies of TME provided strong evidence that distinct biochemical properties of the disease-associated form of the host prion protein (PrPd) could be revealed in two different strains that emerged after serial passages of this disease in hamsters [8]. Studies of a broader panel of hamster-adapted strains, derived from TME or scrapie of small ruminants and involving a conformation-dependent immunoassay (CDI), also suggested that the biological properties of prion strains could be 'enciphered' in the PrPd conformation [9]. Whatever the relationship between the transmissible agents involved in these diseases and the host prion protein, transmission studies in rodents from all the historical studies of scrapie and TME provided the scientific background for characterizing TSEs.

Demonstration of the crucial role of the host prion protein in TSEs [10], including its possible transmission between different species [11], paved the way to the development of novel experimental models with transgenic mice expressing the prion protein of the host of natural TSEs. Thus, a number of prion transgenic mouse lines became available to the scientific community, notably expressing the ovine [12, 13] or bovine prion proteins [14-16], and allowing in-depth studies of the TSE agents involved in these species. The demand for these lines was great as several natural TSE sources fail to transmit the disease in wild-type rodents, thus preventing any characterization of the TSE agents involved in the disease [17-19].

In recent years, considerable efforts have been made in Europe to increase the surveillance of TSEs in ruminants after the discovery in 1996 of a variant form of Creutzfeldt-Jakob disease in humans [20]. Indeed, this novel human disease was rapidly shown to have been caused by the transmissible agent involved in a major food-borne epizooty of bovine spongiform encephalopathy (BSE) in cattle, especially in the UK. Similarities between the TSE agents involved in the two species were ultimately demonstrated by comparative transmission studies in wild-type mice [21]. Due to the greater surveillance, novel forms of TSEs were identified in small ruminants [22, 23] and cattle [24, 25], and could be characterized on the basis of transmission studies performed in rodents in the past and the availability of novel experimental models.

In this review, we will summarize the available data pertaining to characterization of the TSE agents involved in "atypical" forms of TSEs, recently identified in small ruminants and in cattle, by means of transmission studies in rodent models, in the context of background data obtained in the past for the classical BSE agent of the food-borne epizooty and for classical scrapie.

The Cattle BSE Strain in the Scrapie Context in Small Ruminants

When bovine spongiform encephalopathy emerged, the pre-existing background knowledge was based on historical studies of strains derived from rodents, especially in wild-type mice, from the scrapie of small ruminants [26-28]. It rapidly became apparent from transmission studies in wild-type mice that BSE was readily transmissible to wild-type mice, producing consistent features of the disease from different bovine isolates [26, 27], and also after natural or experimental transmission of the disease in other species [4, 29]. This contrasted with the variable behaviour of scrapie in wild-type mice. It also seemed that the relationship between the TSE agents involved in BSE and scrapie, if any, was unclear. Nevertheless, these data provided an experimental basis for the search for cross-species transmissions of BSE, and led to identification in natural conditions of the BSE agent in other species, especially in domestic cats and in humans with variant Creutzfeldt-Jakob disease [21, 30], as well as in a goat [31].

In addition to the transmissibility in inbred wild-type mouse lines, which showed consistent incubation periods of the disease, compared to experimental challenges from cattle BSE, all these reports emphasized the consistent distribution of vacuolation lesions, as demonstrated by the "lesion profiles" used in the approach described by Fraser and Dickinson in scrapie studies [3]. The wild-type mouse lines used for these studies can have distinct *prnp* alleles (*prnp-a* in C57Bl and RIII mouse lines or *prnp-b* allele in VM mouse line), which strongly influence the incubation periods of the disease, depending on the involved strain, and in addition to the influence of the load of TSE agent in the inoculated brain homogenates ("infectious titer"). These two *prnp* alleles differ in their polymorphic residues at amino acids 108 and 189 and, for most scrapie strains, are associated with either short (Leu108/Thr189) or long (Phe108/Val189) incubation periods in mice [32]. Some strains, however, show shorter incubation periods in *prnp-b* mice, as is the case for the BSE agent ("301V strain") and the 22A scrapie strain.

Histopathological characterization relies on the semi-quantitative evaluation, in several mice, of the intensity of vacuolation lesions in a series of selected neurological sites (9 in the grey matter and 3 in the white matter) identified in standardized frontal sections of mouse brains [3, 4]. In studies of the BSE agent in the RIII mouse line, for example, the highest mean vacuolation scores were consistently obtained in the medulla (site 1) and hypothalamus (site 4) and to a lesser extent in the septal nuclei (site) 4), whereas the six other grey matter sites were only poorly vacuolated. However, more recent data showed that a number of sheep scrapie isolates, homozygous for the A_{136} R_{154} Q_{171} allele of the prion gene (*prnp*), also shared this "1.4.7 profile" [33]. Thus, additional criteria were clearly required to identify the BSE agent. These included the identification of vacuolation in other brain regions, such as the cochlear nucleus, and analysis of the localization and features of PrPd deposition by immunohistochemistry or PET-blot analyses [29, 34, 35].

Eventually, the BSE strain associated with the food-borne epizooty in cattle in Europe showed extremely consistent features in mice, contrasting with previous reports which had demonstrated the possible existence of a variety of experimental strains derived from scrapie of small ruminants (reviewed in [36]). The precise origin and significance of this experimental diversity, with regard to a possible genuine variety of TSE agents among natural isolates in small ruminants, remains poorly understood. A number of experimental mouse-adapted scrapie strains have been isolated after a complex history of experimental passages from a same source of scrapie (SSBP/1) through different species [4, 36]. The possibility of isolating multiple prion strains from a single scrapie isolate has also been demonstrated so that it is difficult to say whether this reflects emergence from a single strain during experimental transmissions or co-infection by distinct strains of the natural host of the disease [17]. As a result, at least in the UK, where most studies of scrapie strain typing have been carried out, a varying combination of three strains (ME7 and 87A in *prnp-a* mice and 87V in *prnp-b* mice) would be involved in most natural scrapie cases [4]. Furthermore, recent data indicate that the lesion profiles and immunohistochemical patterns observed after primary transmissions in wild type mice would be correlated with the ovine *prnp* genotype [37, 38].

Unlike wild-type mice, bank voles which are otherwise highly resistant to BSE at primary passage were shown in transmission studies to be highly susceptible to ovine scrapie, and some scrapie sources which were poorly transmissible to wild-type mice, could be readily transmitted in bank voles [39-41]. This provided a useful rodent model for studies of scrapie strains.

Although scrapie in hamsters has been widely used to investigate the pathogenesis of prion diseases, including analysis of the strain phenomenon [8, 42-44], this experimental model has been little used, as compared to mouse models, to investigate the strain diversity of ruminant TSEs. Also, with regard to BSE, this particular TSE agent could not be transmitted to hamster at primary passage from bovine tissues but could be transmitted in this species following inoculation of mouse-passage BSE [45, 46]. Comparisons of BSE with scrapie strains have thus been limited in this experimental model.

Despite intensive investigations of natural scrapie by transmission studies in rodent models, the implementation of active surveillance of scrapie since 2002 and the search for possible BSE by PrPd molecular analysis [47, 48], no scrapie strain in sheep has ever been revealed that could behave as the BSE agent. Transmission studies in mice indicated the presence of the BSE agent in a single French goat in 2002 [31]. Although it was often assumed that recycling of a TSE agent originating from scrapie of small ruminants could have been responsible for the BSE epizooty of cattle [49], the origin of this unusual TSE strain could not be identified by experimental investigations of scrapie strains.

Atypical/Nor98 Scrapie in the Scrapie Context

The increased active surveillance of small ruminants in Europe led to the major discovery that both sheep and goats could be affected by another form of TSE, referred to as "atypical" scrapie or "Nor98" scrapie, that differed in a number of respects from the previously known scrapie, now referred to as "classical" scrapie [22, 23, 50].

The first cases described were identified in Norway in 1998 when five clinical cases of scrapie were reported in sheep with genotypes rarely affected by classical scrapie (sheep with the A_{136} H_{154} Q_{171} *prnp* allele), and which were also characterized by an unusual distribution of brain lesions and PrPd [22]. Western blot tests had already indicated molecular features of PrPd that were distinctly different from both BSE and classical scrapie, revealing a low molecular mass band (~ 12 kDa) in comparison to the usual three-band pattern between 18-30 kDa typically observed in classical scrapie or BSE.

Surprisingly, the first atypical cases in other European countries were identified during active surveillance of TSEs following the observation of discrepancies between the different tests used for the initial or confirmatory diagnosis of TSEs (ELISA, Western blot or immunohistochemistry)[23]. These data became still more intriguing when similar cases were identified in different European countries in sheep homozygous for A_{136} R_{154} R_{171} which, at the time, were believed to be highly, if not entirely, resistant to TSEs [51, 52]. In some of these cases, the presence of the ~ 12 kDa band was reported following PrPres detection by Western blot [51], as in the early observations of Nor98 isolates in Norway [22].

The most crucial unresolved question was whether these cases represented a genuine and previously unknown form of TSE or a biochemical disorder of the prion protein that was not necessarily transmissible [53]. Interestingly, experimental transmission studies of such cases failed to transmit any disease within the lifetime of intra-cerebrally inoculated animals, in wild-type mice (C57BL/6, RIII and VM) or in bank voles [54-56]. To the best of our knowledge, no attempts to transmit to hamsters have been reported.

Thus the answer to the question of experimental transmissibility of such cases was initially only obtained thanks to the availability of transgenic mouse models overexpressing the sheep prion protein [13, 53], prior to the demonstration of transmissibility in sheep [57]. When a series of French cases were subjected to transmission studies in ovine transgenic mice (tg338), they indeed demonstrated that i) such a pathological condition from both sheep and goats allowed experimental transmission of a prion disease after intra-cerebral inoculation, thereby revealing a truly transmissible agent, including from A_{136} R_{154} R_{171} homozygous sheep ii) cases identified through discrepancies in diagnosis tests behaved similarly to the Nor98 isolates from Norway, and iii) no evidence of distinct strains was obtained. The unique features observed after transmission of the disease in ovine transgenic mice involved the same unusual PrPres molecular profile initially described in Nor98 scrapie cases in Norway (Figure), as well as a similar distribution of vacuolar lesions and PrPd deposits in the mouse brains. More recently, these unique features have been confirmed after transmission of atypical scrapie cases from the UK [55].

Interestingly, these results were obtained in a mouse model expressing the V_{136} R_{154} Q_{171} ovine prion protein, which, unlike classical scrapie, does not predispose to transmission of Nor98 scrapie in sheep [58-60]. Such transmission in this ovine transgenic mouse model could however be facilitated by the high levels of expression of the prion protein (8 to 10 fold higher than in the sheep brain). Transmission studies in another transgenic mouse model (TgOvPrP4) expressing the A_{136} R_{154} Q_{171} ovine prion protein indeed showed a strong influence of the protein expression level, which exhibits significant individual variability in this mouse line [56]. Although this study fully confirmed the transmissibility of atypical scrapie, it showed that transmission was much more influenced by the individual levels of prion protein expression than was observed during the transmission of classical scrapie or BSE in this mouse model. The biochemical and histopathological investigations associated with these experiments also confirmed the consistent features obtained from different isolates in sheep, including with different *prnp* genotypes, and goats [60, 61] and that PrPres exhibited unique features by Western blot that were similar to those described in sheep or goat brains affected by the disease [60, 62].

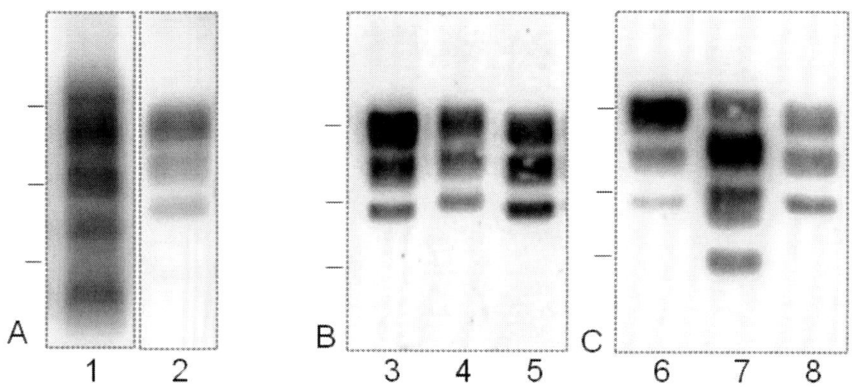

Figure. Western blot identification of PrPres in classical and atypical TSEs of cattle and small ruminants. A – Atypical/Nor98 (lane 1) or classical scrapie (lane 2) in sheep. B and C – Classical (lanes 3 and 6), H-type (lanes 4 and 7) and L-type (lanes 5 and 8) BSEs in cattle. PrPres was detected using Sha31 (panel A and B) or SAF84 (panel C) antibodies against the YEDRYYRE and RPVDQY PrP sequences respectively (amino-acids 156-163 and 175-180 in bovine PrP respectively). Bars to the left of each panel indicate the 29.0, 20.1 and 14.3 kDa molecular mass markers.

Comparison of the experimental data obtained from transmission studies with atypical/Nor98 scrapie with the strain phenomenon identified from classical scrapie is difficult because the data for classical scrapie were largely based on transmission experiments in wild-type mouse models. Transgenic mouse models have only recently become available and have received much less investigation, although some new studies suggested that distinct prion strains could also emerge following transmission of classical scrapie in ovine transgenic mice [63-66]. Nevertheless, there was no indication of the possibility of strain variation following transmission of atypical/Nor98 scrapie in such homologous transgenic mouse models.

However, intriguing results were obtained when attempts were made to transmit a prion disease from atypical scrapie in a transgenic mouse model expressing the porcine prion protein [67]. Whereas no evidence of prion disease was found in any of the mice intra-cerebrally inoculated with 7 classical scrapie isolates, two (2/12) mice inoculated with an atypical scrapie isolate did develop disease. Surprisingly, characterization of the disease, including after a second passage in this transgenic mouse model, revealed phenotypic features similar to those observed following transmission of BSE, from cattle or from experimentally-infected sheep, in this model, although some differences were noted in the lesion profiles or following PET-blot analysis of PrPd distribution. The significance of this finding, obtained from a single isolate of atypical scrapie, is unclear. The theoretical possibility of co-infection of the sheep by atypical scrapie and BSE, as already shown for atypical scrapie and classical scrapie [68] cannot be fully excluded and transmission of this particular isolate in other mouse models typically used to identify the BSE agent, such as wild-type mice or bovine transgenic mice, has not been reported yet. This might also reflect a phenotypic convergence between atypical scrapie and BSE in this transgenic model, with a similar prion conformation dictated by the model in both cases. This indicates that although the diverse rodent models available for risk assessment of transmission barriers in prion diseases are very useful, interpretation of the experimental data is complex.

The increased surveillance of TSEs in small ruminants in Europe was initially justified by the possible presence of BSE in sheep or goats. The demonstration that BSE was experimentally transmissible to sheep and goats, including by oral route, was obtained long before any increase of surveillance [69]. This was followed by the demonstration that BSE could be transmitted in natural conditions to non ruminants, including humans with variant Creutzfeldt-Jakob disease [20, 21, 30]. However, it was not considered practical to base research for BSE in small ruminants on transmission studies in rodents, which was the only method available at that time. This encouraged the development of molecular methods to identify possible BSE in small ruminants, based on the characterization of PrPres, [18, 70-73], and detection of the distinct PrPd molecular features existing between different prion strains, as revealed in earlier findings with experimental models [8, 74, 75]. The feasibility of using molecular methods to identify cross-species transmission of BSE in other species was first established in humans with variant CJD, which showed distinct PrPres features by Western blot, compared to those found in the other forms of Creutzfeldt-Jakob disease [76]. This molecular typing approach proved very successful in the veterinary field since consistent features of BSE were also identified in small ruminants, clearly distinct from the vast majority of scrapie cases [47, 48]. Nevertheless, a single case of BSE was confirmed by transmission studies in mouse models [31], together with the retrospective finding of a probable other case identified by PrPd immunohistochemical analyses of the goat brain [77]. A few unusual cases were reported in sheep, following characterization of PrPres by Western blot [47, 67, 78, 79], which resembled an experimental isolate of scrapie initially derived from a scrapie case (CH1641) in the UK [18]. Whereas these scrapie isolates clearly differ from both BSE [48, 67, 78, 80] and atypical/Nor98 scrapie [48], their significance in the context of natural scrapie variability remains to be established [65, 66, 80-82]. Finally, however, the major finding linked to the implementation of active surveillance in small ruminants, using molecular methods based on PrPd identification for diagnosis and characterization of TSEs, was the discovery of atypical/Nor98 scrapie in these species, and its broad distribution in Europe [48, 58]. As a result, the presence of this novel form of prion disease was confirmed in other regions of the world [83, 84], including in sheep from countries previously believed to be free of prion diseases in ruminants [85].

Atypical BSEs in the Context of BSE

One of the most important findings in the veterinary field, linked to the development of molecular typing of prion diseases for detecting possible BSE in small ruminants, was the identification of two novel forms of BSE in cattle, when it was believed that BSE was a unique disease [24, 25, 86]. The search for possible BSE in sheep was essentially based on the identification of a low apparent molecular mass of PrPres, whereas Western blot revealed a few cattle which showed a high molecular mass of PrPres, compared to most BSE cases, and were therefore described as H-type BSE (Figure)[25, 87]. Similarly, whereas a high level of diglycosylated PrPres was a major feature of BSE, notably after cross-species transmission [76, 88, 89], identification of the other atypical form of BSE was essentially based on lower levels of diglycosylated PrPres, in addition to a slightly lower apparent molecular mass of PrPres (L-type BSE or BASE for Bovine Amyloidotic Spongiform Encephalopathy) (Figure) [24, 87]. These data questioned the transmissibility of these novel pathological conditions and the possible existence of several strains of BSE at a time when BSE was believed to have been caused by a single strain transmitted by contaminated meat-and-bone meal, following recycling of a TSE agent of unknown origin.

Transmissibility in mice was demonstrated for both H-type and L-type BSEs after intra-cerebral challenge in a large panel of rodent models including wild-type mice, bank voles and hamsters, as well as ovine and bovine transgenic mouse lines [23, 46, 90-94]. After detailed investigations, it was eventually demonstrated that H-type and L-type BSEs exhibited different transmissibility and distinct biological and molecular features in these experimental models, both forms of BSE also differing from the well-known strain isolated from classical BSE [14-16;18;37;41]. In particular, the distinct properties of PrPres identified in the cattle brain by Western blot were maintained following transmission to transgenic mice expressing bovine PrP, in association with distinct incubation periods of the disease, as well as different distributions and features of PrPd deposits in the mouse brains [14-16;18;37;41]. Transmission of H-type BSE into C57BL/6 wild-type mice also confirmed the presence of a second, more C-terminally cleaved, form of PrPres (PrPres #2) [95], which, in unglycosylated form, migrates at ~ 14 kDa and can be specifically detected using C-terminal antibodies, as in the cattle brain (Figure)[86] or after transmission in bovine transgenic mice [46, 96]. Overall, these data clearly indicate that the three phenotypes of BSE in cattle are associated with three different major strains of transmissible agents, although their precise interrelationships require more thorough investigation.

Transmission studies of the two atypical forms of BSE, using different transgenic mouse lines expressing the ovine prion protein and differing by the encoded ovine *prnp* alleles or/and expression levels of the transgene, produced less straightforward conclusions. Although experimental transmission of H-type BSE has not yet been reported in sheep, it was transmitted in tg338 transgenic mice expressing high levels of the V_{136} R_{154} Q_{171} protein [91], but failed to transmit to the TgOvPrP4 mouse line expressing moderately high levels of the A_{136} R_{154} Q_{171} protein [97]. In this latter study, the features of transmission of L-type BSE clearly differed from those described in this model for classical BSE. This was shown by the distinct glycoform patterns, but also by the absence of florid plaques that had previously been identified in the mouse brain with all classical BSE sources examined in this model [98-101]. The phenotypic features of L-type BSE in fact revealed similarities with transmission of the Stetsonville isolate of Transmissible Mink Encephalopathy (TME), after a first passage in cattle. These similarities were further confirmed after transmission in Syrian hamsters of both L-type BSE and TME-in-cattle, as well as in bovine transgenic mice, whereas classical and H-type BSEs failed to transmit from bovine brains in this model [46]. This implied that the disease in mink could have been caused by an exposure to L-type BSE, in line with the historical hypothesis of a food-borne transmission in mink of a bovine TSE [102]. Another study of L-type BSE transmitted to the tg338 ovine transgenic mouse line however showed similar molecular and lesion features to those observed in the same mouse line following transmission of classical BSE in this model [92]. These results suggested that one possible origin of classical BSE could have been the recycling of an atypical, putatively sporadic, form of BSE following interspecies transmission. Nevertheless, the origin of the phenotypic shift in tg338 mice has been questioned, since back-passage from tissues of these mice in bovine transgenic mice fully restored the L-type phenotypic features, suggesting that the initial observations in tg338 mice might reflect a phenotypic convergence between L-type and classical BSE in this particular experimental model rather than a genuine strain change or selection[103]. Further studies in sheep that could be infected experimentally with L-type BSE [104], at least after intra-cerebral challenge, should help to clarify this issue.

The experimental evidence supporting the hypothesis that classical BSE could have emerged from L-type BSE was not unprecedented, however. Inoculations of a L-type BSE isolate in C57Bl/6 and SJL mice had indeed produced biochemical and lesion features similar to classical BSE in some mice, but contrary to the study in tg338 mice, this was only observed at the second passage in wild-type mice, whereas no clinical or molecular evidence of prion disease had been found at the first passage [105]. This suggested a possible conversion of L-type BSE into classical BSE or that the classical BSE was initially present in the bovine brain affected with L-type BSE. Intriguingly, very similar conclusions have recently been obtained following serial passages of H-type BSE in C57BL/6 mice, with some mice showing phenotypic features of classical BSE only at the second passage [106]. Similarities with classical BSE were here confirmed by a third passage in this mouse line, which is also able to propagate a prion disease corresponding to H-type BSE for at least three successive passages in other animals. This emergence of two distinct strains by serial passages in an experimental model from a unique TSE source is strikingly reminiscent of previous observations of TME transmissions in hamsters [8], but in this case only one of the two strains (DY) maintained its pathogenicity for mink, the original host of the disease, after serial passages in hamsters [5]. In another experimental situation in C57BL mice, in which the emergence of a ME7-like strain (7D) was consistently observed during serial passages of the 87A scrapie strain, the hypothesis of a possible mutation of the scrapie agent was raised [107]. However, in the case of H-type BSE, the most recent studies demonstrated that cross-species transmission was not required to identify the emergence of classical BSE, since this was also observed after transmission from cattle to bovine transgenic mice in some of the animals, as early as the first passage [108]. As in wild-type mice, this emergence is not consistently observed from each bovine isolate or in all experiments. However these observations strongly support the hypothesis that the food-borne epizooty could have originated from rare cases of atypical BSEs, which would thus identify the currently unknown reservoir of this TSE agent.

Transmissibility of atypical BSE was finally assessed in transgenic mice expressing the human prion protein. Following the discovery that the classical BSE agent had caused variant CJD in humans [21], the question was also raised for atypical BSEs, when the first cases of L-type BSE revealed some molecular and lesion similarities to a sub-type of sporadic CJD (M/V type 2). It needs to be emphasized that some molecular similarities between H-type BSE and some sporadic CJD sub-types with comparable C-terminally cleaved PrPres products have also been noted [109], in a context where the existence of H-type and L-type BSEs in cattle resemble the molecular types 1 and 2 encountered in sporadic CJD cases in humans. Classical BSE was shown to be poorly transmissible to human transgenic mice following intracerebral inoculations of bovine brain tissues [110, 111]. In contrast, transmission of L-type BSE has been obtained from cattle with a 60 % transmission rate after intracerebral challenge in a transgenic mouse line expressing normal levels of the human Met129 PrP protein [112]. Another study confirmed this transmissibility in a transgenic mouse model overexpressing (~ 6-fold) Met129 human PrP but also concluded that, unlike classical BSE, there was no significant species barrier between cattle and humans for this particular bovine strain, as an attack rate of 100 % was observed and the incubation time was not reduced upon secondary passage [113]. In contrast, and to the best of our knowledge, transmission of H-type BSE has not yet been obtained in human transgenic mouse models [113]. Taken together the data obtained in human transgenic mice are consistent with the demonstrations that L-type BSE can be readily transmitted, at least after intra-cerebral challenge, in non human primates [114-116].

Transmission studies of atypical BSEs thus show complex results and, although they clearly demonstrate the existence of at least three strains in cattle in natural conditions, interpretation of experimental data remains difficult in many respects so far. The current stage of these data and their interpretation are briefly summarized in Table.

Table. Summary of transmission studies of bovine spongiform encephalopathies and transmissible mink encephalopathy from cattle, in bovine (Tg Bov), ovine (Tg Ov) or human (Tg Hu) transgenic mice or in wild-type mice and hamsters. When transmission has been achieved, conclusions regarding the phenotypic features are indicated. +/-: limited attack rate, –: no transmission. NR: not reported

		BSE-C	BSE-H	BSE-L	TME	Références
Tg Bov		C	H or C-like	L	L-like	46, 87, 91, 92, 96, 108
Tg Ov	tg338 (VRQ)	C	H	C-like	NR	91, 92, 103
	TgOvPrP4 (ARQ)	C	-	L	L-like	65, 80, 97-99
Tg Hu		+/- , C	-	L	NR	112,113
Wild-type mice		C	H or C-like*	- or +**, C-like	-	17, 19, 26-29, 90, 95, 105, 106
Hamster		- or +***, C	-	TME-like	TME	5, 45, 46, 93

* mice with C-like features observed after second passage

** transmission reported only at second passage with C-like phenotype, whereas mice are negative at first passage

*** transmissible only after passage from wild-type infected mice

CONCLUSION

Transmission studies have proved to be invaluable tools for characterizing the diversity of transmissible agents involved in TSEs. The discovery of the crucial role of the prion protein in these diseases has been a key finding for their diagnosis and has allowed a great increase of surveillance in ruminants in recent years. Experimental transmissions of prion diseases have been considerably facilitated by the development of a number of transgenic mouse models. The importance of these models was confirmed by the recent demonstration that ruminants could be affected by several previously unknown prion diseases. This new landscape of prion diseases in animals raises a number of unresolved questions regarding possible relationships between the different forms of animal and prion diseases. Our understanding is still limited by current uncertainties regarding the precise molecular events producing the biological differences between strains involved in these diseases.

REFERENCES

[1] R.L. Chandler, *Lancet.* 1, 1378 (1961).
[2] R.L. Chandler, *Lancet.* 1, 232 (1971).
[3] H. Fraser, A.G. Dickinson, *J Comp Pathol.* 83, 29 (1973).
[4] M.E. Bruce, Humana Press (1996)
[5] R.A. Bessen, R.F. Marsh, *J Gen Virol.* 73 (Pt 2), 329 (1992).
[6] S.B. Prusiner, *Science.* 216, 136 (1982).
[7] B. Oesch, D. Westaway, M. Walchli, et al., *Cell.* 40, 735 (1985).
[8] R.A. Bessen, R.F. Marsh, *J Virol.* 66, 2096 (1992).
[9] J. Safar, H. Wille, V. Itri, et al., *Nat Med.* 4, 1157 (1998).
[10] H. Bueler, A. Aguzzi, A. Sailer, et al., *Cell.* 73, 1339 (1993).
[11] R.E. Race, S.A. Priola, R.A. Bessen, et al., *Neuron.* 15, 1183 (1995).
[12] C. Crozet, F. Flamant, A. Bencsik, D. Aubert, J. Samarut, T. Baron, *J Virol.* 75, 5328 (2001).
[13] J.L. Vilotte, S. Soulier, R. Essalmani, et al., *J Virol.* 75, 5977 (2001).
[14] M.R. Scott, J. Safar, G. Telling, et al., *Proc Natl Acad Sci U S A.* 94, 14279 (1997).
[15] J. Castilla, A. Gutierrez Adan, A. Brun, et al., *Arch Virol.* 148, 677 (2003).
[16] Buschmann, E. Pfaff, K. Reifenberg, H.M. Muller, M.H. Groschup, *Arch Virol Suppl.* 75 (2000).
[17] M.E. Bruce, A. Boyle, S. Cousens, et al., *J Gen Virol.* 83, 695 (2002).
[18] J. Hope, S.C. Wood, C.R. Birkett, et al., *J Gen Virol.* 80 (Pt 1), 1 (1999).
[19] D.M. Taylor, A.G. Dickinson, H. Fraser, R.F. Marsh, *Neuropathol Appl Neurobiol.* 12, 207 (1986).
[20] R.G. Will, J.W. Ironside, M. Zeidler, et al., *Lancet.* 347, 921 (1996).
[21] M.E. Bruce, R.G. Will, J.W. Ironside, et al., *Nature.* 389, 498 (1997).
[22] S.L. Benestad, P. Sarradin, B. Thu, J. Schonheit, M.A. Tranulis, B. Bratberg, *Vet Rec.* 153, 202 (2003).
[23] A. Buschmann, A.G. Biacabe, U. Ziegler, et al., *J Virol Methods.* 117, 27 (2004).
[24] C. Casalone, G. Zanusso, P. Acutis, et al., *Proc Natl Acad Sci U S A.* 101, 3065 (2004).
[25] A.G. Biacabe, J.L. Laplanche, S. Ryder, T. Baron, *EMBO Rep.* 5, 110 (2004).
[26] H. Fraser, I. McConnell, G.A. Wells, M. Dawson, *Vet Rec.* 123, 472 (1988).
[27] H. Fraser, M.E. Bruce, A. Chree, I. McConnell, G.A. Wells, *J Gen Virol.* 73 (Pt 8), 1891 (1992).
[28] M. Bruce, A. Chree, I. McConnell, J. Foster, G. Pearson, H. Fraser, *Philos Trans R Soc Lond B Biol Sci.* 343, 405 (1994).
[29] R. Green, C. Horrocks, A. Wilkinson, S.A. Hawkins, S.J. Ryder, *J Comp Pathol.* 132, 117 (2005).
[30] H. Fraser, G.R. Pearson, I. McConnell, M.E. Bruce, J.M. Wyatt, T.J. Gruffydd-Jones, *Vet Rec.* 134, 449 (1994).
[31] M. Eloit, K. Adjou, M. Coulpier, et al., *Vet Rec.* 156, 523 (2005).

[32] D. Westaway, P.A. Goodman, C.A. Mirenda, M.P. McKinley, G.A. Carlson, S.B. Prusiner, *Cell.* 51, 651 (1987).
[33] K.E. Beck, M. Chaplin, M. Stack, et al., *Brain Pathol.* 20, 313.
[34] D.A. Brown, M.E. Bruce, J.R. Fraser, *Neuropathol Appl Neurobiol.* 29, 262 (2003).
[35] S. Lezmi, A. Bencsik, T. Baron, *J Histochem Cytochem.* 54, 1087 (2006).
[36] V. Beringue, J.L. Vilotte, H. Laude, *Vet Res.* 39, 47 (2008).
[37] K.E. Beck, R.E. Sallis, R. Lockey, M.M. Simmons, J. Spiropoulos, *J Neuropathol Exp Neurol.* 69, 483.
[38] K.E. Beck, S. Cawthraw, G.C. Saunders, R. Ellis, J. Spiropoulos, *Arch Virol.* 156, 903.
[39] N. Piening, R. Nonno, M. Di Bari, et al., *J Biol Chem.* 281, 9373 (2006).
[40] U. Agrimi, R. Nonno, G. Dell'Omo, et al., *PLoS Pathog.* 4, e1000113 (2008).
[41] M.A. Di Bari, F. Chianini, G. Vaccari, et al., *J Gen Virol.* 89, 2975 (2008).
[42] R.H. Kimberlin, C.A. Walker, *J Gen Virol.* 39, 487 (1978).
[43] R.H. Kimberlin, S. Cole, C.A. Walker, *Neuropathol Appl Neurobiol.* 12, 197 (1986).
[44] R.H. Kimberlin, C.A. Walker, H. Fraser, *J Gen Virol.* 70 (Pt 8), 2017 (1989).
[45] A. Thomzig, S. Spassov, M. Friedrich, D. Naumann, M. Beekes, *J Biol Chem.* 279, 33847 (2004).
[46] S. Nicot, T. Baron, *J Virol.* 85, 1906.
[47] M. Stack, M. Jeffrey, S. Gubbins, et al., *J Gen Virol.* 87, 2099 (2006).
[48] J. Vulin, A.G. Biacabe, G. Cazeau, D. Calavas, T. Baron, *Emerg Infect Dis.* 17, 55.
[49] J.W. Wilesmith, J.B. Ryan, M.J. Atkinson, *Vet Rec.* 128, 199 (1991).
[50] T. Baron, A.G. Biacabe, J.N. Arsac, S. Benestad, M.H. Groschup, *Vaccine.* 25, 5625 (2007).
[51] A. Buschmann, G. Luhken, J. Schultz, G. Erhardt, M.H. Groschup, *J Gen Virol.* 85, 2727 (2004).
[52] G.C. Saunders, S. Cawthraw, S.J. Mountjoy, J. Hope, O. Windl, *J Gen Virol.* 87, 3141 (2006).
[53] A. Le Dur, V. Beringue, O. Andreoletti, et al., *Proc Natl Acad Sci U S A.* 102, 16031 (2005).
[54] S.L. Benestad, J.N. Arsac, W. Goldmann, M. Noremark, *Vet Res.* 39, 19 (2008).
[55] P.C. Griffiths, J. Spiropoulos, R. Lockey, et al., *J Gen Virol.* 91, 2132.
[56] J.N. Arsac, D. Betemps, E. Morignat, et al., *PLoS One.* 4, e7300 (2009).
[57] M.M. Simmons, T. Konold, H.A. Simmons, et al., *BMC Vet Res.* 3, 20 (2007).
[58] A. Fediaevsky, S.C. Tongue, M. Noremark, D. Calavas, G. Ru, P. Hopp, *BMC Vet Res.* 4, 19 (2008).
[59] T. Moum, I. Olsaker, P. Hopp, T. Moldal, M. Valheim, S.L. Benestad, *J Gen Virol.* 86, 231 (2005).
[60] J.N. Arsac, O. Andreoletti, J.M. Bilheude, C. Lacroux, S.L. Benestad, T. Baron, *Emerg Infect Dis.* 13, 58 (2007).
[61] A. Bencsik, T. Baron, *Prion,* Salzbourg, Austria (2010).
[62] M. Klingeborn, L. Wik, M. Simonsson, L.H. Renstrom, T. Ottinger, T. Linne, *J Gen Virol.* 87, 1751 (2006).
[63] A.M. Thackray, L. Hopkins, J. Spiropoulos, R. Bujdoso, *J Virol.* 82, 11197 (2008).
[64] A.M. Thackray, L. Hopkins, R. Lockey, J. Spiropoulos, R. Bujdoso, *J Gen Virol.* 92, 1482.
[65] T. Baron, C. Crozet, A.G. Biacabe, et al., *J Virol.* 78, 6243 (2004).

[66] T. Baron, A. Bencsik, E. Morignat, *PLoS One.* 5, e10310.
[67] J.C. Espinosa, M.E. Herva, O. Andreoletti, et al., *Emerg Infect Dis.* 15, 1214 (2009).
[68] M. Mazza, B. Iulini, G. Vaccari, et al., *Res Vet Sci.* 88, 478.
[69] J.D. Foster, J. Hope, H. Fraser, *Vet Rec.* 133, 339 (1993).
[70] A.F. Hill, K.C. Sidle, S. Joiner, et al., *Neurosci Lett.* 255, 159 (1998).
[71] T.G. Baron, J.Y. Madec, D. Calavas, *J Clin Microbiol.* 37, 3701 (1999).
[72] T.G. Baron, J.Y. Madec, D. Calavas, Y. Richard, F. Barillet, *Neurosci Lett.* 284, 175 (2000).
[73] M.J. Stack, M.J. Chaplin, J. Clark, *Acta Neuropathol.* 104, 279 (2002).
[74] R.J. Kascsak, R. Rubenstein, P.A. Merz, et al., *J Virol.* 59, 676 (1986).
[75] R.A. Bessen, D.A. Kocisko, G.J. Raymond, S. Nandan, P.T. Lansbury, B. Caughey, *Nature.* 375, 698 (1995).
[76] J. Collinge, K.C. Sidle, J. Meads, J. Ironside, A.F. Hill, *Nature.* 383, 685 (1996).
[77] M. Jeffrey, S. Martin, L. Gonzalez, et al., *J Comp Pathol.* 134, 171 (2006).
[78] S. Lezmi, S. Martin, S. Simon, et al., *J Virol.* 78, 3654 (2004).
[79] L. Gonzalez, S. Siso, E. Monleon, et al., *J Gen Virol.* 91, 2630.
[80] T. Baron, A. Bencsik, J. Vulin, et al., *PLoS Pathog.* 4, e1000137 (2008).
[81] T. Yokoyama, K. Masujin, M.J. Schmerr, et al., *PLoS One.* 5, e15450.
[82] T. Baron, A.G. Biacabe, *J Virol.* 81, 7230 (2007).
[83] G.B. Mitchell, K.I. O'Rourke, N.P. Harrington, et al., *J Vet Diagn Invest.* 22, 408.
[84] C.M. Loiacono, B.V. Thomsen, S.M. Hall, et al., *J Vet Diagn Invest.* 21, 454 (2009).
[85] R. Kittelberger, M.J. Chaplin, M.M. Simmons, et al., *J Vet Diagn Invest.* 22, 863.
[86] J.G. Jacobs, J.P. Langeveld, A.G. Biacabe, et al., *J Clin Microbiol.* 45, 1821 (2007).
[87] A. Buschmann, A. Gretzschel, A.G. Biacabe, et al., *Vet Microbiol.* 117, 103 (2006).
[88] R.A. Somerville, A. Chong, O.U. Mulqueen, C.R. Birkett, S.C. Wood, J. Hope, *Nature.* 386, 564 (1997).
[89] T. Kuczius, I. Haist, M.H. Groschup, *J Infect Dis.* 178, 693 (1998).
[90] T.G. Baron, A.G. Biacabe, A. Bencsik, J.P. Langeveld, *Emerg Infect Dis.* 12, 1125 (2006).
[91] V. Beringue, A. Bencsik, A. Le Dur, et al., *PLoS Pathog.* 2, e112 (2006).
[92] V. Beringue, O. Andreoletti, A. Le Dur, et al., *J Neurosci.* 27, 6965 (2007).
[93] Y. Shu, K. Masujin, H. Okada, et al., *Prion.* 5, 103.
[94] R. Nonno, M Di Bari, L Pirisinu, S Marcon, et al., *Prion,* Thessalonilki, Greece (2009).
[95] AG Biacabe, JG Jacobs, A bencsik et al., *Prion. 1, 61 (2007).*
[96] H. Okada, K. Masujin, Y. Iwamaru, et al., *Vet Pathol.* 48, 942.
[97] T. Baron, A. Bencsik, A.G. Biacabe, E. Morignat, R.A. Bessen, *Emerg Infect Dis.* 13, 1887 (2007).
[98] C. Crozet, A. Bencsik, F. Flamant, S. Lezmi, J. Samarut, T. Baron, *EMBO Rep.* 2, 952 (2001).
[99] C. Cordier, A. Bencsik, S. Philippe, et al., *J Gen Virol.* 87, 3763 (2006).
[100] A. Bencsik, T. Baron, *J Infect Dis.* 195, 989 (2007).
[101] Bencsik, S. Debeer, T. Petit, T. Baron, *PLoS One.* 4, e6929 (2009).
[102] R.F. Marsh, R.A. Bessen, S. Lehmann, G.R. Hartsough, *J Gen Virol.* 72 (Pt 3), 589 (1991).
[103] V Beringue, O Andreoletti, L Herzog et al., *Prion,* Salzbourg, Austria (2010).
[104] R Nonno, C Casalone, M Di Bari et al., *Prion,* Madrid, Spain (2008).

[105] R. Capobianco, C. Casalone, S. Suardi, et al., *PLoS Pathog.* 3, e31 (2007).
[106] T. Baron, J. Vulin, A.G. Biacabe, et al., *PLoS One.* 6, e15839.
[107] M.E. Bruce, A.G. Dickinson, *J Gen Virol.* 68 (Pt 1), 79 (1987).
[108] JM Torres, JC Espinosa, *Emerg Infect Dis.* 17, 1636 (2011).
[109] S. Notari, R. Strammiello, S. Capellari, et al., *J Biol Chem.* 283, 30557 (2008).
[110] E.A. Asante, J.M. Linehan, M. Desbruslais, et al., *EMBO J.* 21, 6358 (2002).
[111] D. Padilla, V. Beringue, J.C. Espinosa, et al., *PLoS Pathog.* 7, e1001319.
[112] Q. Kong, M. Zheng, C. Casalone, et al., *J Virol.* 82, 3697 (2008).
[113] V. Beringue, L. Herzog, F. Reine, et al., *Emerg Infect Dis.* 14, 1898 (2008).
[114] E.E. Comoy, C. Casalone, N. Lescoutra-Etchegaray, et al., *PLoS One.* 3, e3017 (2008).
[115] F. Ono, N. Tase, A. Kurosawa, et al., *Jpn J Infect Dis.* 64, 81.
[116] F. Ono, K. Terao, N. Tase, et al., *Jpn J Infect Dis.* 64, 50.

In: Prions and Prion Diseases: New Developments
Editor: Jean-Michel Verdier
ISBN: 978-1-62100-027-3
© 2012 Nova Science Publishers, Inc.

Chapter 7

PRE-MORTEM DIAGNOSTIC SCREENING FOR TRANSMISSIBLE SPONGIFORM ENCEPHALOPATHIES BY PROTEOMIC APPROACHES

Nandini Falisse-Poirrier, Olivier Thellin, Ingrid Dupiereux, Willy Zorzi, Ernst Heinen and Benaïssa Elmoualij*
Department of Human-Histology-CRPP, University of Liège,
Sart Tilman, Liège, Belgium

ABSTRACT

Within the vast family of neurodegenerative disorders, sub-acute transmissible spongiform encephalopathies (TSEs), or prion diseases, constitute a group of rare diseases affecting the central nervous system of humans and animals. They are characterised by a long asymptomatic phase that can last several months up to many years. This phase is then followed by a short clinical period where neurological disorders are commonly manifested in the form of cerebellar ataxia and dementia. Throughout its duration, the disease remains transmissible and infectious, causing no immune response and ultimately leading to the progressive neuronal death and fated demise of the affected animal or patient. Presently, although clinical signs of disease can provide strong evidence of the presence of TSE, final confirmation of disease is achieved following the post-mortem examination of brain tissue. TSEs share common histopathological features that include the classical diagnostic triad of spongiform vacuolation, astrogliosis and neuronal loss. In experimental models, the definitive presence of a TSE disease is confirmed by performing tissue bioassays in mice and directly measuring the infectivity titre. In this chapter we revisit the key milestones that laid the foundations for our current knowledge of the prion protein, agent responsible for transmissible spongiform encephalopathies and discuss the relevance of proteomic techniques for uncovering specific prion disease biomarkers for future pre-mortem diagnosis.

---

* Correspondence should be addressed to: Benaïssa Elmoualij, Department of Human Histology, CRPP, University of Liège, 1, avenue de l'Hôpital, Sart Tilman, 4000 Liège Belgium, Telephone: (32) 4 366 43 28, Fax: (32) 4 366 43 21, Email: b.elmoualij@ulg.ac.be

INTRODUCTION

Proteinopathies are an atypical group of diseases caused by misconformed proteins. These proteins are able to replicate in their host, transconforming normal proteins produced by the host into new misconformed proteins. In higher organisms, this leads mainly to neuronal diseases through neuronal cell death, resulting in the death of the host. The detection of misconformed proteins ante-mortem in the patient is therefore critical to reach a diagnostic. Classical detection techniques are limited by their sensitivity, as such misconformed proteins are rare outside the central nervous system. A solution is to increase the sensitivity of detection techniques. Another is to use proteomics to identify new easier-to-detect biomarkers of such proteinopathies.

In this paper, we will first present an overview of proteomics, after which we will introduce the key milestones of our current knowledge of the transmissible spongiform encephalopathies. We will then review several ways proteomics can help prion research.

PROTEOMICS: AN OVERVIEW OF A GROWING FIELD

The last decades have seen a huge surge in the field of genomics, aiming to map the genetic composition of individual organisms. Since the first publication of the complete sequence of a genome [1], the progress made in this field have been phenomenal. Presently, researchers are shifting their focus to the next challenge: using the wealth of genetic information to study the functional expression of genes, in other words, proteins. The elucidation of the structure, function, regulation and interaction of proteins expressed by the genome of an organism, is invaluable to comprehend the dynamic and complex biological processes occurring at a cellular and molecular level, how they differ in various cell types and how they are altered in different disease states. This Herculean task forms the aims of the proteomics field.

Proteomics can be defined as the study of the proteome: the entire set of proteins expressed from a genome including all isoforms, polymorphisms and post-translational modifications [2]. The phenotype of a cell is dependent on protein interaction networks that are involved in complex biological pathways and the biological basis of multigenic processes such as ageing, disease and stress cannot be identified solely on the basis of the genome. The analysis of the proteome thus presents certain advantages such as providing information on ongoing biological processes occurring at a given time point, that in turn, reflect the current physiological state of the cell. It also has a certain advantage to mRNA expression studies, that have previously been shown to be ambiguous, as the expression level does not always reflect the amount of active protein in a cell [3], due notably to the presence of post-transcriptional regulators such as miRNA. Built on the foundations of genomics, the development of the proteomics field owes a lot to recent improvements in advanced bio-informatic databases and analytical software [4]. Moreover the impressive development of methods to identify large numbers of cellular proteins and detect differences in their levels in different cell states, have contributed to the growth of this field.

Currently in proteomics there are many available techniques to study protein profiling and differential protein abundance [5,6]. Protein separation is typically carried out by classical two-dimensional gel electrophoresis (2-DE). Originally described by O'Farrell in 1975 [7], this technique separates proteins by isoelectric focusing (according to their isoelectric point or pI) followed by SDS-PAGE (according to their relative molecular mass) in second dimension. Numerous publications have shown the powerful potential of this technique to visualize and analyse protein differentials between biological states. Research is constantly being conducted to improve the imaging analysis techniques and make significant changes to classical 2-DE in order to eliminate some of its weaknesses [8].

Parallel to gel-based systems, many liquid chromatography techniques such as size exclusion, ion exchange, affinity and reversed phase along with electrophoretic separation in liquid phase techniques have been extensively studied and used in the field of protein separation. The growing need for speed and sensitivity, indispensable for scaling up, is encouraging researchers to improve two-dimensional liquid chromatography (2DLC) systems [9] as this could promote the rapid development of this area of research, owing to their high potential for automation and flexibility at being interfaced with gel or liquid array-based immunological techniques and analytical systems such as tandem mass spectrometry (MS/MS) [10,11]. In 2DLC, almost any combination of columns with different retention properties is available. However, since most current 2DLC techniques are interfaced with mass spectrometry, the choice for the first dimension fractionation has to be followed by reverse phase chromatography (RP) in the second dimension as samples eluted from the RP column are in an ideal state to be injected into the mass spectrometer. RP-HPLC techniques have gone a long way since its application for peptide separation in 1976. Since then advances have improved peptide recovery, selectivity, and resolution through discovery of ion pairing agents and high porosity of silica particles. The introduction of non-porous RP systems has greatly improved separation speed by avoiding the problem of protein adsorption within pores of traditional porous RP-LC systems that had the consequence of peak tailing, loss of resolution and low protein recovery [12]. Despite being a powerful tool in resolving peptides and proteins of low molecular mass, the peak capacity of a single RP column is generally not enough for separation of complex cell extracts [13]. By coupling a first dimension chromatographic separation technique to the RP column, 2DLC systems have thus the powerful potential of resolving complex protein mixtures. The choice for the first dimension column is either size exclusion or ion exchange chromatography techniques such as chromatofocusing (CF) [9]. This is a liquid separation method for protein fractionation according to pI. CF being essentially an ion-exchange technique, proteins are bound to an anion exchanger and eluted by a continuous decrease of the buffer pH. Proteins are thus eluted in order of their isoelectric points. The principle of buffer elution involves the use of amphoteric buffers titrated to a lower pH to generate a linear gradient. In CF separation, proteins sharing identical pI focus and elute as a single peak. Although CF has been used as a preparative method for fractionating proteins, recent analytical columns allow loading up to 5mg of protein facilitating proteomic studies. The main advantage of CF as compared to the classical ion-exchange technique is that it mainly avoids the presence of large amounts of salt which could interfere with downstream mass spectrometry analysis. Another advantage is that it can readily be automated and interfaced to other liquid separations. A more recently commercialised 2DLC technique, the ProteomeLab PF-2D, couples CF in first dimension to RP in second dimension). The system utilizes a self-contained liquid flow path, thereby reducing the risk of sample contamination during transfer between dimensions. In addition to its user-friendly work procedures, the resulting liquid protein fractions can either be analysed on-line by MS/MS after trypsin digestion or can be used for gel and immunological-based characterisations accounting for the high versatility of this technique. In this context, we have previously shown the 2DLC system, integrated in the ProteomeLab PF-2D platform, as a tool of reference for antigen targeting in immunoproteomic applications [10,14].

In recent years, the coupling of protein separation systems with different mass spectrometry technologies has evolved as the dominant tools in the field of protein identification and post-translational modifications [15]. The key developments that have facilitated the analysis of proteins and peptides have probably been the invention of the 'time-of-flight' (TOF) MS and two 'soft-ionization' methods, namely the matrix-assisted laser desorption ionization (MALDI) and the electrospray ionization (ESI) [16]. Their development of the last years allows them now to enter the field of clinical research and diagnostics [6].

Prion Diseases: The Agent and the Resulting Proteinopathies

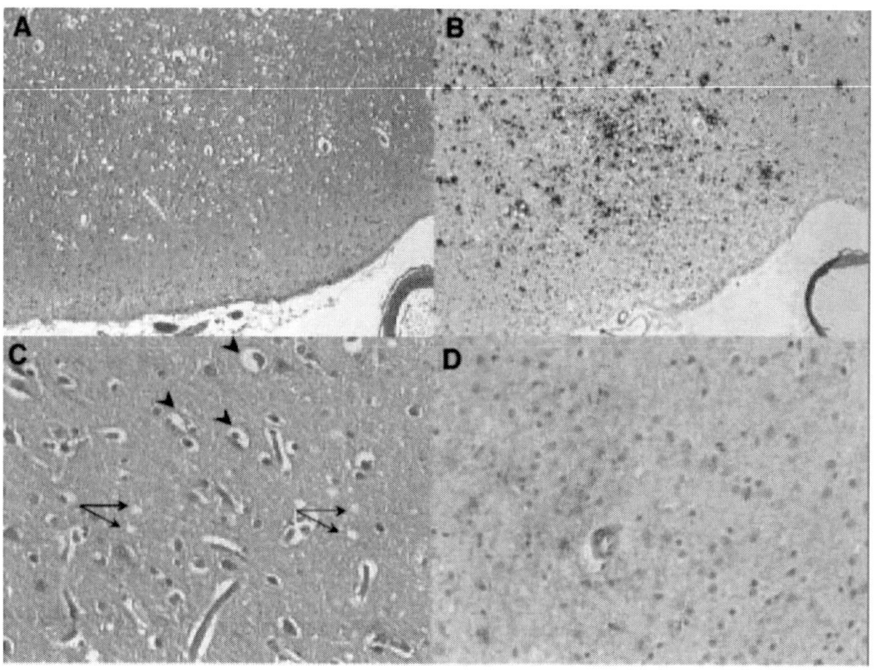

Figure 1. Histopathological changes in the frontal cortex of CJD-infected human brain, showing the typical spongiform degeneration and neuronal loss. Tissue from patient CJD1 showed severe changes indicating spongiform encephalopathy after staining with hematoxylin and eosin (A) as well as abundant perivacuolar PrPRes deposits after staining with antibody 3F4 (B; original magnification, x50), leading to the obvious diagnosis of prion disease. In patient CJD4 (C), spongiform changes were mild/moderate, as visualized by staining with hematoxylin and eosin: true spongiosis (arrows) can be distinguished from vacuolar artifacts (arrowheads). Sparse deposits of PrPRes (original magnification, x200) were detected with antibody 3F4 (D).

Within the vast family of neurodegenerative disorders, sub-acute transmissible spongiform encephalopathies (TSEs), or prion diseases, constitute a group of rare diseases affecting the central nervous system of humans and animals [17,18]. They are characterised by a long asymptomatic phase that can last several months up to many years. This phase is then followed by a short clinical period where neurological disorders are commonly manifested in the form of cerebellar ataxia and dementia [19,20]. Throughout its duration, the disease remains transmissible and infectious, causing no immune response and ultimately leading to the progressive neuronal death and fated demise of the affected animal [21]. Presently, although clinical signs of disease can provide strong evidence of the presence of TSE, final confirmation of disease is achieved following the post-mortem examination of brain tissue [19]. TSEs share common histopathological features that include the classical diagnostic triad of spongiform vacuolation (figure 1), astrogliosis and neuronal loss [17,21]. In experimental animal models, the definitive presence of a TSE disease is confirmed by performing tissue samplings and directly measuring the infectivity titre [19].

THE NATURE OF THE INFECTIOUS AGENT

Several hypotheses, concerning the nature of the agent responsible for TSEs, have been proposed by the scientific community [18] among which the most popular ones include the viral hypothesis, the virino hypothesis, the 'protein-only' hypothesis and the holoprotein hypothesis [22]. However, after 30 years of research, the existence of TSE virino or virus has not been demonstrated and the 'protein-only' hypothesis is the currently admitted model of the TSE agent.

The 'protein-only' hypothesis was proposed in 1982 when Prusiner introduced the concept of the 'PRION', for *pro*teinaceous *in*fectious particle, in order to distinguish the TSE agent from all the classical infectious agents (viruses or viroids emitted previously) [18]. The prion is described as being composed of an infectious protein particle, designated as '***PrPsc***' following the prototype 'scrapie', devoid of nucleic acids and resulting from a structural modification of a normal constituent of cells called the cellular prion protein or '***PrPc***'. The possibility of having two thermodynamically stable protein conformations for a single primary structure met with a lot of scepticism. However, since 1998, numerous experimental data have reinforced the concept of the prion: one of the strongest evidence in favour of the prion hypothesis was the observation that mice lacking the prion gene were resistant to scrapie infection, neither developing the signs of scrapie nor propagating the disease [23]. The *Prnp gene,* coding for the cellular prion protein or PrPc [24], was first identified in 1985. The nucleotide and amino acid sequence of PrPc is highly conserved in the primate family with degrees of homology varying between 97.8%-99.7% for the former and between 98%-99.6% for the latter [25]. The *Prnp* gene contains two exons in hamster and human and three exons in mouse and sheep [26]. However the open reading frame, in primates and other mammals, is entirely contained within a single exon [25] (figure 2).

This feature eliminates the possibility that PrPsc could arise from alternative splicing. Mainly present as a monomer, the cellular prion protein (PrPc) differs from its infectious isoform by its physicochemical properties namely its high solubility in detergents, its alpha helix rich content and its susceptibility to proteolytic digestion by proteases such as proteinase K [28]. Alternatively, PrPsc exists as an aggregate, is rich in beta sheets, is insoluble in detergents and is partially resistant to proteolytic digestion by proteinase K giving rise to 27-30 kDa residues called PrP27-30 or PrPres for the 'proteinase resistant' region of PrPsc. Several models have been designed to explain the way PrPc is transconformed into PrPsc, but none of them has been definitely proved as of today [29,30].

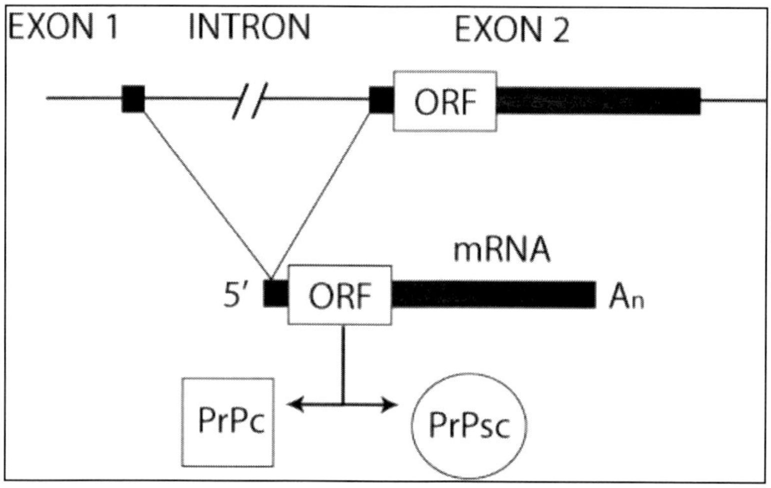

Figure 2. Organisation and expression of the hamster prion protein gene. Untranslated regions of the mRNA are indicated by black boxes. An open reading frame (ORF) or protein coding region is indicated by the open box. The two diagonal lines show a splicing event that joins the 5' leader sequences to the remainder of the coding sequences [27].

Animal Prionopathies

Historically, the earliest known form of TSE dates back to the 18th century where 'scrapie' (Sc), considered today as the prototype of this group of diseases, was first described in sheep and goat [31] (figure 3). Since then, TSEs in other animals have been discovered such as the chronic wasting disease affecting wild deer, elk and moose populations of North America, the transmissible mink encephalopathy, the feline spongiform encephalopathy, the exotic ungulate encephalopathy affecting Nyala and Greater Kudu and the bovine spongiform encephalopathy [20]. A unique property of TSEs is that their aetiology may be sporadic, inherited, or acquired [32,31]. In animals, only the sporadic and acquired forms seem to be predominant although predisposed genetic susceptibility has been recognised [33]. By definition, the origin of sporadic forms is not clear [32]. Typical sporadic forms of TSE in animals are scrapie in sheep and goat. Scrapie is also classified as an acquired disease as its transmission is believed to occur from ewe to offspring *in utero* [34] and to other lamb members by ingestion of infected placenta or cutaneously through abraded skin. Chronic wasting disease in captive herds of mule, deer and elk could occur after oral consumption of prion-infected sheep by-products [27].

Other examples of the acquired forms of animal TSEs include the bovine spongiform encephalopathy (BSE) and scrapie in experimental models of mice. Commonly known as the 'mad cow disease', BSE was detected in more than 280,000 bovines mainly across the United Kingdom but also in the other European Union countries as well as the United States of America and Canada [35,36,37]. Despite a highly debated aetiology [38,39,40,41,42], it is commonly admitted that the origin of the BSE epidemic was linked to cattle feed that was mainly composed of a meat and bone meal prepared from the carcasses of TSE deceased cattle, allowing the infectious agent to propagate.

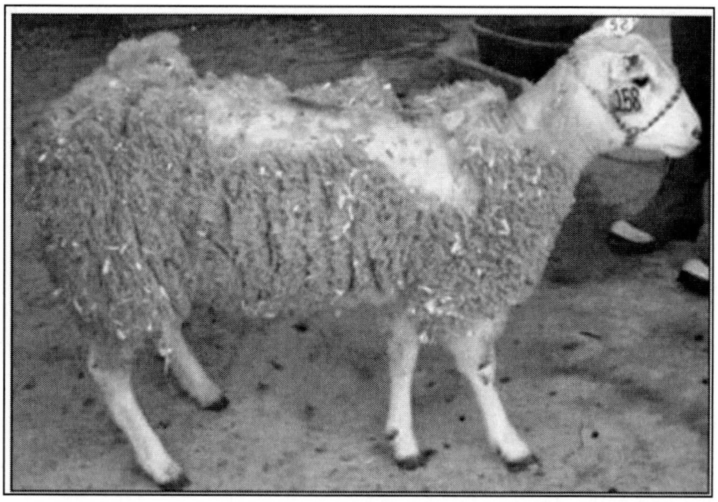

Figure 3. Sheep infected with scrapie.

HUMAN PRIONOPATHIES

In humans, the sporadic form of Creutzfeldt-Jakob disease (sCJD) was the first discovered form of TSE, described by Creutzfeldt, in 1920, and Jakob, in 1921. Soon after, other human TSEs such as Kuru, the Gertsmann-Sträussler-Scheinker syndrome (GSS), Fatal Familial Insomnia (FFI) and the variant form of CJD (vCJD) surfaced. All three aetiological forms of TSEs (sporadic, inherited and acquired) have been described in humans [27]. The sporadic form of the Creutzfeldt-Jakob disease (sCJD) constitutes the most common form of human TSE, responsible for about 85% of all the cases. Interestingly, in humans, common polymorphisms occurring at codons 117 (Ala-Val) and 129 (Met-Val) seem to play a role in the susceptibility to sporadic TSEs. Indeed, a homozygosity for Met or Val at codon 129 appears to increase the vulnerability of an individual to succumb to the sporadic form of CJD [43,25]. The inherited forms of TSE are genetic in nature and are linked to as many as 30 genetic mutations of the causative agent, especially linked to the number of octapeptide repeat copies in the N-terminal domain. These mutations have been shown to be responsible for the inherited or familial forms of prion diseases [26] and account for about 15% of total human TSE cases [17]. These include the familial form of CJD (fCJD), GSS and FFI (table 1). The acquired transmission of TSE accounts for less than 5% of all cases and results either from the ingestion or the iatrogenic transmission of infected tissue [17]. In humans, cases arising from the ingestion of infected tissues have been observed in two cases: that of vCJD and Kuru. The history of Kuru dates back to 1957 where it was endemic among the Fore tribe of Papua New Guinea who were involved in cannibalistic rituals upon the death of a tribe member [37]. The disease was characterized by headaches, joint pains and shaking of the limbs. The incidence of the disease decreased rapidly with the cessation of the ritual. In animals, the most popular case of infection by ingestion of contaminated tissue has been the bovine spongiform encephalopathy, and its transmission to humans as vCJD has been the cause of great health, economic and scientific concern over the recent years. Iatrogenic cases have been reported in human pituitary derived infected hormones and direct contact or inoculation with cerebral tissue such as corneal [44] and dura mater grafts.

Table 1. List of known human TSE, their aetiological origin and frequency [17]. sCJD, sporadic Creutzfeldt-Jakob disease; iCJD, iatrogenic Creutzfeldt-Jakob disease; fCJD, familial Creutzfeldt-Jakob disease; vCJD, variant Creutzfeldt-Jakob disease; GSS, Gerstmann-Staussler-Sheinker syndrome; sFI, sporadic fatal insomnia; FFI, familial fatal insomnia

Aetiology	Phenotype	Frequency
Sporadic	sCJD, sFI	~85%
Inherited	GSS, fCJD, FFI	~10-15%
Acquired	iCJD, Kuru, vCJD	<5%

PROTEOMIC AND PRION: A PROMISING PARTNERSHIP

Pre-Mortem Prion Diagnostic: Screening of Body Fluids and Tissues through Detection of PrP or Surrogate Biomarkers, the Need for Proteomics

Independently of their origin, all TSE diseases are known to be infectious and can be transmissible horizontally [44,45,46]. Recently, transmission of prion diseases from blood transfusion has been reported [47,48,45] and combined with observations of prion infectivity in the urine of scrapie infected mice [49] is a cause of major concern worldwide. The transmissibility of the infectious agent, within a same species, was first demonstrated in 1936 by the accidental transmission of scrapie to sheep, using a brain extract of an infected animal [31]. In 1986, the discovery of the bovine spongiform encephalopathy (BSE) [37,50] and its transmission to humans as variant CJD (vCJD) marked a turning point in the history of TSEs. The first cases of vCJD in humans were reported in 1996 and, since then, about 190 deaths were recorded in 2006 [36]. In 2007, a fourth case of transfusion-associated vCJD infection was reported in the UK [51]. Emerging 10 years after the first BSE cases, molecular studies examining strain typing and migration patterns on gel and *in vivo* experiments [52,53,54], consisting in injecting the BSE and vCJD strain to macaques and mice, raised the possibility of a trans-species transmission of the agent and triggered a wide concern across the scientific community, the economy, political and public health sectors.

Presently, the emergence of new atypical cases such as the sporadic fatal insomnia (sFI), bovine amyloid spongiform encephalopathy (BASE) and Nor98 of sheep, have sparked discussions in the medical and veterinary communities on the complexity of these diseases, their propagation, structure and molecular status [55].

The danger to public health due to dietary and medical exposure to infectious prions has driven huge efforts in the prion domain to develop highly sensitive methods of detection of prions to control its spread among animals and humans. Since the presence of the proteinase K residue PrP27-30 was found to be often proportional to infectivity in numerous infectious preparations [20], its direct detection forms the basis of all commercially available diagnostic kits for TSEs. PrPsc, unfortunately, cannot be used as a diagnostic tool due to its very low presence in tissues as well as body fluids such as blood, cerebrospinal fluid urine and saliva. In 1994, a significant milestone achieved was the observation that the infectious protein could catalyze the cell-free conversion of PrPc into PrPres [56,57]. Firstly developed by Caughey and co-workers [56], another new *in vitro* conversion system, called PMCA (protein misfolding cyclic amplification) transformed large quantities of PrPc using minute quantities of PrPres [57]. Resulting quantities of PrPres were then detectable by western blot or ELISA. Conceptually analogous to DNA amplification by polymerase chain reaction, the PMCA technique has important implications for sensitive biochemical diagnosis and research in the prion domain [58] such as detection of the infectious agent in body fluids and tissues.

As prion diseases are characterised by a long asymptomatic phase that can last several months up to as many as 40 years and since events of transfusion-associated vCJD infection have been reported in the UK [51], there is an increasing demand for the development of tests to screen blood. Unfortunately, as mentioned above, the detection of PrPres in the blood is very difficult, considering its low concentration and its hydrophobicity making its purification a problem. A way to get round this problem is to look for surrogate biomarkers using proteomics [59]. As an example, Wei and colleagues [60] used lectins to isolate and study 708 glycoproteins and found 111 proteins presenting more than a 2-fold modulation in concentration, some of them already known to be associated with neurodegenerative diseases. Other recent research for neurodegenerative disease blood-based biomarkers have been reviewed by Noelker and colleagues [61]. In prion diseases, proteomic tools are also being applied to identify specific prion strain disease biomarkers. Indeed, pre-mortem diagnosis of prion diseases is not available and confirmation of a TSE disease is only possible after post-mortem histopathological tests and eventual bioassays. A proteomic study conducted on vCJD infected cerebrospinal fluid revealed the presence of two proteins, p130 and p131, that seemed absent in other dementias [62]. Based on their sequence, the proteins were identified as belonging to the 14-3-3 family and have since been shown to be potential targets for discriminating vCJD from other dementias [63,64], although its clinical use in vCJD has yet to be confirmed [65,66]. Inversely, cell surface proteomics also implicated PrPc as a potential biomarker for non-neurodegenerative diseases such as carcinoma [4].

APPLICATION OF PROTEOMICS IN NEURODEGENERATIVE DISEASES

Proteomics is increasingly becoming a tool of choice to gain insight into the pathological mechanisms of a wide variety of neurodegenerative disorders [67]. The common biological materials that are investigated in the field consist of cerebrospinal fluid, brain tissue, cell cultures and animals models. The most important human neurodegenerative diseases consist of the Huntington's disease, Prion diseases (TSE), amyotrophic lateral sclerosis, Alzheimer's disease (AD), frontotemporal dementia and Parkinson's disease (PD) [68]. Increasing evidence seems to show an overlap of these neurodegenerative disorders, with a contribution of environmental, epigenetic and genetic factors. Moreover, these neurodegenerative disorders seem to share a common feature: that of being associated with oxidative stress occurring in the mitochondria [69]. Post-mortem analyses have indeed revealed overall oxidative damage to proteins, lipids and DNA. Presently, altered metal homeostasis is being discussed as constituting a common aetiological factor in PD, AD and TSE diseases. Extensive reviews on the application of proteomics in the field of neurodegenerative disorders were provided by David, Hoerndli and colleagues [70,67] and by Noelker and colleagues [71].

The most common form of dementia to affect humans worldwide is Alzheimer's disease. Proteomic tools have previously been used to compare different affected and un-affected regions of the AD brain. In this way, it has allowed the identification of 411 proteins that were present at differential levels between one or more cerebral regions from AD and non-AD brains [67]. Moreover the molecular identity of 37 proteins with significantly altered expression was determined. Most of these proteins belonged to functional groups involved in synaptic transmission, stress response, lipid transport, glycolysis and roles in the pathogenesis of diabetes. In other post-mortem proteomic studies, GFAP, G protein beta subunit, 60kDa heat shock protein, internexin, mitochondrial ATP synthase alpha and calpain were shown to be differentially present and thus involved in the pathogenesis of AD. The amino acid sequencing and identification of β-amyloid as being the major extracellular component of the senile plaques observed in both Down's disease and Alzheimer's disease, subsequently formed the basis for the cloning of the amyloid precursor protein (APP) gene. This was crucial in highlighting the involvement of this protein in the Alzheimer's disease. Both immunochemical and electrophoretic analyses have contributed to show that tau, a major protein component of neurofibrillary tangles, differs biochemically in Alzheimer's disease as compared to the normal physiological cases. Indeed, the pathological tau has been shown to undergo post-translational modifications including ubiquitination, glycosylation, glycation and hyperphosphorylation, although the influence of these changes remains unknown. In the future, proteomic approaches investigating protein-protein interactions and post-translational modifications involved will more than likely remain and contribute to the progression of this field.

Parkinson's disease is the next most prevalent human neurodegenerative disorder. An important feature of this disease is the presence of cytoplasmic inclusions of misfolded proteins, called Lewy bodies, in affected brain regions [72]. The major proteinaceous component of these is alpha-synuclein [67]. As in AD, oxidative stress seems to be a key factor in the pathogenesis of this disease. A comparative proteomic study was thus undertaken to investigate alterations in protein levels associated with AD and PD. This study revealed three human brain UCH-L1 (ubiquitin carboxyl-terminal hydrolase L1) isoforms and it is presently believed that the full length UCH-L1 is a key target in both PD and AD.

Prionologists are occupied with another question: what are the interacting partners of PrPc [73] ? Interestingly, two studies, performed on rabbit epithelial cells [74] and SH-SY5Y [75], have shown the protective effect of PrPc towards toxicity induced by paraquat. The mechanism of paraquat toxicity itself is thought to involve mitochondrial dysfunction resulting from the inhibition of the activity of complex 1 by the high production rate of $O_2^{\circ -}$ in the redox cycling of paraquat [76,77]. This mechanism has, however, been debated by others [78]. An inhibition of the mitochondrial complex 1 could lead to a lower ATP synthesis, induce membrane depolarisation and favour Ca^{2+} deregulation [79]. Interestingly, we have previously shown, using human neuroblastoma cells, that following exposure to paraquat there was a mitochondrial membrane depolarization and reduction in ATP content in the treated cells [75]. Using MTS, LDH, ATP and mitochondrial membrane depolarisation assays, we showed that over-expression of PrPc protected cells against paraquat toxicity. The apparent anti-oxidant characteristic of PrPc has been attributed to a Cu/Zn-SOD function [80,81], supported by *in vivo* findings that have shown Prnp°/° mice to express reduced brain copper levels, Cu/Zn-SOD activity and hence greater susceptibility to oxidative stress [82,83]. However, the Cu/Zn-SOD role of PrPc has lately been a subject of heated debate [84,85] and the mechanism, by which PrPc-mediated protection against paraquat occurs, currently remains a mystery.

Although efforts have been made to highlight certain protein partners both *in vivo* and *in vitro* [86,87,88], an understanding of the physiological function of the prion protein and its interaction partners is still an ongoing quest [73,89]. That subject will be developed here below. Nevertheless, prion proteins are able not only to interact with proteins already present in the cells, but are also able to modify the expression of other proteins. For example, an overexpression of PrPc in the SH-SY5Y cell line upregulates a series of proteins, such as annexin V [90]. Also, infection of a neuroblastoma N2a cell line with PrPsc induced a downregulation of several proteins involved in protein folding [91]. This is particularly interesting considering that the transconformation of PrPc into PrPsc involved prion protein misfolding. This could lead to new therapies targeting proteinopathies.

In the past, one of the most publicly debated iatrogenic person-to-person transmission of the CJD agent occurred via injection of cadaver-derived human growth hormone (hGH) administered as a treatment for growth failure secondary to hGH deficiency [92]. It happened that the CJD agent was co-purified with hGH. Therefore, co-purification of prion protein with other biological products used in human therapy must be placed under strict supervision. Indeed, using a classical proteomic approach, Van Dorsselaer and colleagues recently detected PrPc among other non-gonadotropin proteins in urinary human chorionic gonadotropin and in highly-purified urinary human menopausal gonadotropin products [93]. While PrPc and PrPsc isolates differently, this illustrates that prion proteins can still be found in actual biological products.

Functions of the Native PrPc

More than two decades after its discovery, one of the questions that remain largely unexplained in the field of prion diseases concerns the physiological function of the normal prion isoform or PrPc. Its high conservation in the animal kingdom as well as its ubiquitous presence could lead us to suppose that it plays a central role in the cell. Nevertheless, *in vivo* studies performed on PrPc knock-out (PrP°/°) mice, homozygote for the deletion of the Prnp gene (Prnp°/°), show that these mice are not only perfectly viable but that they present no detectable global anatomic, developmental or behavioural disorder. These observations suggest that PrPc does not constitute an indispensable factor to cellular survival [23,94]. Interestingly, however, physiological studies have revealed electrophysiological and structural abnormalities in the hippocampus [95,96,97], loss of Purkinje cells [98,99] and alterations in the circadian rhythm and sleep patterns in Prnp°/° mice [100]. Moreover, other *in vivo* studies have shown an increase in cellular oxidative damage in the brains from Prnp°/° mice [101,102]. Following the above observations, it could be argued that the function of PrPc in cell survival mechanisms is of such importance that it is redundant in the cell [103].

PrPc is mainly expressed at the cell membrane and in neurons, is primarily located in presynaptic domains. Its implication regarding synaptic transmission has hence been investigated [97,104,105,106] as well as its role in copper metabolism, cellular adhesion, signalling pathways [107], cellular redox state and cell survival against oxidative stress [80].The investigation methods involves notably proteomic techniques.

1. Synaptic Transmission

Synaptic degeneration represents a fundamental and consistent change in prion diseases [108]. Predominantly present in presynaptic domains, the co-localisation of PrPc with synapsin I and Grb2 [109], proteins associated with synaptic vesicles, suggests that it could be implicated in vesicle recycling or execute a more direct role in synaptic activity. It has thus been postulated that the loss of PrPc function could lead to synapse or synaptic process deterioration [106]. Indeed some *in vitro* studies, carried out on Prnp°/° mouse hippocampal sections, show a weakening of the fast post-synaptic potential mediated by the $GABA_A$ (γ-aminobutyric acid) receptors as well as a deregulation of the long term potential implicated in the processes of learning and memory [97]. Moreover, the situation can be re-established by re-introducing large numbers of copies of the transgene encoding the human PrPc in the Prnp°/° mice [106]. Nevertheless, other studies realised in this domain haven't reproduced these results [105,110] implying that the role of PrPc in synaptic transmission remains controversial.

Synaptic vesicles are not the only vesicle to involve prion proteins. Affinity proteomic studies have recently shown that PrPc can bind to Rab7a, which is involved in vesicle trafficking, suggesting the involvement of endosomal compartments in the trafficking and regulation of PrPc [111].

2. Regulation of Copper Metabolism in Vivo and In Vitro

In this field of study, it has been proposed that by fixing copper, PrPc could play a crucial role in its uptake, thus regulating its concentration at the synapse and distribution in the cell [112]. Indeed, a 50% reduction of copper concentration in synaptosomal preparations of Prnp°/° mice as compared to wild-type preparations has been reported [104]. A similar observation on endosomal, synaptosomal and membrane preparations from Prnp°/° mice has shown an 80% reduction in copper concentration as compared to control levels [113]. However, others have not reproduced these results: Rachidi and his collaborators observed that there was no uptake of extracellular divalent copper at physiological concentrations of this metal [114] ; the total concentration of copper was not significantly different in Prnp°/° and Tga 20 mice, despite a ten fold overexpression of PrPc in the latter [115]. Other observations, reported in this chapter, show that there was no significant change in the activity of the cupro-enzymes, Cu/Zn-superoxide dismutase and cytochrome C oxidase, in Prnp°/°, Tga 20 and wild-type mice. Furthermore, the reduction of copper in infected brain homogenates of mice would not be specific to copper as this effect is observed for other cations as well namely zinc, magnesium and calcium [83]. From these observations, the physiological relevance of the interaction between PrPc and copper and its role in the uptake of copper in neurons and/or its trafficking/transport towards neuronal cupro-enzymes remains enigmatic. Another hypothesis is that PrPc present on astrocytes could collect Cu from the extracellular environment and store it inside the astrocytes, protecting the neurons from copper toxicity [116,117].

3. Cell Adhesion and Signalling

The membrane localisation of PrPc, by the intermediary of its GPI anchor, has triggered an interest to study the role that the PrPc plays as a receptor in cellular adhesion and signalling [107]. An *in vitro* study, investigating the state of cellular aggregation in neuroblastoma cells of mice expressing different levels of PrPc, has shown that cells over-expressing PrPc tend to aggregate more [107]. It has been proposed that PrPc could interact with several ligands such as laminin [118], the receptor of laminin [119], the precursor of the laminin receptor [120], NCAM (neural cell adhesion molecule) [88] and STI-1(stress inducible protein 1) [121]. Cellular aggregation is an event that could thus result from an interaction between PrPc and a ligand such as laminin [87,118]. Indeed, by interacting with its membrane receptors, laminin could intervene in the proliferation, death and differentiation of neurons. Recent studies have shown that the interaction of PrPc with NCAM could also be implicated in neuritogenesis. This response would require the recruitement of NCAM by PrPc and activation of the tyrosine kinase p59fyn [122]. STI-1, which, as mentioned above, is a direct interacting partner of PrPc, could also induce the growth of neurites in hippocampal neurons via the activation of the extracellular regulated kinase (ERK) [121]. An *in vitro* study showed also that infection with PrPsc could modify the expression of the laminin receptor [123]. Taken together, these data reveal the implication of PrPc in neuritogenesis by its contribution to cellular adherence on a laminin rich matrix.

4. Apoptotic Pathways

Experiments using neuronal cell cultures derived from Prnp°/° mice seem to indicate that PrPc imparts a resistance to apoptosis induced under conditions of serum deprivation [124]. In these cells, an expression of PrPc, like that of the anti-apoptotic Bcl2, identified as a possible interaction partner of PrPc, is capable to restore resistance to apoptosis [86]. These data therefore suggest the implication of PrPc in the regulation of the Bax/Bcl2 dependent apoptotic pathway which is preponderant in neurons. The anti-apoptotic function of PrPc is also suggested by the observation, *in vitro* on mouse retinal explants, that the protein STI-1, that is a direct interacting partner of PrPc, exerces a neuroprotective role by activating the cAMP dependent protein kinase [125,126]. Also, studies performed on tissue slices have revealed that the binding of PrPc with specific antibodies could induce extensive apoptosis in cerebellar and hippocampal neurons [127]. Inversely, however, other anti-PrPc antibodies would not have the same effect. The discordance between these results and the preceding ones could be a consequence of using antibodies that recognised distinct epitopes. Indeed, certain antibodies could induce the activation of PrPc by miming an interaction with its physiological ligand, whereas others could inhibit its physiological activation. Moreover, the models used in the studies [125,127] were also different. Others also argue against an anti-apoptotic role of PrPc: for example, the apoptotic response following treatment with staurosporine (dependent on p53 and caspase 3) of kidney embryonic cells and primary cultured neurons [128] is positively regulated by the expression of PrPc. It is thus impossible, at this stage, to definitely designate PrPc as an anti-apoptotic or pro-apoptotic protein as its implication on cellular survival seems to depend on the cell type and apoptotic pathway involved. In addition, apoptosis is not the only cell death pathway that can be modulated by PrPc. A recent study showed that while PrPc downregulation does not induce apoptosis in glioma cells, it increases autophagy-dependent cell death in these cells [129].

5. Redox State of the Cell

The role of PrPc in redox signalling has previously been highlighted [125,122]. An indirect interaction of PrPc with NADPH oxidase (nicotinamide adenine dinucleotide phosphate-oxidase), leading to the production of reactive oxygen species (ROS), has been reported in serotonergic and noradrenergic neurons [130]. Moreover, in these cells, the binding and aggregation of PrPc by specific antibodies has been shown to induce the activation of the MAP-kinase ERK pathway, via protein kinase Fyn whose role in cell survival has been largely documented [122]. We could therefore assume that the NADPH dependent activation of ERK, observed in both neuronal and non-neuronal cells, could constitute a response implicating the participation of PrPc in maintaining the redox state of the cell [131]. Conversely, pathogenic PrP could induce an oxidative stress in N2a cells expressing mutant D177N/Met-128 PrP, in animal model of inherited prion disease or in prion-infected mice, leading to an upregulation of proteins implicated in protection against oxidative stress, such as peroxiredoxin 4 [132].

6. Cell Survival: Protection against Oxidative Stress

Among the speculated functions of PrPc, one that rapidly gained interest is the copper dependent anti-oxidant function that the protein could exert in situations of cellular oxidative stress [133]. A compelling observation supporting the anti-oxidant role of PrPc has been the comparative study of neurons derived from Prnp°/° and wild-type mice treated with oxidative stress inducing agents such as hydrogen peroxide, xanthine oxidase and copper ions. In this study, the Prnp°/° neurons were shown to be much more susceptible to the induced oxidative stress as compared to their wild-type counterparts. Susceptibility to oxidative stress and hence to ROS was correlated with a reduction in superoxide dismutase activity [134]. Moreover, brain tissue derived from Prnp°/° mice, was shown to accumulate oxidative stress markers, namely lipid peroxidation products and protein carbonylation. Also, hypoxia and ischemia, known to cause neuronal death by oxidative damage, induced brain lesions that were much more important in the Prnp°/° mice as compared to the wild-type mice. In a set of experiments that involved comparing the biological state of cells over-expressing PrPc with cells having a low level of expression, we and others have shown a relationship between PrPc expression and the cellular defence against toxicity induced by pesticide molecules such as paraquat (1,1'-dimethyl-4,4' bipyridium dichloride) [75,74]. Paraquat (PQ) is a quaternary nitrogen herbicide, well characterized for its pneumotoxicant properties and bears structural similarity to 1-methyl-4-phenyl pyridinium (MPP^+), an active toxin implicated in Parkinson's disease [79]. The two studies carried out showed that cells over-expressing the cellular form of the prion protein were more resistant to PQ toxicity than cells expressing low levels of the protein.

The mechanism by which PrPc could protect cells against oxidative stress is either by activating the Cu/Zn superoxide dismutase (Cu/Zn-SOD) enzyme [80] or by directly activating an intrinsic SOD-like antioxidant characteristic when copper is bound to the octapeptide repeat region [81,133,135]. Interestingly, PrP isolated from scrapie-infected mice, shows reduced SOD activity compared to PrP isolated from control mice and this was shown to match the low copper levels seen in the brains of the infected mice [82]. Moreover, Prnp°/° mice have been shown to suffer late-stage oxidative degradation in the neuronal synaptic regions where PrPc is localised in wild-type controls [101,136]. The activities of the cellular antioxidant machinery also seem to be affected. Indeed levels of glutathione (GSH) and the enzymatic activities of glutathione reductase (GR), glutathione peroxidase (GPx) and SOD have been reported to be disturbed in the Prnp°/° cell models.

In infected cell models, similar observations have been made where the PrPsc infected cells show higher susceptibility to oxidative stress than uninfected cells. Although the exact mechanism is far from being understood, it is hypothesised that PrPc participates in the cellular SOD activity by catalysing the conversion of superoxide anions to hydrogen peroxide and by helping maintain GSH levels [137]. GSH is an important anti-oxidant that helps convert the toxic hydrogen peroxide to water, in turn getting oxidised to glutathione disulphide (GSSG). This reaction is catalysed by the enzyme GPx. Finally, GSH is regenerated by the reduction of GSSG, reaction catalysed by glutathione reductase (GR). Prion protein deficient neurons have been shown to present low levels of GR. This has the consequence of rendering the Prnp°/° cells susceptible to toxicity induced by hydrogen peroxide. Moreover, GSH being an important copper chelator, any deficiency in GR would lead to a metabolic imbalance of copper. The Cu/Zn-SOD-like anti-oxidant activity of PrPc has become the subject of a heated debate [84,85].

Furthermore, ever since the affinity for copper was discovered [138], the interaction of PrPc with other transition metals has also been investigated. Recombinant prion protein, in addition to fixing Cu^{2+}, has been shown to bind manganese [139] (Mn^{2+}) at both the octapeptide repeat region, along the residues 60-90, and along a C-terminal site spanning the residues 93-111 [140]. Other metals such as cobalt, nickel and Zn^{2+} [141] have also been shown to bind to PrPc, although with a lower affinity. This suggested that PrPc could contribute to cellular protection against toxic levels of such metallic ions [113].

Supporting these *in vitro* data, differences in the concentrations of metals, mainly copper, manganese and iron have been observed in Prnp°/° models, as well as in mice infected by the scrapie agent, [142,82,83]. Indeed there is a general decrease in copper levels and an increase in manganese levels in the brains of scrapie infected mice [82,83].

A disturbance in iron homeostasis has also been shown in scrapie-infected mouse neuroblastoma cells [143,142]. These cells presented elevated levels of free iron and reactive oxygen species markers suggesting that scrapie alters iron metabolism and decreases the capacity of the cell to deal with excessive iron [144].

CONCLUSION

Research on TSEs is becoming more and more dependent on proteomic techniques. Indeed, while single protein investigations can answer specific questions, they show two main limitations. Firstly, even if improvements such as quantitative immuno-PCR have been made, they fail to detect very low concentrations of pathological proteins in body fluids such as blood and urine, which is of paramount importance for the safety of both blood transfusion and purification of bioproducts to be administered in human therapy. Secondly, they are not appropriate for the study of numerous or undetermined target proteins. Proteomic techniques bring ways to get round these problems. By targeting numerous proteins at the same time, they have the capability to identify specific biomarkers associated with each type of TSE. Identification of such biomarkers, easier to detect and quantify because present in higher concentration in body fluids, will allow more reliable testing of bioproducts and the creation of routine pre-mortem diagnostic kits, hence earlier detection of diseases and better response to potential treatments. Also, proteomic techniques make it much easier to link apparently unrelated proteins, in case of TSEs or in *in vitro* or *in vivo* models related to TSEs research. Considering its potential, proteomic is expected to play a major role in the future of proteinopathies research.

REFERENCES

[1] Zhu, H., Bilgin, M., And Snyder, M., *Annu. Rev. Biochem.*, 72, 783 (2003)

[2] Graham, D. R., Elliott, S. T., And Van Eyk, J. E., *J. Physiol*, 563, 1 (2005)

[3] Anderson, L. And Seilhamer, J., *Electrophoresis*, 18, 533 (1997)

[4] De, Wit M., Jimenez, C. R., Carvalho, B., Belien, J. A., Is-Van Diemen, P. M., Mongera, S., Piersma, S. R., Vikas, M., Navani, S., Ponten, F., Meijer, G. A., And Fijneman, R. J., *Gut* (2011)

[5] Steel, L. F., Haab, B. B., And Hanash, S. M., *J. Chromatogr. B Analyt. Technol. Biomed. Life Sci.*, 815, 275 (2005)

[6] Walsh, G. M., Rogalski, J. C., Klockenbusch, C., And Kast, J., *Expert. Rev. Mol. Med.*, 12, E30 (2010)

[7] O'Farrell, P. H., *J. Biol. Chem.*, 250, 4007 (1975)

[8] Unlu, M., Morgan, M. E., And Minden, J. S., *Electrophoresis*, 18, 2071 (1997)

[9] Neverova, I. And Van Eyk, J. E., *J. Chromatogr. B Analyt. Technol. Biomed. Life Sci.*, 815, 51 (2005)

[10] Falisse-Poirrier, N., Ruelle, V., Elmoualij, B., Zorzi, D., Pierard, O., Heinen, E., De Pauw, E., And Zorzi, W., *J. Microbiol. Methods*, 67, 593 (2006)

[11] Yan, F., Sreekumar, A., Laxman, B., Chinnaiyan, A. M., Lubman, D. M., And Barder, T. J., *Proteomics.*, 3, 1228 (2003)

[12] Itoh, H., Nimura, N., Kinoshita, T., Nagae, N., And Nomura, M., *Anal. Biochem.*, 199, 7 (1991)

[13] Wagner, K., Racaityte, K., Unger, K. K., Miliotis, T., Edholm, L. E., Bischoff, R., And Marko-Varga, G., *J. Chromatogr. A*, 893, 293 (2000)

[14] Ruelle, V., Falisse-Poirrier, N., Elmoualij, B., Zorzi, D., Pierard, O., Heinen, E., De Pauw, E., And Zorzi, W., *J. Proteome. Res.*, 6, 2168 (2007)
[15] Zhu, H., Bilgin, M., And Snyder, M., *Annu. Rev. Biochem.*, 72, 783 (2003)
[16] Mann, M., Hendrickson, R. C., And Pandey, A., *Annu. Rev. Biochem.*, 70, 437 (2001)
[17] Collinge, J., *J. Neurol. Neurosurg. Psychiatry*, 76, 906 (2005)
[18] Prusiner, S. B., *Science*, 216, 136 (1982)
[19] Manson, J. C., Cancellotti, E., Hart, P., Bishop, M. T., And Barron, R. M., *Biochem. Soc. Trans.*, 34, 1155 (2006)
[20] Prusiner, S. B., *Proc. Natl. Acad. Sci. U. S. A*, 95, 13363 (1998)
[21] Weissmann, C., *Nat. Rev. Microbiol.*, 2, 861 (2004)
[22] Weissmann, C., *Nature*, 352, 679 (1991)
[23] Bueler, H., Aguzzi, A., Sailer, A., Greiner, R. A., Autenried, P., Aguet, M., And Weissmann, C., *Cell*, 73, 1339 (1993)
[24] Oesch, B., Westaway, D., Walchli, M., Mckinley, M. P., Kent, S. B., Aebersold, R., Barry, R. A., Tempst, P., Teplow, D. B., Hood, L. E., And ., *Cell*, 40, 735 (1985)
[25] Schatzl, H. M., Da Costa, M., Taylor, L., Cohen, F. E., And Prusiner, S. B., *J. Mol. Biol.*, 245, 362 (1995)
[26] Prusiner, S. B., *Philos. Trans. R. Soc. Lond B Biol. Sci.*, 343, 447 (1994)
[27] Prusiner, S. B., *Annu. Rev. Microbiol.*, 43, 345 (1989)
[28] Zahn, R., Liu, A., Luhrs, T., Riek, R., Von Schroetter, C., Lopez, Garcia F., Billeter, M., Calzolai, L., Wider, G., And Wuthrich, K., *Proc. Natl. Acad. Sci. U. S. A*, 97, 145 (2000)
[29] Eichner, T. And Radford, S. E., *Mol. Cell*, 43, 8 (2011)
[30] Norrby, E., *J. Intern. Med.*, 270, 1 (2011)
[31] Collinge, J., *Annu. Rev. Neurosci.*, 24, 519 (2001)
[32] Aguzzi, A., *J. Neurochem.*, 97, 1726 (2006)
[33] Goldmann, W., *Vet. Res.*, 39, 30 (2008)
[34] Foster, J. D., Mckelvey, W. A., Mylne, M. J., Williams, A., Hunter, N., Hope, J., And Fraser, H., *Vet. Rec.*, 130, 341 (1992)
[35] Aguzzi, A. And Heikenwalder, M., *Nat. Rev. Microbiol.*, 4, 765 (2006)
[36] Collee, J. G., Bradley, R., And Liberski, P. P., *Folia Neuropathol.*, 44, 102 (2006)
[37] GAJDUSEK, D. C. And ZIGAS, V., *N. Engl. J. Med.*, 257, 974 (1957)
[38] Bounias, M. And Purdey, M., *Sci. Total Environ.*, 297, 1 (2002)
[39] Chatterjee, S. And Van Marck, E., *J. Postgrad. Med.*, 52, 223 (2006)
[40] Colchester, A. C. And Colchester, N. T., *Lancet*, 366, 856 (2005)
[41] Purdey, M., *Med. Hypotheses*, 60, 797 (2003)
[42] Shankar, S. K. And Satishchandra, P., *Lancet*, 366, 790 (2005)
[43] Prusiner, S. B., *Trends Biochem. Sci.*, 21, 482 (1996)
[44] Hogan, R. N., Brown, P., Heck, E., And Cavanagh, H. D., *Cornea*, 18, 2 (1999)
[45] Ricketts, M. N. And Brown, P., *Clin. Lab Med.*, 23, 129 (2003)
[46] Zobeley, E., Flechsig, E., Cozzio, A., Enari, M., And Weissmann, C., *Mol. Med.*, 5, 240 (1999)
[47] Brown, P., *Vox Sang.*, 89, 63 (2005)
[48] Brown, P., *Dev. Biol. (Basel)*, 120, 27 (2005)
[49] Seeger, H., Heikenwalder, M., Zeller, N., Kranich, J., Schwarz, P., Gaspert, A., Seifert, B., Miele, G., And Aguzzi, A., *Science*, 310, 324 (2005)

[50] Wells, G. A., Scott, A. C., Johnson, C. T., Gunning, R. F., Hancock, R. D., Jeffrey, M., Dawson, M., And Bradley, R., *Vet. Rec.*, 121, 419 (1987)

[51] , *Euro. Surveill*, 12, E070118 (2007)

[52] Bruce, M. E., Will, R. G., Ironside, J. W., Mcconnell, I., Drummond, D., Suttie, A., Mccardle, L., Chree, A., Hope, J., Birkett, C., Cousens, S., Fraser, H., And Bostock, C. J., *Nature*, 389, 498 (1997)

[53] Collinge, J., Sidle, K. C., Meads, J., Ironside, J., And Hill, A. F., *Nature*, 383, 685 (1996)

[54] Hill, A. F., Desbruslais, M., Joiner, S., Sidle, K. C., Gowland, I., Collinge, J., Doey, L. J., And Lantos, P., *Nature*, 389, 448 (1997)

[55] Watts, J. C., Balachandran, A., And Westaway, D., *Plos. Pathog.*, 2, E26 (2006)

[56] Kocisko, D. A., Come, J. H., Priola, S. A., Chesebro, B., Raymond, G. J., Lansbury, P. T., And Caughey, B., *Nature*, 370, 471 (1994)

[57] Saborio, G. P., Permanne, B., And Soto, C., *Nature*, 411, 810 (2001)

[58] Saa, P., Castilla, J., And Soto, C., *Methods Mol. Biol.*, 299, 53 (2005)

[59] Huzarewich, R. L., Siemens, C. G., And Booth, S. A., *J. Biomed. Biotechnol.*, 2010, 613504 (2010)

[60] Wei, X., Herbst, A., Ma, D., Aiken, J., And Li, L., *J. Proteome. Res.*, 10, 2687 (2011)

[61] Noelker, C., Hampel, H., And Dodel, R., *Mol. Diagn. Ther.*, 15, 83 (2011)

[62] Harrington, M. G., Merril, C. R., Asher, D. M., And GAJDUSEK, D. C., *N. Engl. J. Med.*, 315, 279 (1986)

[63] Beaudry, P., Cohen, P., Brandel, J. P., Delasnerie-Laupretre, N., Richard, S., Launay, J. M., And Laplanche, J. L., *Dement. Geriatr. Cogn Disord.*, 10, 40 (1999)

[64] Zerr, I., Bodemer, M., Gefeller, O., Otto, M., Poser, S., Wiltfang, J., Windl, O., Kretzschmar, H. A., And Weber, T., *Ann. Neurol.*, 43, 32 (1998)

[65] Hill, A. F., Butterworth, R. J., Joiner, S., Jackson, G., Rossor, M. N., Thomas, D. J., Frosh, A., Tolley, N., Bell, J. E., Spencer, M., King, A., Al Sarraj, S., Ironside, J. W., Lantos, P. L., And Collinge, J., *Lancet*, 353, 183 (1999)

[66] Zeidler, M., Stewart, G. E., Barraclough, C. R., Bateman, D. E., Bates, D., Burn, D. J., Colchester, A. C., Durward, W., Fletcher, N. A., Hawkins, S. A., Mackenzie, J. M., And Will, R. G., *Lancet*, 350, 903 (1997)

[67] Hoerndli, F., David, D. C., And Gotz, J., *Prog. Neurobiol.*, 76, 169 (2005)

[68] Kurosinski, P., Guggisberg, M., And Gotz, J., *Trends Mol. Med.*, 8, 3 (2002)

[69] Lopez, M. F. And Melov, S., *Circ. Res.*, 90, 380 (2002)

[70] David, D. C., Hoerndli, F., And Gotz, J., *Prog. Neurobiol.*, 76, 153 (2005)

[71] Noelker, C., Hampel, H., And Dodel, R., *Mol. Diagn. Ther.*, 15, 83 (2011)

[72] Olanow, C. W. And Mcnaught, K., *Mov Disord.*, 26, 1056 (2011)

[73] Aguzzi, A., Sigurdson, C., And Heikenwalder, M., *Annu. Rev. Pathol.* (2007)

[74] Senator, A., Rachidi, W., Lehmann, S., Favier, A., And Benboubetra, M., *Free Radic. Biol. Med.*, 37, 1224 (2004)

[75] Dupiereux, I., Falisse-Poirrier, N., Zorzi, W., Watt, N. T., Thellin, O., Zorzi, D., Pierard, O., Hooper, N. M., Heinen, E., And Elmoualij, B., *J. Neurosci. Res.* (2007)

[76] Cocheme, H. M. And Murphy, M. P., *J. Biol. Chem.*, 283, 1786 (2008)

[77] Fukushima, T., Yamada, K., Hojo, N., Isobe, A., Shiwaku, K., And Yamane, Y., *Exp. Toxicol. Pathol.*, 46, 437 (1994)

[78] Ramachandiran, S., Hansen, J. M., Jones, D. P., Richardson, J. R., And Miller, G. W., *Toxicol. Sci.*, 95, 163 (2007)

[79] Dinis-Oliveira, R. J., Remiao, F., Carmo, H., Duarte, J. A., Navarro, A. S., Bastos, M. L., And Carvalho, F., *Neurotoxicology*, 27, 1110 (2006)

[80] Brown, D. R. And Besinger, A., *Biochem. J.*, 334 (Pt 2), 423 (1998)

[81] Brown, D. R., Wong, B. S., Hafiz, F., Clive, C., Haswell, S. J., And Jones, I. M., *Biochem. J.*, 344 Pt 1, 1 (1999)

[82] Thackray, A. M., Knight, R., Haswell, S. J., Bujdoso, R., And Brown, D. R., *Biochem. J.*, 362, 253 (2002)

[83] Wong, B. S., Brown, D. R., Pan, T., Whiteman, M., Liu, T., Bu, X., Li, R., Gambetti, P., Olesik, J., Rubenstein, R., And Sy, M. S., *J. Neurochem.*, 79, 689 (2001)

[84] Hutter, G., Heppner, F. L., And Aguzzi, A., *Biol. Chem.*, 384, 1279 (2003)

[85] Jones, S., Batchelor, M., Bhelt, D., Clarke, A. R., Collinge, J., And Jackson, G. S., *Biochem. J.*, 392, 309 (2005)

[86] Bounhar, Y., Zhang, Y., Goodyer, C. G., And Leblanc, A., *J. Biol. Chem.*, 276, 39145 (2001)

[87] Gauczynski, S., Peyrin, J. M., Haik, S., Leucht, C., Hundt, C., Rieger, R., Krasemann, S., Deslys, J. P., Dormont, D., Lasmezas, C. I., And Weiss, S., *EMBO J.*, 20, 5863 (2001)

[88] Schmitt-Ulms, G., Legname, G., Baldwin, M. A., Ball, H. L., Bradon, N., Bosque, P. J., Crossin, K. L., Edelman, G. M., Dearmond, S. J., Cohen, F. E., And Prusiner, S. B., *J. Mol. Biol.*, 314, 1209 (2001)

[89] Damberger, F. F., Christen, B., Perez, D. R., Hornemann, S., And Wuthrich, K., *Proc. Natl. Acad. Sci. U. S. A* (2011)

[90] Weiss, E., Ramljak, S., Asif, A. R., Ciesielczyk, B., Schmitz, M., Gawinecka, J., Schulz-Schaeffer, W., Behrens, C., And Zerr, I., *Neuroscience*, 169, 1640 (2010)

[91] Provansal, M., Roche, S., Pastore, M., Casanova, D., Belondrade, M., Alais, S., Leblanc, P., Windl, O., And Lehmann, S., *Prion.*, 4, 292 (2010)

[92] Belay, E. D. And Schonberger, L. B., *Annu. Rev. Public Health*, 26, 191 (2005)

[93] Van, Dorsselaer A., Carapito, C., Delalande, F., Schaeffer-Reiss, C., Thierse, D., Diemer, H., Mcnair, D. S., Krewski, D., And Cashman, N. R., *Plos. One.*, 6, E17815 (2011)

[94] Sailer, A., Bueler, H., Fischer, M., Aguzzi, A., And Weissmann, C., *Cell*, 77, 967 (1994)

[95] Colling, S. B., Collinge, J., And Jefferys, J. G., *Neurosci. Lett.*, 209, 49 (1996)

[96] Colling, S. B., Khana, M., Collinge, J., And Jefferys, J. G., *Brain Res.*, 755, 28 (1997)

[97] Collinge, J., Whittington, M. A., Sidle, K. C., Smith, C. J., Palmer, M. S., Clarke, A. R., And Jefferys, J. G., *Nature*, 370, 295 (1994)

[98] Katamine, S., Nishida, N., Sugimoto, T., Noda, T., Sakaguchi, S., Shigematsu, K., Kataoka, Y., Nakatani, A., Hasegawa, S., Moriuchi, R., And Miyamoto, T., *Cell Mol. Neurobiol.*, 18, 731 (1998)

[99] Sakaguchi, S., Katamine, S., Nishida, N., Moriuchi, R., Shigematsu, K., Sugimoto, T., Nakatani, A., Kataoka, Y., Houtani, T., Shirabe, S., Okada, H., Hasegawa, S., Miyamoto, T., And Noda, T., *Nature*, 380, 528 (1996)

[100] Tobler, I., Gaus, S. E., Deboer, T., Achermann, P., Fischer, M., Rulicke, T., Moser, M., Oesch, B., Mcbride, P. A., And Manson, J. C., *Nature*, 380, 639 (1996)

[101] Klamt, F., Dal Pizzol, F., Conte Da Frota ML JR, Walz, R., Andrades, M. E., Da Silva, E. G., Brentani, R. R., Izquierdo, I., And Fonseca Moreira, J. C., *Free Radic. Biol. Med.*, 30, 1137 (2001)
[102] Wong, B. S., Liu, T., Li, R., Pan, T., Petersen, R. B., Smith, M. A., Gambetti, P., Perry, G., Manson, J. C., Brown, D. R., And Sy, M. S., *J. Neurochem.*, 76, 565 (2001)
[103] Roucou, X. And Leblanc, A. C., *J. Mol. Med.*, 83, 3 (2005)
[104] Herms, J., Tings, T., Gall, S., Madlung, A., Giese, A., Siebert, H., Schurmann, P., Windl, O., Brose, N., And Kretzschmar, H., *J. Neurosci.*, 19, 8866 (1999)
[105] Herms, J. W., Kretzchmar, H. A., Titz, S., And Keller, B. U., *Eur. J. Neurosci.*, 7, 2508 (1995)
[106] Whittington, M. A., Sidle, K. C., Gowland, I., Meads, J., Hill, A. F., Palmer, M. S., Jefferys, J. G., And Collinge, J., *Nat. Genet.*, 9, 197 (1995)
[107] Mange, A., Milhavet, O., Umlauf, D., Harris, D., And Lehmann, S., *FEBS Lett.*, 514, 159 (2002)
[108] Clinton, J., Forsyth, C., Royston, M. C., And Roberts, G. W., *Neuroreport*, 4, 65 (1993)
[109] Spielhaupter, C. And Schatzl, H. M., *J. Biol. Chem.*, 276, 44604 (2001)
[110] Lledo, P. M., Tremblay, P., Dearmond, S. J., Prusiner, S. B., And Nicoll, R. A., *Proc. Natl. Acad. Sci. U. S. A*, 93, 2403 (1996)
[111] Zafar, S., Von, Ahsen N., Oellerich, M., Zerr, I., Schulz-Schaeffer, W. J., Armstrong, V. W., And Asif, A. R., *J. Proteome. Res.*, 10, 3123 (2011)
[112] Pauly, P. C. And Harris, D. A., *J. Biol. Chem.*, 273, 33107 (1998)
[113] Brown, D. R., Qin, K., Herms, J. W., Madlung, A., Manson, J., Strome, R., Fraser, P. E., Kruck, T., Von Bohlen, A., Schulz-Schaeffer, W., Giese, A., Westaway, D., And Kretzschmar, H., *Nature*, 390, 684 (1997)
[114] Rachidi, W., Vilette, D., Guiraud, P., Arlotto, M., Riondel, J., Laude, H., Lehmann, S., And Favier, A., *J. Biol. Chem.*, 278, 9064 (2003)
[115] Waggoner, D. J., Drisaldi, B., Bartnikas, T. B., Casareno, R. L., Prohaska, J. R., Gitlin, J. D., And Harris, D. A., *J. Biol. Chem.*, 275, 7455 (2000)
[116] Brown, D. R., *Neurobiol. Dis.*, 15, 534 (2004)
[117] Tiffany-Castiglioni, E., Hong, S., And Qian, Y., *Int. J. Dev. Neurosci.* (2011)
[118] Graner, E., Mercadante, A. F., Zanata, S. M., Forlenza, O. V., Cabral, A. L., Veiga, S. S., Juliano, M. A., Roesler, R., Walz, R., Minetti, A., Izquierdo, I., Martins, V. R., And Brentani, R. R., *Brain Res. Mol. Brain Res.*, 76, 85 (2000)
[119] Simoneau, S., Haik, S., Leucht, C., Dormont, D., Deslys, J. P., Weiss, S., And Lasmezas, C., *Biol. Chem.*, 384, 243 (2003)
[120] Rieger, R., Edenhofer, F., Lasmezas, C. I., And Weiss, S., *Nat. Med.*, 3, 1383 (1997)
[121] Lopes, M. H., Hajj, G. N., Muras, A. G., Mancini, G. L., Castro, R. M., Ribeiro, K. C., Brentani, R. R., Linden, R., And Martins, V. R., *J. Neurosci.*, 25, 11330 (2005)
[122] Mouillet-Richard, S., Ermonval, M., Chebassier, C., Laplanche, J. L., Lehmann, S., Launay, J. M., And Kellermann, O., *Science*, 289, 1925 (2000)
[123] Provansal, M., Roche, S., Pastore, M., Casanova, D., Belondrade, M., Alais, S., Leblanc, P., Windl, O., And Lehmann, S., *Prion.*, 4, 292 (2010)
[124] Kim, B. H., Lee, H. G., Choi, J. K., Kim, J. I., Choi, E. K., Carp, R. I., And Kim, Y. S., *Brain Res. Mol. Brain Res.*, 124, 40 (2004)
[125] Chiarini, L. B., Freitas, A. R., Zanata, S. M., Brentani, R. R., Martins, V. R., And Linden, R., *EMBO J.*, 21, 3317 (2002)

[126] Zanata, S. M., Lopes, M. H., Mercadante, A. F., Hajj, G. N., Chiarini, L. B., Nomizo, R., Freitas, A. R., Cabral, A. L., Lee, K. S., Juliano, M. A., De Oliveira, E., Jachieri, S. G., Burlingame, A., Huang, L., Linden, R., Brentani, R. R., And Martins, V. R., *EMBO J.*, 21, 3307 (2002)
[127] Solforosi, L., Criado, J. R., Mcgavern, D. B., Wirz, S., Sanchez-Alavez, M., Sugama, S., Degiorgio, L. A., Volpe, B. T., Wiseman, E., Abalos, G., Masliah, E., Gilden, D., Oldstone, M. B., Conti, B., And Williamson, R. A., *Science*, 303, 1514 (2004)
[128] Paitel, E., Sunyach, C., Alves, Da Costa, Bourdon, J. C., Vincent, B., And Checler, F., *J. Biol. Chem.*, 279, 612 (2004)
[129] Barbieri, G., Palumbo, S., Gabrusiewicz, K., Azzalin, A., Marchesi, N., Spedito, A., Biggiogera, M., Sbalchiero, E., Mazzini, G., Miracco, C., Pirtoli, L., Kaminska, B., And Comincini, S., *Autophagy.*, 7, 840 (2011)
[130] Schneider, B., Mutel, V., Pietri, M., Ermonval, M., Mouillet-Richard, S., And Kellermann, O., *Proc. Natl. Acad. Sci. U. S. A*, 100, 13326 (2003)
[131] Schneider, B., Pietri, M., Ermonval, M., Mouillet-Richard, S., And Kellermann, O., *Med. Sci. (Paris)*, 20, 21 (2004)
[132] Massignan, T., Biasini, E., Lauranzano, E., Veglianese, P., Pignataro, M., Fioriti, L., Harris, D. A., Salmona, M., Chiesa, R., And Bonetto, V., *Mol. Cell Proteomics.*, 9, 611 (2010)
[133] Brown, D. R., Clive, C., And Haswell, S. J., *J. Neurochem.*, 76, 69 (2001)
[134] Brown, D. R., Schulz-Schaeffer, W. J., Schmidt, B., And Kretzschmar, H. A., *Exp. Neurol.*, 146, 104 (1997)
[135] Wong, B. S., Venien-Bryan, C., Williamson, R. A., Burton, D. R., Gambetti, P., Sy, M. S., Brown, D. R., And Jones, I. M., *Biochem. Biophys. Res. Commun.*, 276, 1217 (2000)
[136] Sakudo, A., Lee, D. C., Yoshimura, E., Nagasaka, S., Nitta, K., Saeki, K., Matsumoto, Y., Lehmann, S., Itohara, S., Sakaguchi, S., And Onodera, T., *Biochem. Biophys. Res. Commun.*, 313, 850 (2004)
[137] White, A. R., Collins, S. J., Maher, F., Jobling, M. F., Stewart, L. R., Thyer, J. M., Beyreuther, K., Masters, C. L., And Cappai, R., *Am. J. Pathol.*, 155, 1723 (1999)
[138] Pan, K. M., Stahl, N., And Prusiner, S. B., *Protein Sci.*, 1, 1343 (1992)
[139] Brown, D. R., Hafiz, F., Glasssmith, L. L., Wong, B. S., Jones, I. M., Clive, C., And Haswell, S. J., *EMBO J.*, 19, 1180 (2000)
[140] Jackson, G. S., Murray, I., Hosszu, L. L., Gibbs, N., Waltho, J. P., Clarke, A. R., And Collinge, J., *Proc. Natl. Acad. Sci. U. S. A*, 98, 8531 (2001)
[141] Deloncle, R., Guillard, O., Bind, J. L., Delaval, J., Fleury, N., Mauco, G., And Lesage, G., *Neurotoxicology*, 27, 437 (2006)
[142] Fernaeus, S., Halldin, J., Bedecs, K., And Land, T., *Brain Res. Mol. Brain Res.*, 133, 266 (2005)
[143] Fernaeus, S. And Land, T., *Neurosci. Lett.*, 382, 217 (2005)
[144] Fernaeus, S., Reis, K., Bedecs, K., And Land, T., *Neurosci. Lett.*, 389, 133 (2005)

In: Prions and Prion Diseases: New Developments
Editor: Jean-Michel Verdier
ISBN: 978-1-62100-027-3
© 2012 Nova Science Publishers, Inc.

Chapter 8

ADDED VALUE OF BIOCHEMICAL TOOLS FOR THE DIAGNOSIS OF HUMAN PRION DISEASE

Armand Perret-Liaudet and Isabelle Quadrio
University Hospital Center of Lyon, Department of Neurobiology,
Human Prion Diseases Laboratory, Lyon, France

ABSTRACT

Human prion diseases (PrDs) are transmissible fatal nervous system disorders with major public health implications. They are characterized by the presence of a disease-associated form of the physiological cellular prion protein. Development of diagnostic procedures is important to avoid human to human transmission through blood products and medical devices. To date, although diagnostic performance was increased since introduction of a CSF biomarker, there is no marker ensuring a definite diagnosis before death and post-mortem analysis of brain is still the gold standard. Biochemical methods used for the detection of disease-associated PrP in frozen brain have clearly participated to the increase of the knowledge in the description of the different phenotypes of PrDs. To ensure the diagnosis, we need at least a panel of two kinds of markers: a surrogate marker correlated with the clinical evolution of the disease and a specific marker, hallmark of the brain deposits of disease-associated PrP. The detection of protein 14-3-3 in cerebrospinal fluid, the surrogate marker, associated to clinical signs, electro-encephalogram, cranial MRI and prion protein gene examination, together have increased the specificity and sensitivity of in vivo diagnostics. New developments in the detection of specific disease-associated PrP in biological fluids as CSF or blood are promising for diagnosis in vivo; but for the moment, they still keep in research context and are not yet available for the diagnostic. As mixed neurodegenerative pathologies are current situations, the new markers would be included in a panel able to ensure the etiological diagnosis of dementia.

INTRODUCTION

Human prion diseases (PrDs) are fatal but rare disorders with relative low incidence. Transmissibility of the agent responsible of the disease was reported in animal models as a major feature, and was the basis of human-to-human and animal-to-human transfers of disease. PrDs are characterized by : rapid and progressive loss of neurons associated with vacuolation in the neuropil, termed spongiform change, in nearly all types of disease; and deposition in the brain of an abnormal conformer of the physiological cellular prion protein (PrPC) termed PrPSc (Sc indicates scrapie of sheep). Thus, PrDs are transmissible spongiform encephalopathies belonging to the group of misfolding neurodegenerative diseases [1]. Owing to these features, PrDs have public health implications and require the earliest possible diagnosis, in spite of the lack of specific therapy. For diagnostic tools availability, three categories of diagnostic levels have been defined: possible, probable and definite, the two last being considered as CJD cases by the different surveillance national networks [2, 3].

PrDs may be acquired most frequently by yet unidentified events that produce PrPSc, secondly through germ-line mutations in the prion protein gene (PRNP), finally and more historically through infection (inoculation or dietary exposure). PrDs include Kuru, Creutzfeldt-Jakob disease (CJD), Gerstmann-Straüssler-Scheinker disease (GSS) and fatal familial or sporadic insomnia (FFI or sFI) [4,5]. A further subtype of genetic PrD is associated with deposition of amyloid in vessel walls, thus termed PrP cerebral amyloid angiopathy (PrP-CAA) [5]. A recently described new form is the variably protease-sensitive prionopathy (VPSPr) [6,7]. According to etiology, PrDs are grouped as follows.

I) Sporadic:

Sporadic CJD (sCJD) is the most frequent form of human PrDs whereas sporadic fatal insomnia has common characteristics of FFI. VPSPr has been discussed as being the sporadic representative of GSS [7].

II) Genetic human PrDs comprise a wide spectrum of phenotypes that are associated with mutation in the PRNP, including CJD, FFI, GSS, PrP-CAA and atypical forms not fitting any of the above:

1) Mostly missense but rarely also insertional mutations are associated with spongiform encephalopathy compatible with CJD (gCJD).

2) A specific point mutation (D178N associated with methionine at codon 129) is associated with highly selective thalamic neurodegeneration and characteristic clinical symptoms, hence the name FFI [8]. The same mutation associated with valine at codon 129 leads to a gCJD phenotype.

3) GSS is a form of brain (PrP) amyloidosis characterized by the appearance of (multi-centric) amyloid plaques in the brain [5]. Biochemically, GSS is characterized by the presence of N- and C-terminal truncated proteinase K (PK)-resistant PrP degradation products that range from ~ 7 to 15 kDa and a low-molecular mass band in western blot (WB), although very rarely a CJD-like pattern has been also reported. GSS is mainly associated with point mutations in the PRNP. A GSS-like phenotype has been described in cases with long insertional mutations and also with stop codon mutations. The latter may be associated with PrP CAA as well [5,9].

4) Base pair insertions in the PRNP may cause atypical diseases (on both a clinical and neuropathological level) and cannot always be interpreted as a CJD or GSS phenotype [10]. Base pair deletions are also described and suggested to be pathogenic [11,12], however, this merits further studies.

III) Acquired [13]:

1) Kuru: related to ritualistic cannibalism.

2) Variant CJD (vCJD): associated with consuming bovine spongiform encephalopathy (BSE)-infected tissue or with receiving transfusion from blood donors carrying the vCJD agent.

3) Iatrogenic CJD (iCJD): associated mostly with the application of human growth hormone and dura transplant; gonadotrophin hormone, neurosurgery, cornea transplants and deep electrodes were sources of very occasional cases of transmission.

Diagnostic Strategy of PrDs

1. Clinical Features

CJD was for the first time described by Creutzfeldt [14] and Jakob [15]. Whereas, these first descriptions of CJD concerned young people, rapidly the classical form was recognized as Creutzfeldt-Jakob disease.

The diagnosis of sCJD is first suggested by particular combinations of symptoms reflecting the involvement of various areas of the brain. The most frequent sign is dementia found in 98 %, followed by myoclonus (87%), cerebellar symptoms (75%) and visual complaints (60%). Further neurological symptoms include movement disorders (Parkinsonism, dystonia, as well as chorea), pyramidal signs and in the terminal phase akinetic mutism. In its typical form, the disease presentation consists in a brutal cognitive impairment with a rapid progressive course associating visual disturbance (mainly cortical cecity and visual agnosia), myoclonus and cerebellar syndrome. The disease course is generally 4-7 months.

In Kuru and iCJD linked to the application of contaminated batches of hGH, ataxic presentation at onset is frequently found, whereas others iCJD do not show significant difference with sCJD.

The Variant CJD is characterized by early psychiatric and sensory symptoms, which are soon followed by dementia, extrapyramidal symptoms, ataxia and myoclonus, the course of disease is higher than in sCJD [16].

Genetic CJD does not show significant deviation from sCJD. In GSS, the spectrum includes ataxia, pseudobulbar signs, spastic paraparesis, parkinsonism and slowly progressing cognitive decline [17]. FFI is characterized by insomnia, dysautonomia, motor deficits (dysarthria, limb ataxia), myoclonus and dementia [8].

Accordingly, a case of CJD is suspected in presence of rapidly progressive dementia (< 2 years) and one neurological sign after elimination of other neurological disease. Brutal appearance of neurological sign in a patient with a risk known factor, genetic or iatrogenic, needs to be treated as a suspicion of CJD.

At this moment of the suspicion, the neurologist will start investigation involving imaging, electroencephalogram and CSF analysis.

2. Electroencephalogram

The electroencephalogram (EEG) has been a gold standard for diagnosing PrD. Periodic sharp wave complexes (PSWCs) with triphasic morphology in the correct clinical context are an important component of the in vivo diagnostic procedure but sensitivity remains low [2].

3. Neuroimaging

Although cranial CT may be used to exclude some other disorders, MRI is more specific and sensitive for the diagnosis of PrD. Proposed radiological criteria include either cortical gyriform changes (more than three gyri) in diffusion-weighted (DW) and FLAIR images, or a hyperintense signal in the head of the caudate nucleus or striatum uni- or bilateral in T2, DW, or FLAIR images [18]. A uni- or bilateral striatal high signal with one ribbon-like signal in more than one gyrus in the cerebral cortex on DW and FLAIR images also supports the diagnosis of sCJD.

Variant CJD is represented by a different pattern. The so-called 'pulvinar sign' on MRI brain scan is defined as hyperintensity of the posterior thalamus relative to the signal intensity of the anterior putamen. In the appropriate clinical context, the pulvinar sign and hyperintensity in the dorsomedial thalamic nuclei (the hockey stick sign) are sensitive and specific features of vCJD [19]. Only one VV type 1 and one MV type 2 sCJD case have been reported to show a 'pulvinar sign' compatible with that seen in vCJD; furthermore, it was described in E200K gCJD [20].

4. Cerebrospinal Fluid: Currently Used in Vivo Biomarkers

Immunodetection by western-blot (WB) (figure 1) of protein 14-3-3 (p14-3-3) was originally demonstrated to have an excellent sensitivity and specificity for human PrD [21], and was soon introduced in the international diagnostic criteria. p14-3-3 is not specific for PrD but, although it remains unclear, the main explanation to the high increase in CSF is its release linked to the neuronal damage. Various other pathological conditions leading to a positive detection of p14-3-3 include viral or paraneoplastic encephalitis, recent stroke, Hashimoto encephalitis, metabolic encephalopathy, epilepsy, vascular dementia, rapid forms of Alzheimer's disease, Lewy body dementia, or Wernicke encephalopathy [2,22]. Overall specificity depends on the controls and has been estimated from 74 to 84% [22-24]. Interestingly, when only dementing disorders are considered as controls, the specificity was higher, reaching 88 to 96% [21,24,25].

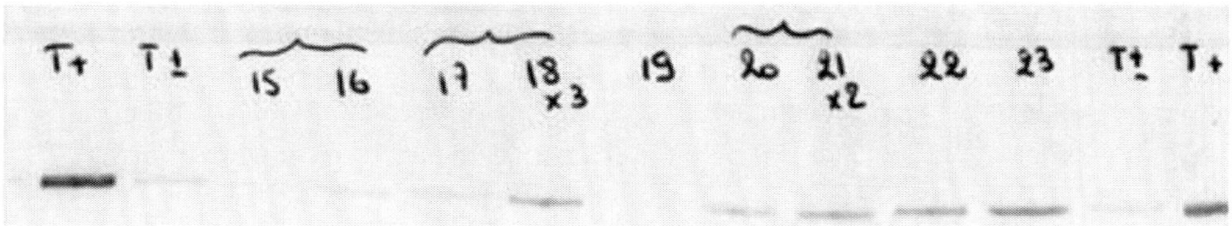

Figure 1. detection of protein 14-3-3 in CSF by western-blot. Immunoblot analysis of protein 14-3-3 in CSF obtained from patients with a suspicion of CJD is shown. Protein 14-3-3 (p14-3-3) band is revealed using a polyclonal antibody raised against all the isoforms of p14-3-3. Each patient is analysed neat and concentrated to give a total proteinorachia near 1 g/L. The concentrated sample is only analysed as an internal control to confirm the relative intensity seen with the native CSF. The result is expressed as positive, negative or doubtful, in comparison to 2 CSF controls with positive and doubtful signals (T+ and T+/- respectively). In this run, the samples 15, 17 and 19 were considered negative, the sample 20 was doubtful and finally one CSF patient (lanes 22 and 23, neat CSF with proteinorachia at 1g/L) gave positive signal.

The use of p14-3-3 is highly different among the countries. For example, after the first publication of Hsich, it was rapidly introduced in 1997 in France and UK but its diffusion as a routine tool in these two countries was absolutely different. In France, with a large network of neurologists it largely contributed to the increase of referrals and sCJD cases numbers between the period 1994-1996 and 1997-2008, since the clinical chemists involved in p14-3-3 assay (Bordeaux, Lyon, Montpellier, Paris and Reims), need to refer any suspicion with CSF p1433 to the French Surveillance Network of CJD [26]; in UK, its slowest diffusion as a routine tool leading to a 10 fold less number of referrals, could be one of the major factor explaining why the numbers of cases of sCJD in UK is 30 to 40 % less than in France, with about the same number of inhabitants. The annual mortality mean rates per million is as follow for the four most populated European countries: UK: 1.02; Germany: 1.21; Italy: 1.24; France 1.48 [3].

5. Genetic Analysis

The PRNP (20p12-ter) encodes a product of 253 amino acids, including octapeptide repeats. Genetic forms are linked either to point mutations in the open reading frame or insertions in the PRNP octapeptide repeat region between codons 51 and 91 [10,27]. DNA sequencing of the coding region of the PRNP should be performed in all suspected cases mainly to exclude pathogenic mutations. Clinicopathological phenotypes of inherited PrDs are summarized in [10,28]. It must be noted that all genetic cases do not present with a clear familial history, thus lack of proven inheritance pattern does not exclude a genetic disorder. The interest of the codon 129 polymorphism determination will be discussed further.

6. Tissue-Based Diagnosis

This includes evaluation of surgical biopsy material or post-mortem examination of the brain. For definite diagnosis, widespread sampling is required because the distribution of tissue-lesioning varies considerably. Cautious interpretation of tiny surgical biopsy samples is needed when evaluated only by histopathology. The diagnostic hallmark of nearly all disease forms is spongiform degeneration in the gray matter accompanied by neuronal loss and reactive astrogliosis. This is completed by the examination of the distribution and morphology of disease-associated PrP by immunohistochemistry (see chapter before).

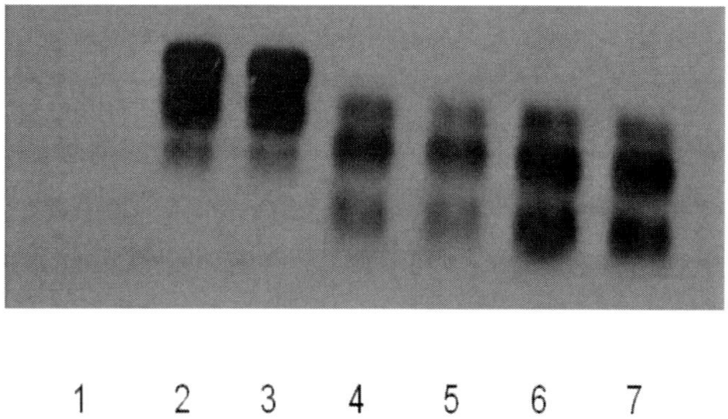

Figure 2. Detection of PrPres in human brain by western-blot. Immunoblot analysis of brain homogenates were obtained from patients died with a suspicion of CJD is shown. Total PrP is revealed using 3F4, a monoclonal antibody raised against a short size epitope of Prion protein, as 3 bands with different apparent molecular weight (MW) before proteinase K (PK) treatment, without clear separation between PrPc and PrPsc (lanes 2-3). After PK treatment, the digested PrPc is not recognized by the 3F4 antibody (lane 1) giving negative signal. When PrPsc is present, signal of 3 bands remains but these bands shift near lower MW than non digested bands, indicating that PK only cut a part of PrPsc (lanes 4-7). Lane 1 (T-): 10 mg equivalent of PK digested brain homogenate from a patient without PrD. Lanes 2-3 (T- sans PK): same than lane 1, but without PK digestion. Lanes 4-5 (4ST): 10 mg equivalent of PK digested striatum homogenate from a patient with sCJD. Lanes 6-7 (5CO): 10 mg equivalent of PK digested frontal cortex homogenate from a patient with sCJD.

In association with the neuropathological examination, detection of PrPres using WB completes the diagnostic procedure. Biochemical characterization has been based on the relative resistance of PrPSc to protease; thus, treatment with PK is used to digest PrPC present in all homogenates. The residual C-terminal resistant core of the pathological form is then called PrPres (where res indicates resistant to protease) [29]. After denaturation of the tissue extract by heating with sodium dodecyl sulfate (SDS), it is analyzed by acrylamide gel electrophoresis and the denaturated proteins are transferred into solid support and detected with an enzyme-labeled antibody. The resulting signals of PrPres showed typical bands corresponding to the three glycosylation states (figure 2).

In addition to the brain, detection of PrPSc (and/or PrPres) has been reported in various human peripheral tissues. To understand its reliability, one must be aware of the different tissue distribution of disease-associated PrP in different etiological PrD forms [30], and furthermore, that detectability might require sophisticated biochemical methods. Some tissues were proposed as promising for routine application, but at the moment tonsil is the only validated tissue used in the field of diagnosis (figure 3) [31].

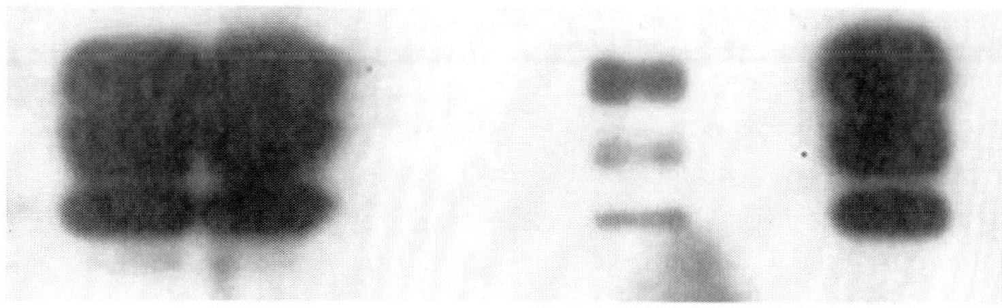

Figure 3. detection of PrPres in human tonsil by western-blot. Immunoblot analysis of tonsil homogenates after ultracentrifugation were obtained from patients with a high suspicion of vCJD, is shown. PrPres is revealed using 3F4. When PrPsc is present, signal of 3 bands remains and shows a characteristic molecular pattern in vCJD very similar to those obtained in BSE. In sCJD, no signal is detected indicating that in sporadic forms, the agent is not accumulating in this peripheral organ. Lane 1: 10 μg equivalent of PK digested brain homogenate from a patient with vCJD. Lanes 2: 10 μg equivalent of PK digested brain homogenate from a patient with vCJD, spiked in 20 mg of tonsil homogenate. Lane 3: 20 mg equivalent of PK digested tonsil homogenate from a control patient. Lane 4: 20 mg equivalent of PK digested tonsil homogenate from a sCJD patient. Lanes 5 and 6: 2 and 20 mg respectively of PK digested tonsil homogenate from a vCJD patient.

7. Diagnosis Criteria of CJD

Diagnosis criteria were modified all along increase of knowledge and validation of new tools for in vivo diagnosis. Criteria are different depending of the etiological form of PrDs. Clinical diagnostic criteria for sCJD were first formulated 30 years ago, using a combination of distinctive clinical features and electroencephalography (EEG) [32]. In recent years, clinical diagnostic criteria have been amended, including useful surrogate biomarkers in the cerebrospinal fluid (CSF) [33, 34]. The clinical criteria can be found in the EUROCJD website [3]. Since diagnostic criteria require the detection of rapidly progressive dementia (< 2 years) and at least two more of the symptoms mentioned above [1,2], atypical presentation of CJD at onset can delay the diagnosis at least before the dementia appears. Increase of the knowledge of phenotype variability of PrDs would improve the performance of diagnostic criteria.

The Molecular Diversity of PrD, Background of Phenotypic Variability

1. Clinical Variability of Human PrDs

Many clinical forms are described in sCJD. These forms are mainly linked to the order of appearance of signs. The Hendenheim's form is characterized by visual agnosia and cortical cecity associated to the dementia, representing the main form of sCJD (35). The cerebellar form is characterized by ataxia at onset (36). Panencephalopathic forms, thalamic presentation were also reported (37, 38). Additionally, the disease course can be increased up to 2 years, leading to misdiagnosis during the follow up of the patient. Using these clinical criteria, the minor clinical phenotypes can be excluded of sCJD definition, at least during the period where rapid decline is absent.

However, the sensitivity of periodic sharp wave complexes (PSWCs) with triphasic morphology is best for the Hendenheim's cases, less for other molecular subtypes of sCJD and not for vCJD. As for other markers, the value of MRI differs according to the molecular subtype [39]. Recently, for long disease sCJD forms, a thalamic hyperintense signal has been reported. MRI was proposed to be included in the diagnostic criteria for sCJD [40].

The overall sensitivity of p1433 is highest for sCJD, but depends also on PRNP codon 129 polymorphism and molecular typing of PrPSc [24]. In addition, the sensitivity increases in the end stage of the disease, and is highest for cases with shorter course of the disease [41]. For inherited forms, overall sensitivity can be estimated ~ 76 to 78% but is highly linked to the genetic anomaly: only 20% for FFI, 50% for GSS, but ~ 90% for E200K and V210I gCJD mutations [24,42,43]. For iCJD, overall sensitivity of p14-3-3 reaches 77% but is only 70% for growth hormone-related iCJD, whereas for dura mater graft-associated iCJD the sensitivity is ~ 88% [44,45]. For vCJD, sensitivity is reported as between 40 and 58%, with an increase during the disease course [24,46].

2. Molecular Diversity of PrD

The concept of strains of the PrDs pathogen agent has been proposed to explain the diversity of clinical and neuropathological profiles of PrD both in humans and in animals. Strains were originally defined in experimental transmission studies by their incubation time and neuropathology lesion profile persisting during serial transmission [47].

Few years after, distinct PrPSc profiles or types have been found in both humans and animals. They can be distinguished by specific physicochemical properties such as molecular size after PK treatment, relative PK resistance, conformational stability and glycoform ratio [48-54]. The hypothesis that strain properties are enciphered in the structure of PrPSc subtypes has not been solved completely. However, it is suggested that particular PrPSc types partially correlate with phenotypes of the disease. Molecular typing of PrPSc is done by WB analysis and focuses both on the fragment size after PK treatment and the glycosylation pattern. This molecular typing associated with PRNP codon 129 polymorphism provides the molecular basis for the disease classification [52, 53, 55, 56]. Based on the electrophoretic mobility of PK-treated fragments, two major conformers were distinguished (Figure 1): type 1 corresponds to a cleavage at residue 82 and an electrophoretic mobility of 21 kDa whereas type 2 has a cleavage site at residue 97 and a mobility of 19 kDa [52]. Moreover, these types correlate with principal types of neuropathogical deposits, where type 1 seems to more associated to the diffuse synaptic deposit whereas type 2 was majorly found when focal and or plaques were described [57]. These different types were identified in CJD, whatever the etiology, sporadic, iatrogenic and gCJD [51, 56-62]. High variability was also reported in relative percentage of glycosylation of PrPsc. It must be emphasized that molecular typing revealed that vCJD is different (abundant high-molecular-mass glycoform together with a relative molecular mass of 19 kDa) [48, 51]. Significant differences in glycosylation status between gPrDs and sCJD were also reported (59).

In parallel to mutations in the PRNP gene, polymorphisms are known [10, 27]. Codon 129 is the best-known influential polymorphism. Here either methionine (M) or valine (V) is encoded: individuals may be MV heterozygotes, or MM/VV homozygotes. This polymorphism influences susceptibility to disease (related to homozygosity) and also phenotypic variability. To date, all the v-CJD patients were found to be MM homozygotes, although PrPres 2b was found in spleen of a heterozygote patient who was transfused with blood products obtained from a v-CJD patient. Importantly, the codon 129 polymorphism also has a role in genetic forms, exemplified by mutation (D178N) giving FFI or gCJD clinical presentation depending on this polymorphism [60].

When combining PrPSc types 1 or 2 and PRNP codon 129 polymorphism, six sCJD phenotypes were defined previously, which represents the basis of the most frequently used disease classification [53]. Phenotypically indistinguishable, MM and MV type 1 were classified as the same group, whereas MM type 2 was divided into two (MM-2C and MM-2T) according to distinctive histopathological features (cortical or thalamic predominance, respectively). MM-2T sCJD is the molecular subtype that is also called sFI. MV-2K is clearly associated with plaque-like deposits, exhibiting ataxia and long clinical duration whereas the clinical duration of VV-2 with focal deposits is more rapid; the last and rare subtype is VV1-1 in younger patients than others sCJD correlates with focal synaptic IHC [63]. An alternative classification, taking into account three different electrophoretic mobilities of PrPSc, has also been proposed [48, 55, 64]. Experimental conditions such as pH, EDTA and copper or zinc content influence the PK activity and consequently the molecular typing [64-67]. In a recent multi-centric study operating with strict and standardized conditions of pH and EDTA concentrations for preparing brain homogenates, exact correlations were obtained with characterization of the same molecular typing by the different participants [68].

A further issue relates to the observation that PrPSc type 1 and type 2 can co-occur in the same brain, in the same region, or separately (Figure 4). This phenomenon has been reported for sporadic, iatrogenic and genetic cases [49, 57, 59, 69-71]. In a large series of sCJD, the presence of both types appears significant: 15% of the VV, 43% of the MM, 23% of the MV cases analyzed and 35% of all cases regardless of the codon 129 genotype harbour both types of PrPSc [72]. Recently, a particular ladderlike molecular pattern with lower bands ranging from 29 to 6 kDa has been detected in sporadic cases with PrD-like morphology (VPSPr) [6]. This particular PrPSc has been reported as having lower protease resistance, being in lower quantity in the brain and specifically being probed by the 1E4 rather than by the 3F4 anti-PrP antibody after PK treatment. This pattern has been associated with all the three codon 129 phenotypes [6, 7, 73-75].

It has become clear that the clinicopathologic variability of PrDs parallels that of animal diseases such as scrapie or BSE in which phenotypic heterogeneity has been related to both agent strain variation and host genetic factors. Recent progress identified four discrete transmission human PrD strains, including: M1CJD to sCJD (MM1 and MV1); V2CJD to sCJD (MV2 and VV2); V1CJD to sCJD (VV1); and M2CJD to sCJD (MM2) [76].

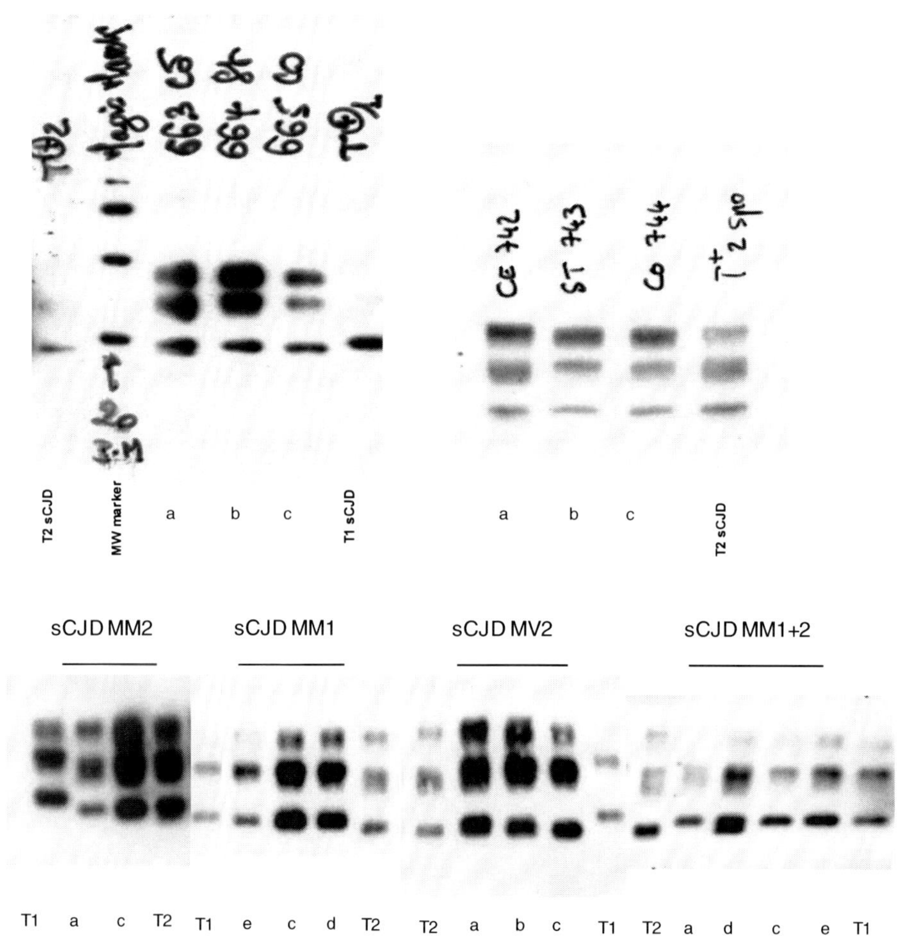

Figure 4. Demonstration of the molecular diversity of PrPres in human brain samples from individuals affected by prion disease. Immunoblot analysis of brain homogenates were obtained from patients died with a suspicion of CJD, is shown.. PK-resistant fragments of PrPSc were revealed 3F4 anti-PrP antibody. Sources of brain area homogenates are: a: cerebellum; b: striatum; c: frontal cortex; d: thalamus; e: occipital cortex. T1 control: type 1 PrPres control from sCJD; T2 control: type 2 PrPres control from sCJD. 1: PrPres type 1; 2: PrPres type 2; 1 + 2: coexistence of type 1 and type 2 in the same patient. M: Methionine; sCJD: Sporadic Creutzfeldt-Jakob disease; V: Valine; vCJD: Variant CJD. Fig 4a PrPres from different areas of a brain in a patient exhibiting E200K mutation of PRNP. We often note a particular glycosylation pattern in this E200K-gCJD, distinct of those of PrPres seen in sCJD and distinct also to the molecular signature of vCJD PrPres 2b. This particular pattern consists in a high percentage of bi glycosylated band comparatively to the 2 others and was fully described in reference 59. Fig 4b. PrPres from different areas of a brain in a vCJD patient. The characteristic molecular pattern of PrPres 2b is illustrated in all the 3 brain areas presented of one vCJD patient. Whereas sCJD and gCJD present high variability of PrPres pattern, vCJD is characterized by an unique molecular pattern. Fig 4c. PrPres from different areas of brains in different sCJD patients. Two types of molecular pattern of PrPres are shown : type 1 and type 2 depending on the MW of unglycosylated band. Variability can occur in the same patient and in the same area as it is illustrated in this figure for the patient sCJD MM1+2. Associated to codon 129 polymorphism, typing PrPres provides the basis for phenotypes classification in association with neuropathological deposits and in correlation with clinical presentation and course evolution of the disease. This classification supports the concept of prions strains.

Detecting Disease-Associated PrP in Periphery: The Future?

It is widely assumed that detection of the pathological isoforms (PrPSc) is crucial for the diagnosis. So far, the definitive diagnosis of PrD still requires neuropathologic and biochemical examination using brain tissue obtained by biopsy or after autopsy.

The major aim of different approaches is to detect PrPSc in vivo in a relatively non-invasive way by increasing sensitivity without losing specificity when detecting a low amount of PrPSc in peripheral tissue or body fluid. It has to be noticed that screening tests used for the large-scale diagnosis of animal PrD (mainly ELISA protocols) are not routinely used for human diagnosis, mostly owing to the small number of cases analyzed simultaneously; meanwhile, few of them have been adapted and validated for human diagnosis [77-78].

1. Optimisation of Biochemical Detection of Disease-Associated PrP

Different adaptations of the detection of PrP by western blot technique were developed to improve sensitivity, robustness or simplification of the process. Alternatively, others immunologic principles were also proposed. In this paragraph, we present the most principal possibilities.

Concentration of PrP

Successive centrifugation steps with detergent, high-speed cold centrifugation or ultracentrifugation with detergent of the brain homogenates prepared after PK treatment permitted selective concentration of PrPres in the pellet [79-81]. Precipitation techniques using isopropanol or polyoxometalates have also been proposed [82, 83].

Partial Purification and/or Concentration of PrPsc

In a search of precipitation procedures that preferentially act on PrPSc, sodium phosphotungstate (NaPTA) has emerged as a very sensitive technique [54, 84]. Indeed, NaPTA has been used extensively and appeared particularly useful for peripheral tissue where PrPSc is in much lower quantity than in the brain [85-87].

Different ligand molecules have been reported to bind specifically to PrPSc. Whereas blood fibrinogen was reported able to bind both PrPsc and PrPc, blood plasminogen is the first endogenous ligand to have been described to interact with PrPSc but not PrPc [88]. This natural binding appears to be dependent on the denaturating conditions of the extraction medium and is more efficient when aggregated conditions for PrPSc are performed [89]. Streptomycin has been described to interact with PrPSc with a higher affinity than for PrPc. However, PK treatment seems to be needed to concentrate the pathological form more accurately [90]. In a comparative study, streptomycin precipitation was shown to exhibit a sensitivity as high as the already well established and accepted NaPTA precipitation [91].

Another strategy was based on the screening of synthetic polymeric ligands to identify compounds having specificity for PrPSc. Designated as ‘Seprion’ ligands, they have been claimed to bind PrPSc from different species (human, bovine, small ruminant) without PK treatment. Bound on microplate wells, the ligand capturs PrPSc with comparable results to the immunometric sandwich ELISA assay on a panel of bovine brain samples [92].

The known property of PrP to bind nucleic acid has been used to select artificial ligand (aptamer) in vitro from a large randomized library of 2-fluoro-modified RNA. One of these ligands (aptamer SAF-93) had > 10-fold higher affinity for PrPSc than for recombinant PrPC [93].

Denaturation of brain homogenates with guanidine salt followed by phenol extraction has also been proposed to extract PrPSc selectively. The obtained migration pattern in WB seems to be sufficiently different between non-CJD and CJD samples, notably with bands at lower molecular mass [94].

A recent study used a new misfolded protein assay that detects PrP aggregates independently from their protease resistance and showed that, in some PrDs disease-associated PrP aggregates may conspicuously accumulate in the CNS, yet they do not appear to acquire much PK resistance [95].

Alternative Enzymatic Digestion

Although the central point in the biochemical detection is the distinction of PrPc from PrPSc, the PK resistance of PrPSc seems to be relative, as a part of PrPSc is thought to be sensitive to the protease action [6, 54, 96]. To address this issue, alternatives to PK treatment have been proposed. One uses a specific enzymatic digestion of PrPC with thermolysin. Unable to access to its cleavage site in the PrPSc, thermolysin has no activity on PrPSc and permits detection in its fulllength form [97, 98].

Specific Antibodies to PrPsc

So far, only a few anti-PrP antibodies have been claimed to be able to distinguish between PrPSc and PrPC [99-102]. Although none of them is used in routine diagnosis, possibly owing to a lack of affinity, a sandwich assay has recently been described to be efficient at detecting a low quantity of brain PrPSc spiked in human plasma [103].

Conformation-Dependent Immunoassay

Another assay able to distinguish both forms has been also proposed. The conformation-dependent immunoassay measures the relative amounts of b-sheet and a-helix content of samples. It is based on the principle that the reactivity of PrPc and PrPsc in denaturating conditions against a specific antibody is different. Fluorescence signals, linked to a europium-labeled detection antibody, are compared between a denaturated and a native portion of each sample, and allow quantification of PrPsc [54]. To increase sensitivity, a conformation-dependent immunoassay has been successfully associated with NaPTA precipitation in various tissue samples [100, 104, 105].

Protein Misfolded Cyclic Amplification (PMCA)

This technique uses a principle analogous to PCR for nucleic acid, which mimics in vitro the replication of PrPSc in vivo [106]. Samples are submitted to cycles of incubation and sonication in the presence of a large amount of PrPc, which does not amplify (theoretically) in the absence of PrPSc. One drawback of PMCA is the nature of the PrPc used as a substrate for the conversion process, which originally resulted from brain tissue. Efforts have been undertaken to replace it by recombinant PrP, to provide an automatized version of PMCA and to simplify by shifting from the sonication step to a «shaking» step.

Progress in the analytical methods has given rise to new questions about the pathophysiology of PrDs. One example is the description of partially PK-resistant PrP found in brains of patients without clinical and histological hallmarks of CJD [107]. This raises the issue of a hypothetical existence of stable intermediates of PrP in preclinical states or other PrP strains without clinical expression. Also, the recent description of VPSPr phenotype [6] raises a further question of how exactly the spectrum and incidence of disorders with alterations of the PrP can be defined.

Optimization of analytical procedures allows detection of atypical strains of human PrDs so that the public health threats from potential new forms of infectious prion disease can be investigated. It is still to be proved that sCJD MV type 2 is linked to BASE, the atypical form of BSE [108-111], or that VPSPr qualifies as a true strain.

2. What is Promising for Diagnostic Levels Using PrP Detection?

2.1. Peripheral Tissues

In addition to the brain, detection of PrPSc (and/or PrPres) has been reported in various human peripheral tissues. To understand its reliability, one must be aware of the different tissue distribution of disease-associated PrP in different etiological PrD forms [30], and furthermore, that detectability might require sophisticated biochemical methods. Some tissues were proposed as promising for routine application. Only detection of PrPsc in tonsil is used currently in suspicion of v-CJD when MRI is not possible or not contributive [31]. On the other hand, a cross-sectional opportunistic survey of tonsil tissue, and a previous one examining the appendix, suggested that the prevalence of the vCJD agent in UK may be higher than previously thought [112,113]. But, as appendicectomy seems to be more invasive than tonsillectomy, the appendix was not proposed as a routine test as tonsil for vCJD diagnosis. Based on its high sensitivity and specificity, detection in the olfactory mucosa has been also proposed [114, 115]. However, owing to its invasive approach, it is usually not applied in the clinical setting. Less invasive, skeletal muscle and peripheral nerves biopsies could be used in the future as they are currently used for myopathies and neuropathies diagnostic and that PrPsc was detected in these tissues. Effectively, skeletal muscle may harbor disease-associated PrP in vCJD as well as in sCJD (in the latter usually associated with a longer disease course) [116]. Similarly, peripheral nerves have also shown disease-associated PrP [117, 118]. However, the sensitivity is not high enough now, so that these biopsies provide added diagnostic value compared to current diagnostic procedures.

2.2. Biological fluids : CSF, Blood and Urine

CSF

Studies attempting to detect disease-associated PrP in CSF have been run since 1992 [119]. Later, a technique using microscopy and fluorescence permitted the detection of PrP aggregates in CSF, but although its specificity was excellent (100%), sensitivity was only 20% [120]. In the last 2 years, the presence of total PrP was reported in human CSF in various neurological diseases. As reported for peptides amyloid Ab1-42 levels in AD, decrease of PrP was expected in CJD. If a significant decrease of the total amount was observed among the group of neurodegenerative diseases tested (CJD, Alzheimer's disease, a synucleopathies) compared with non-degenerative and healthy controls, no significant difference was observed within the neurodegenerative group [121]. Interestingly, the codon 129 polymorphism seems to have no influence on the amount of total PrP in CSF [122]. Recently, using a PMCA derived method, called real-time quaking-induced conversion (RT-QUIC), the limit of detection of > 1 fg of PrPsc in diluted CJD brain was obtained. In a first cohort of a 30 CSF, promising results were done using RT-QUIC with sensitivity and specificity of 80 and 100 % respectively [123].

Blood

The development of most of the PrPSc blood detection techniques has been boosted in the last few years since it was reported that transfused blood from individuals incubating vCJD has transmitted infection to recipients in the UK [124-128]. The most suitable blood compartment to detect the agent should be defined, as several studies indicate that the bulk of the infectious material is in white cells, but the plasma is also clearly infectious [129, 130].

Different methods underdevelopment and validation can be mentioned.

The ELISA based technique without PK treatment developed by AMORFIX was tested in a large-scale study in plasma specimens [131]. Although the sensitivity could not be given owing to a lack of vCJD samples, specificity was evaluated as 99.9%, but further validation is in progress with a larger cohort using this test.

The second technique involves the principle of PMCA which has been improved by automation and optimized to high-efficiency detection in blood samples from experimentally affected animals [132-134]. These results open avenues for validation of this technique as a confirmatory test for PrPSc detection in human plasma.

Recently, Edgeworth and co-workers reported a solid-state binding matrix to capture and concentrate disease-associated prion proteins coupled to direct immunodetection of surface-bound material using serial and high dilutions of v-CJD brain samples but now further work is expected to develop this assay into a practical blood-screening test with increased sensitivity (in this paper 71.4%) [135].

In parallel, sensitivity and applicability of RT-QuIC method was improved for detecting PrPsc from a complex matrix as plasma using prior immunoprecipitation with 15B3 antibody. This technique, called «enhanced» QuIC (eQuIC) was able to detect near the attogram level of brain PrPrcs, improving the detection of PrPsc in plasma and serum of scrapie infected hamsters; further application to human plasma is waited [136].

Despite all efforts focusing on the tracking of vCJD agent in blood, there is still no routine test that delivers an early and specific diagnosis of human PrD. However, due to economical reasons, low incidence of PrDs and the difficulty in increasing sensitivity in a reproducible manner, for companies, there seems to be no priority anymore to develop a specific and sensitive marker for clinically typical forms of CJD. Indeed, many companies decided to abandon this research after loss of expenses.

The same and more difficult point is the issue of asymptomatic carriers of PRNP mutations. Bloodbased detection of disease-associated PrP in these carriers (genetic or vCJD agent) with lack of specificity would be very difficult to manage ethically. Detecting hallmarks in PRNP mutation carriers is a major point for two reasons: first, families of genetic PrD are highly aware of a need for preclinical detection; and second, validating tools in the preclinical state will boost the research in therapy because only those initiated before clinical symptoms may have relevant efficacy.

For suspected patients of sCJD, sensitivity seems to be more critical than specificity because the final diagnosis will be done by evaluating different investigations and probably confirmed or excluded by autopsy. Such a sensitive assay will increase safety for surgical procedures with reusable medical devices.

Urine

PrPSc-like signals were initially reported in the urine of patients with E200K gCJD [137]. The PrP signal in WB was reported as a unique band after PK treatment and concentration step of PrP in urine. In a contradictory study, this band was claimed to be unrelated to CJD, but rather would correspond to outer membrane proteins of enterobacteria [138].

Another study identified this band as an Ig-like chain in scrapie-affected hamster [139]. The authors also confirmed the presence of a PrP band in urine collected from experimental scrapie-affected hamster (263K), vCJD, sCJD and gCJD patients, whereas urine from Alzheimer's disease patients and healthy subjects were negative. Unfortunately, although the presence of this band seems to be specific in our hands, there is a lack of sensitivity because this band appears only at very late stages of the disease. Whatever the exact nature of this band, other groups confirmed the presence of infectivity in urine from scrapie-affected mice with lymphocytic nephritis or independently of the inflammatory status in a hamster model [140, 141]. Using the PMCA technique, WB identification of PrPSc in urine of hamster experimentally affected with scrapie was also observed [142]. A recent study using a bidimensional gel electrophoresis coupled with a mass spectrometry analysis of healthy human urine has proved and characterized the presence of PrP in normal urine [143].

Finally, there is no actual consensus on the usefulness of peripheral tissue or biological fluid as CSF, blood and urine to detect in routine PrPsc in suspected PrDs patients. A difficulty remains in the fact that the exact structure and localization of the disease-associated PrP in blood, CCSF and urine has not been clearly identified.

Moreover, in absence of validated routine test for the detection of PrPsc in suspected PrDs patients, we cannot assume that, whatever its excellent specificity, a biomarker representative of cerebral deposits would be enough to ensure the diagnosis. Effectively, in AD where the amyloid and Tau deposits can be present years and years before the onset of disease, the molecular pattern of AD biomarkers in CSF, hallmark of the brain deposits, was only incorporated in clinical criteria diagnosis of AD at the stage of dementia [144]. For mild cognitive impairment presentation, these biomarkers which were reported predictive of the evolution near Alzheimer dementia [145], they were only considered at this moment as research criteria [146]. Consequently, continuous efforts should be done to increase in parallel sensitivity of surrogate markers ensuring at this time the diagnosis of probability of 90 % of all PrDs cases.

Moreover, recent studies indicate that modifications of proteins such as tau, a-synuclein, TDP-43, or amyloid-beta may be found as concomitant protein depositions in most of the neurodegenerative diseases [147]. Indeed, sCJD, VPSPr, some forms of PrP amyloidosis, GSS, as well as gCJD cases may also show cooccurrence of protein depositions [5, 59, 148]. Detection of PrP and/or PrPSc could be included in the panel of systematic biomarker panel testing of neurodegenerative dementia.

POTENTIAL DEVELOPMENT OF SURROGATE MARKERS

1. New Development in Imaging

Development of functional imaging has promising implication for routine diagnostics in disease forms accumulating amyloid plaques (i.e., GSS or vCJD). In addition to methods examining the metabolism, several imaging probes have been shown to target PrP amyloid as it was developed for amyloid in AD using Pittsbirgh Compound B (PIB) [149, 150]. A recent study demonstrated that FDDNP (2-(1-{6-[(2-[F-18] fluoroethyl) (methyl) amino]-2-naphthyl} ethylidene) malononitrile) might be used to correlate clinical symptoms with amyloid load in the brain of individuals with GSS [151]. Thus, although it may be useful to understand the progression of disease or to complement other diagnostic methods in PrP amyloidoses, it seems less relevant in the evaluation of most sCJD cases, where PrP deposits in the brain do not show the amyloid tinctorial properties.

For long disease sCJD forms, introducing the thalamic hyperintense signal seen in MRI technique in the diagnostic criteria for sCJD, will increase significantly diagnosis accuracy was proposed to be included [40].

2. Biological Surrogate Markers: Others Candidates?

It has to be kept in mind that in the correct clinical context (i.e., neurodegenerative disease) specificity of p14-3-3 is the highest of all the surrogate markers. Regarding other surrogate markers in CSF, tau protein presents a comparable level of sensitivity and specificity in sCJD [24, 152-154]. In the other etiological forms, data are needed to evaluate the exact analytical performances and the added value of tau protein compared with p14-3-3. The most interesting test for the future seems to be the ratio of total tau and phosphorylated tau, due to the overlapping clinical features with atypical Alzheimer's disease and the exponential development of those tests for Alzheimer's disease diagnosis [23, 155-159]. Neuronal specific enolase (NSE), a glycolytic enzyme, and S100beta protein, a glial protein, have no added value for diagnostic use in CSF [22-24, 159]. Ubiquitin has been proposed as a new tool for CJD diagnosis after being identified in a systematic proteomic study of CSF [160]. Performances of ubiquitin are comparable to tau protein in that study, showing a sensitivity of 94% and a specificity of 97%. These preliminary results have to be confirmed on a larger scale in particular in comparison to others neurodegenerative diseases as FTLD with positive inclusions [161] and subtypes of AD exhibiting high CSF ubiquitine levels [162].

In blood and urine, no surrogate biomarker with high accuracy is available at this moment for diagnostic purpose.

CONCLUSION

PrDs are rare but fatal disorders with considerable public health implications. The central event in the pathogenesis is the conformational change of the physiological protein PrPC into the pathological conformer PrPSc. Research has helped in the understanding of the phenotypic variability indicating that combination of codon 129 and molecular type PrPSc is the major factor of phenotypic diversity [71, 76, 163, 164]. These analytical progresses would be important to define reproducible conformational differences for each human prion strain that goes beyond the type 1/type 2 distinction and can be used for diagnostic purposes.

These are also of crucial importance in predicting survival and thus are a starting point for the assessment of potential therapies [165]. Importantly, sCJD subtypes are both qualitatively and regionally distinct in the predominance of apoptosis-related proteins, confirming regional vulnerabilities of sCJD subtypes that potentially reflect distinct responses to pathogenetic events, and suggesting that cell-protective therapeutic strategies also would have to consider distinct sCJD subtypes [166].

In spite of the lack of specific tests to detect disease-associated PrP in body fluids, the added value of clinical symptoms and results of CSF p14-3-3, EEG, cranial MRI and PRNP examinations have increased the specificity and sensitivity of in vivo diagnostics.

It seems to be utopist to believe that one unique biomarker could give the accurate diagnostic with 100 % of sensitivity and specificity.

Therefore, efforts must be done in two directions. For safety problem linked to transfusion or use of invasive medical devices, developing a PrPsc blood test to reject suspected donors is a priority. For this, the most suitable blood compartment to detect the agent remains to be defined and high level of accuracy needs to be reached; a specificity of 99 % is unacceptable because a high percentage of blood donors would be excluded from donors program. For diagnostic purpose, continuous efforts should be made to increase sensitivity and specificity of surrogate markers in less common subtypes of PrDs and to develop a PrPsc biological fluid-based test in parallel ensuring specificity. Effectively, regarding atypical forms of PrDs, clinicians may lack experience with diagnosing these conditions. Future surrogate markers would be more representative of the clinical evolution of the disease, eventually being a clinical stage disease whereas PrPsc detected in the fluid or peripheral tissue would be the signature of the PrD, whatever the clinical stage. Development of systematic biomarker panels in biological fluids including neuropathological biomarkers of neurodegenerative dementia and biomarkers of the course of the disease is probably the most adequate way to resolve diagnostic problems in diseases with a high rate of neuro-degenerative co-pathology.

REFERENCES

[1] Kovacs GG, Budka H. Molecular pathology of human prion diseases. *Int J Mol Sci* 2009;10:976-99

[2] WHO. WHO manual for surveillance of human transmissible spongiform encephalopathies including variant Creutzfeldt-Jakob disease. *Geneva: WHO,* 2003

[3] European CJD Surveillance Network (EUROCJD) Total cases of CJD/GSS (deaths) and Annual Mortality Rates per Million , updated june 2010. *www.eurocjd.ed.ac.uk/surveillance* [Last accessed Sep 14, 2011]

[4] Budka H, Aguzzi A, Brown P, et al. Neuropathological diagnostic criteria for Creutzfeldt-Jakob disease (CJD) and other human spongiform encephalopathies (prion diseases). *Brain Pathol* 1995;5:459-66
[5] Ghetti B, Piccardo P, Frangione B, et al. Prion protein amyloidosis. *Brain Pathol* 1996;6:127-45
[6] Gambetti P, Dong Z, Yuan J, et al. A novel human disease with abnormal prion protein sensitive to protease. *Ann Neurol* 2008;63:697-708
[7] Zou WQ, Puoti G, Xiao X, et al. Variably protease-sensitive prionopathy: a new sporadic disease of the prion protein. *Ann Neurol* 2010;68:162-72
[8] Medori R, Tritschler HJ, LeBlanc A, et al. Fatal familial insomnia, a prion disease with a mutation at codon 178 of the prion protein gene. *N Engl J Med* 1992;326:444-9
[9] Ghetti B, Bugiani O, Tagliavini F, Piccardo P. Gerstmann-Straussler-:Scheinker disease. In: Dickson DW, editor. *Neurodegeneration: The molecular pathology of dementia and movement disorders.* Basel: ISN Neuropath Press 2003
[10] Kovacs GG, Trabattoni G Hainfellner JA, et al. Mutations of the prion protein gene phenotypic spectrum. *J Neurol* 2002;249:1567-82
[11] Beck JA, Mead S, Campbell TA, et al. Two-octapeptide repeat deletion of prion protein associated with rapidly progressive dementia. *Neurology* 2001;57:354-6
[12] Capellari S, Parchi P, Wolff BD, et al. Creutzfeldt-Jakob disease associated with a deletion of two repeats in the prion protein gene. *Neurology* 2002;59:1628-30
[13] Will RG. Acquired prion disease: iatrogenic CJD, variant CJD, kuru. *Br Med Bull* 2003;66:255-65
[14] Creutzfeldt HG. Uber eine eigenartige herdformige Erkrankung des Zentralen systems. *Z Neurol Psychiat* 1920; 57: 1-18
[15] Jakob A. Uber eigenartige Erkrankungen des central nerven systems mit bemakens wertein anatomischen Befunden. *Z Neurol Psychiat* 1921; 64 : 147-228.
[16] Will RG, Ward HJ. Clinical features of variant Creutzfeldt-Jakob disease. *Curr Top Microbiol Immunol* 2004;284:121-32
[17] Ghetti B, Dlouhy SR, Giaccone G, et al. Gerstmann-Straussler-Scheinker disease and the Indiana kindred. *Brain Pathol* 1995;5:61-75
[18] Tschampa HJ, Zerr I, Urbach H. Radiological assessment of Creutzfeldt-Jakob disease. *Eur Radiol* 2007;17:1200-11
[19] Collie DA, Summers DM, Sellar RJ, et al. Diagnosing variant Creutzfeldt-Jakob disease with the pulvinar sign: MR imaging findings in 86 neuropathologically confirmed cases. *AJNR Am J Neuroradiol* 2003;24:1560-9
[20] Kovacs GG, Horvath S, Strobel T, et al. Genetic Creutzfeldt-Jakob disease mimicking variant Creutzfeldt-Jakob disease. *J Neurol Neurosurg Psychiatry* 2009;80:1410-11
[21] Hsich G, Kenney K, Gibbs CJ, et al. The 14-3-3 brain protein in cerebrospinal fluid as a marker for transmissible spongiform encephalopathies. *N Engl J Med* 1996;335:924-30
[22] Chohan G, Pennington C, Mackenzie JM, et al. The role of cerebrospinal fluid 14-3-3 and other proteins in the diagnosis of sporadic Creutzfeldt-Jakob disease in the UK: a 10-year review. *J Neurol Neurosurg Psychiatry* 2010;81:1243-8
[23] Bahl JM, Heegaard NH, Falkenhorst G, et al. The diagnostic efficiency of biomarkers in sporadic Creutzfeldt-Jakob disease compared to Alzheimer's disease. *Neurobiol Aging* 2009;30:1834-41

[24] Sanchez-Juan P, Green A, Ladogana A, et al. CSF tests in the differential diagnosis of Creutzfeldt-Jakob disease. *Neurology* 2006;67:637-43
[25] Burkhard PR, Sanchez JC, Landis T, Hochstrasser DF. CSF detection of the 14-3-3 protein in unselected patients with dementia. *Neurology* 2001;56:1528-33
[26] Réseau national de surveillance des maladies de Creutzfeldt-Jakob et maladies apparentées ; Nombre de cas décédés certains ou probables de MCJ en France par année de signalement pour les suspicions, par année de décès pour les cas de MCJ décédés.(Last updated mai 2011) *http://www.invs.sante.fr/publications/mcj/donnees_mcj.html* [Last accessed Sep 14, 2011]
[27] Mead S. Prion disease genetics. *Eur J Hum Genet* 2006;14:273-81
[28] Capellari S, Strammiello R, Saverioni D, et al. Genetic Creutzfeldt-Jakob disease and fatal familial insomnia: insights into phenotypic variability and disease pathogenesis. *Acta Neuropathol* 2011;121:21-37
[29] Meyer RK, McKinley MP, Bowman KA, et al. Separation and properties of cellular and scrapie prion proteins. *Proc Natl Acad Sci USA* 1986;83:2310-14
[30] World Health Organization (WHO) Tables on tissue infectivity distribution in transmissible spongiform encephalopathies, updated 2010. *www.who.int/bloodproducts/* tablestissueinfectivity.pdf [Last accessed May 5, 2011]
[31] Hill AF, Butterworth RJ, Joiner S, et al. Investigation of variant Creutzfeldt-Jakob disease and other human prion diseases with tonsil biopsy samples. *Lancet* 1999;353:183-9
[32] Masters CL, Harris JO, Gajdusek DC et al. Creutzfeldt-Jakob disease: patterns of worldwide occurrence and the significance of familial and sporadic clustering. *Ann Neurol* 1979; 5: 177–88
[33] Zerr I, Pocchiari M, Collins S, et al. Analysis of EEG and CSF 14-3-3 proteins as aids to the diagnosis of Creutzfeldt-Jakob disease. *Neurology* 2000;55:811-15
[34] Collins SJ, Sanchez-Juan P, Masters CL, et al. Determinants of diagnostic investigation sensitivities across the clinical spectrum of sporadic Creutzfeldt-Jakob disease. *Brain* 2006;129:2278-87
[35] Heidenhain A. Klinische und anatomische Undersuchungen über eine eigeneratige organische Erkrangkung des Zentralnervensystems in Praesenium. *Zeitschrift für die gest Neurologie und Psychiatrie* 1929; 118 : 49-114
[36] Garcin R, Brion S, Knochneviss A. Le syndrome de Creutzfeldt-Jakob et les syndromes cortico-striés du présenium. *Revue Neurologique* 1963; 109 : 419-441
[37] Mizutani Y, Okumura A, Oda M, Shiraki H. Panencephalopathic type of Creutzfeldt-Jakob disease. *Journal of Neurology, Neurosurgery and Psychiatry* 1981; 44 : 103-115.
[38] Brownell B, Oppenheimer DR. An ataxic form of subacute presenile polioencephalopathy (Creutzfeldt-Jakob disease). *J Neurol Neurosurg Psychiat* 1965; 28 : 350-61.
[39] Meissner B, Kallenberg K, Sanchez-Juan P, et al. MRI lesion profiles in sporadic Creutzfeldt-Jakob disease. *Neurology* 2009;72:1994-2001
[40] Zerr I, Kallenberg K, Summers DM, et al. Updated clinical diagnostic criteria for sporadic Creutzfeldt-Jakob disease. *Brain* 2009;132:2659-68
[41] Sanchez-Juan P, Sanchez-Valle R, Green A, et al. Influence of timing on CSF tests value for Creutzfeldt-Jakob disease diagnosis. *J Neurol* 2007;254:901-6

[42] Kovacs GG, Puopolo M, Ladogana A,et al. Genetic prion disease: the EUROCJD experience. *Hum Genet* 2005;118:166-74
[43] Ladogana A, Sanchez-Juan P, Mitrova E, et al. Cerebrospinal fluid biomarkers in human genetic transmissible spongiform encephalopathies. *J Neurol* 2009;256:1620-8
[44] Brown P, Preece M, Brandel JP, et al. Iatrogenic Creutzfeldt-Jakob disease at the millennium. *Neurolog* 2000;55:1075-81
[45] Noguchi-Shinohara M, Hamaguchi T, Kitamoto T, et al. Clinical features and diagnosis of dura mater graft associated Creutzfeldt Jakob disease. *Neurology2007*;69:360-7
[46] Green AJ, Ramljak S, Muller WE, et al. 14-3-3 in the cerebrospinal fluid of patients with variant and sporadic Creutzfeldt-Jakob disease measured using capture assay able to detect low levels of 14-3-3 protein. *Neurosci Lett* 2002;324:57-60.
[47] Bruce ME, Fraser H. Scrapie strain variation and its implications. *Curr Top Microbiol Immunol* 1991;172:125-38
[48] Collinge J, Sidle KC, Meads J, et al. Molecular analysis of prion strain variation and the aetiology of 'new variant' *CJD. Nature* 1996;383:685-90
[49] Head MW, Bunn TJ, Bishop MT, et al. Prion protein heterogeneity in sporadic but not variant Creutzfeldt-Jakob disease: UK cases 1991-2002. *Ann Neurol* 2004;55:851-9
[50] Kascsak RJ, Rubenstein R, Merz PA, et al. Immunological comparison of scrapie-associated fibrils isolated from animals infected with four different scrapie strains. *J Virol* 1986;59:676-83
[51] Parchi P, Capellari S, Chen SG, et al.Typing prion isoforms. Nature 1997;386:232-4
[52] Parchi P, Castellani R, Capellari S, et al. Molecular basis of phenotypic variability in sporadic Creutzfeldt-Jakob disease. *Ann Neurol* 1996;39:767-78
[53] Parchi P, Giese A, Capellari S, et al.Classification of sporadic Creutzfeldt-Jakob disease based on molecular and phenotypic analysis of 300 subjects. *Ann Neurol* 1999;46:224-33
[54] Safar J, Wille H, Itri V, et al. Eight prion strains have PrP(Sc) molecules with different conformations. *Nat Med* 1998;4:1157-65
[55] Hill AF, Joiner S, Wadsworth JD, et al. Molecular classification of sporadic Creutzfeldt-Jakob disease. *Brain* 2003;126:1333-46
[56] Gambetti P, Kong Q, Zou W, et al. Sporadic and familial CJD: classification and characterisation. *Br Med Bull* 2003;66:213-39
[57] Puoti G, Giaccone G, Rossi G, et al. Sporadic Creutzfeldt-Jakob disease: co-occurrence of different types of PrP(Sc) in the same brain. *Neurology* 1999;53:2173-6
[58] Ironside JW, Ritchie DL, Head MW. Phenotypic variability in human prion diseases. *Neuropathol Appl Neurobiol* 2005;31:565-79
[59] Kovacs GG, Seguin J, Quadrio I, et al. Genetic Creutzfeldt-Jakob disease associated with the E200K mutation: characterization of a complex proteinopathy. *Acta Neuropathol* 2011;121:39-57
[60] Monari L, Chen SG, Brown P, et al. Fatal familial insomnia and familial Creutzfeldt-Jakob disease: different prion proteins determined by a DNA polymorphism. *Proc Natl Acad Sci USA* 1994;91:2839-42
[61] Hill AF, Joiner S, Beck JA, et al. Distinct glycoform ratios of protease resistant prion protein associated with PRNP point mutations. *Brain* 2006;129:676-85
[62] Parchi P, Zou W, Wang W, et al. Genetic influence on the structural variations of the abnormal prion protein. *Proc Natl Acad Sci USA* 2000;97:10168-72

[63] Parchi P, Strammiello R, Giese A, Kretzschmar H. Phenotypic variability of sporadic human prion disease and its molecular basis: past, present, and future. *Acta Neuropathol* 2011;121:91-112

[64] Wadsworth JD, Hill AF, Joiner S, et al. Strain-specific prion-protein conformation determined by metal ions.*Nat Cell Biol* 1999;1:55-9

[65] Cali I, Castellani R, Yuan J, et al. Classification of sporadic Creutzfeldt-Jakob disease revisited. *Brain* 2006;129:2266-77

[66] Notari S, Capellari S, Giese A, et al. Effects of different experimental conditions on the PrPSc core generated by protease digestion: implications for strain typing and molecular classification of CJD. *J Biol Chem* 2004;279:16797-804

[67] Zanusso G, Farinazzo A, Fiorini M, et al. pH-dependent prion protein conformation in classical Creutzfeldt-Jakob disease. *J Biol Chem* 2001;276:40377-80

[68] Parchi P, Notari S, Weber P, et al. Inter-laboratory assessment of PrP(Sc) typing in Creutzfeldt-Jakob disease: a western blot study within the neuroprion consortium. *Brain Pathol* 2009;19:384-91

[69] Cali I, Castellani R, Alshekhlee A, et al. Co-existence of scrapie prion protein types 1 and 2 in sporadic Creutzfeldt-Jakob disease: its effect on the phenotype and prion-type characteristics. *Brain* 2009;132:2643-58

[70] Schoch G, Seeger H, Bogousslavsky J, et al. Analysis of prion strains by PrPSc profiling in sporadic Creutzfeldt-Jakob disease. *PLoS Med* 2006;3:e14

[71] Uro-Coste E, Cassard H, Simon S, et al. Beyond PrP res type 1/type 2 dichotomy in Creutzfeldt-Jakob disease. *PLoS Pathog* 2008;4:e1000029

[72] Parchi P, Strammiello R, Notari S, et al. Incidence and spectrum of sporadic Creutzfeldt-Jakob disease variants with mixed phenotype and co-occurrence of PrPSc types: an updated classification. *Acta Neuropathol* 2009;118:659-71

[73] Head MW, Knight R, Zeidler M, et al. A case of protease sensitive prionopathy in a patient in the UK. *Neuropathol Appl Neurobiol* 2009;35:628-32

[74] Jansen C, Head MW, van Gool WA, et al. The first case of protease-sensitive prionopathy (PSPr) in the Netherlands: a patient with an unusual GSS-like clinical phenotype. *J Neurol Neurosurg Psychiatry* 2010;81:1052-5

[75] Rodriguez AB, Garrido JM, Zarranz JJ, et al. A novel variant of human disease with a protease-sensitive prion protein and heterozygosity methionine/valine at codon 129: Case report. *BMC Neurol* 2010;10:99

[76] Bishop MT, Will RG, Manson JC. Defining sporadic Creutzfeldt-Jakob disease strains and their transmission properties. *Proc Natl Acad Sci USA* 2010;107:12005-10

[77] Ugnon-Cafe S, Dorey A, Bilheude JM, et al. Rapid screening and confirmatory methods for biochemical diagnosis of human prion disease. *J Virol Methods* 2011; 175(2):216-23.

[78] Grassi J, Maillet S, Simon S, Morel N. Progress and limits of TSE diagnostic tools. *Vet Res* 2008;39:33

[79] Brown P, Coker-Vann M, Pomeroy K, et al. Diagnosis of Creutzfeldt-Jakob disease by western blot identification of marker protein in human brain tissue. *N Engl J Med* 1986;314:547-51

[80] Lee DC, Stenland CJ, Hartwell RC, et al. Monitoring plasma processing steps with a sensitive western blot assay for the detection of the prion protein. *J Virol Methods* 2000;84:77-89

[81] Madec JY, Groschup MH, Buschmann A, et al. Sensitivity of the western blot detection of prion protein PrPres in natural sheep scrapie. *J Virol Methods* 1998;75:169-77
[82] Grassi J, Creminon C, Frobert Y, et al. Specific determination of the proteinase K-resistant form of the prion protein using two-site immunometric assays. Application to the post-mortem diagnosis of BSE. *Arch Virol Suppl* 2000;16:197-205
[83] Lee IS, Long JR, Prusiner SB, Safar JG. Selective precipitation of prions by polyoxometalate complexes. *J Am Chem Soc* 2005;127:13802-3
[84] Wadsworth JD, Joiner S, Hill AF, et al. Tissue distribution of protease resistant prion protein in variant Creutzfeldt-Jakob disease using a highly sensitive immunoblotting assay. *Lancet* 2001;358:171-80
[85] Glatzel M, Abela E, Maissen M, Aguzzi A. Extraneural pathologic prion protein in sporadic Creutzfeldt-Jakob disease. *N Engl J Med* 2003;349:1812-20
[86] Notari S, Moleres FJ, Hunter SB, et al. Multiorgan detection and characterization of protease-resistant prion protein in a case of variant CJD examined in the United States. *PLoS One* 2010;5:e8765
[87] Peden AH, Ritchie DL, Head MW, Ironside JW. Detection and localization of PrPSc in the skeletal muscle of patients with variant, iatrogenic, and sporadic forms of Creutzfeldt-Jakob disease. *Am J Pathol* 2006;168:927-35
[88] Fischer MB, Roeckl C, Parizek P, et al. Binding of disease-associated prion protein to plasminogen. *Nature* 2000;408:479-83
[89] Shaked Y, Engelstein R, Gabizon R. The binding of prion proteins to serum components is affected by detergent extraction conditions. *J Neurochem* 2002;82:1-5
[90] Moussa A, Coleman AW, Bencsik A, et al. Use of streptomycin for precipitation and detection of proteinase K resistant prion protein (PrPsc) in biological samples. *Chem Commun* (Camb) 2006;9:973-5
[91] Quadrio I, Ugnon-Cafe S, Dupin M, et al. Rapid diagnosis of human prion disease using streptomycin with tonsil and brain tissues. *Lab Invest* 2009;89:406-13
[92] Lane A, Stanley CJ, Dealler S, Wilson SM. Polymeric ligands with specificity for aggregated prion proteins. *Clin Chem* 2003;49:1774-5
[93] Rhie A, Kirby L, Sayer N, et al. Characterization of 2¢-fluoro-RNA aptamers that bind preferentially to disease-associated conformations of prion protein and inhibit conversion. *J Biol Chem* 2003; 278: 39697-705
[94] Bastian FO, McDermott ME, Perry AS, et al. Safe method for isolation of prion protein and diagnosis of Creutzfeldt-Jakob disease. *J Virol Methods* 2005;130:133-9
[95] Polymenidou M, Prokop S, Jung HH, et al. Atypical prion protein conformation in familial prion disease with PRNP P105T mutation. *Brain* Pathol 2011;21:209-14
[96] Pastrana MA, Sajnani G, Onisko B, et al. Isolation and characterization of a proteinase K-sensitive PrPSc fraction. *Biochemistry* 2006;45:15710-17
[97] Cronier S, Gros N, Tattum MH, et al. Detection and characterization of proteinase K-sensitive disease-related prion protein with thermolysin. *Biochem J* 2008;416:297-305
[98] Owen JP, Maddison BC, Whitelam GC,Gough KC. Use of thermolysin in the diagnosis of prion diseases. *Mol Biotechnol* 2007;35:161-70
[99] Curin Serbec V, Bresjanac M, Popovic M, et al. Monoclonal antibody against a peptide of human prion protein discriminates between Creutzfeldt-Jacob's disease-affected and normal brain tissue. *J Biol Chem* 2004;279:3694-8

[100] Jones M, Wight D, McLoughlin V, et al. An antibody to the aggregated synthetic prion protein peptide (PrP106-126) selectively recognizes disease-associated prion protein (PrP(Sc)) from human brain specimens. *Brain* Pathol 2009;19:293-302

[101] Korth C, Stierli B, Streit P, et al. Prion (PrPSc)-specific epitope defined by a monoclonal antibody. *Nature* 1997;390:74-7

[102] Paramithiotis E, Pinard M, Lawton T, et al. A prion protein epitope selective for the pathologically misfolded conformation. *Nat Med* 2003;9:893-9

[103] Tattum MH, Jones S, Pal S, et al. A highly sensitive immunoassay for the detection of prion-infected material in whole human blood without the use of proteinase K. *Transfusion* 2010;50:2619-27

[104] Safar JG, Geschwind MD, Deering C, et al. Diagnosis of human prion disease. *Proc Natl Acad Sci USA* 2005;102:3501-6

[105] Safar JG, Lessard P, Tamguney G, et al. Transmission and detection of prions in feces. *J Infect Dis* 2008;198:81-9

[106] Saborio GP, Permanne B, Soto C. Sensitive detection of pathological prion protein by cyclic amplification of protein misfolding. *Nature* 2001;411:810-13

[107] Yuan J, Xiao X, McGeehan J, et al. Insoluble aggregates and protease-resistant conformers of prion protein in uninfected human brains. J Biol Chem 2006;281:34848-58

[108] Arsac JN, Biacabe AG, Nicollo J, et al. Biochemical identification of bovine spongiform encephalopathies in cattle. *Acta Neuropathol* 2007;114:509-16

[109] Casalone C, Zanusso G, Acutis P, et al. Identification of a second bovine amyloidotic spongiform encephalopathy: molecular similarities with sporadic Creutzfeldt-Jakob disease. *Proc Natl Acad Sci USA* 2004;101:3065-70

[110] Comoy EE, Casalone C, Lescoutra-Etchegaray N, et al. Atypical BSE (BASE) transmitted from asymptomatic aging cattle to a primate. *PLoS One* 2008;3:e3017

[111] Kong Q, Zheng M, Casalone C, et al. Evaluation of the human transmission risk of an atypical bovine spongiform encephalopathy prion strain. *J Virol* 2008;82:3697-701

[112] Hilton DA, Ghani AC, Conyers L, et al. Prevalence of lymphoreticular prion protein accumulation in UK tissue samples. *J Pathol* 2004;203:733-9

[113] Clewley JP, Kelly CM, Andrews N, et al. Prevalence of disease related prion protein in anonymous tonsil specimens in Britain: cross sectional opportunistic survey. *BMJ* 2009;338:b1442

[114] Tabaton M, Monaco S, Cordone MP, et al. Prion deposition in olfactory biopsy of sporadic Creutzfeldt-Jakob disease. *Ann Neurol* 2004;55:294-6

[115] Zanusso G, Ferrari S, Cardone F, et al. Detection of pathologic prion protein in the olfactory epithelium in sporadic Creutzfeldt-Jakob disease. *N Engl J Med* 2003;348:711-19

[116] Krasemann S, Neumann M, Geissen M, et al. Preclinical deposition of athological prion protein in muscle of experimentally infected primates. *PLoS One* 2010;5:e13906

[117] Favereaux A, Quadrio I, Perret-Liaudet A, et al. Prion protein accumulation involving the peripheral nervous system in a sporadic case of Creutzfeldt-Jakob disease. *Neuropathol Appl Neurobiol* 2003;29:602-5

[118] Favereaux A, Quadrio I, Vital C, et al. Pathologic prion protein spreading in the peripheral nervous system of a patient with sporadic Creutzfeldt-Jakob disease. *Arch Neurol* 2004;61:747-50

[119] Tagliavini F, Prelli F, Porro M, et al. A soluble form of prion protein in human cerebrospinal fluid: implications for prion-related encephalopathies. *Biochem Biophys Res Commun* 1992;184:1398-404
[120] Bieschke J, Giese A, Schulz-Schaeffer W, et al. Ultrasensitive detection of pathological prion protein aggregates by dual-color scanning for intensely fluorescent targets. *Proc Natl Acad Sci USA* 2000;97:5468-73
[121] Meyne F, Gloeckner SF, Ciesielczyk B, et al. Total prion protein levels in the cerebrospinal fluid are reduced in patients with various neurological disorders. *J Alzheimers Dis* 2009;17:863-73
[122] Schmitz M, Schlomm M, Hasan B, et al. Codon 129 polymorphism and the E200K mutation do not affect the cellular prion protein isoforms composition in the cerebrospinal fluid from patients with Creutzfeldt-Jakob disease. *Eur J Neurosci* 2010;31:2024-31
[123] Atarashi R, Satoh K, Sano K et al.Ultrasensitive human prion detection in CSF by real-time quaking-induced conversion. *Nat Med.* 2011 Feb;17(2):175-8.
[124] Hewitt PE, Llewelyn CA, Mackenzie J, Will RG. Three reported cases of variant Creutzfeldt-Jakob disease transmission following transfusion of labile blood components. *Vox Sang* 2006;91:348
[125] HPA. Fourth case of variant CJD infection associated with blood transfusion. [Press release] 2007 2007 01 17 [cited January 2007]; Available from: *http://www.hpa.org.uk/Topics/* InfectiousDiseases/InfectionsAZ/ CreutzfeldtJakobDisease/ VariantCJDAndBlood/ [Last accessed May 5, 2011]
[126] Llewelyn CA, Hewitt PE, Knight RS, et al. Possible transmission of variant Creutzfeldt-Jakob disease by blood transfusion. *Lancet* 2004;363:417-21
[127] Peden AH, Head MW, Ritchie DL, et al. Preclinical vCJD after blood transfusion in a PRNP codon 129 heterozygous patient. *Lancet* 2004;364:527-9
[128] Wroe SJ, Pal S, Siddique D, et al. Clinical presentation and pre-mortem diagnosis of variant Creutzfeldt-Jakob disease associated with blood transfusion: a case report. *Lancet* 2006;368:2061-7
[129] Brown P. Blood infectivity, processing and screening tests in transmissible spongiform encephalopathy. *Vox Sang* 2005;89:63-70
[130] Brown P, Cervenakova L, Diringer H. Blood infectivity and the prospects for a diagnostic screening test in Creutzfeldt-Jakob disease. *J Lab Clin Med* 2001;137:5-13
[131] Guntz P, Walter C, Schosseler P, et al. Feasibility study of a screening assay that identifies the abnormal prion protein PrPTSE in plasma: initial results with 20,000 samples. *Transfusion* 2010;50:989-95
[132] Castilla J, Saa P, Soto C. Detection of prions in blood. *Nat Med* 2005;11:982-5 107.
[133] Saa P, Castilla J, Soto C. Presymptomatic detection of prions in blood. *Science* 2006;313:92-4
[134] Saa P, Castilla J, Soto C. Ultra-efficient replication of infectious prions by automated protein misfolding cyclic amplification. *J Biol Chem* 2006;281:35245-52
[135] Edgeworth JA, Farmer M, Sicilia A, et al. Detection of prion infection in variant Creutzfeldt-Jakob disease: a blood-based assay. *Lancet* 2011;377:487-93
[136] Orrú CD, Wilham JM, Raymond LD et al. Prion disease blood test using immunoprecipitation and improved quaking-induced conversion. *MBio.* 2011 May 10;2(3):e00078-11

[137] Shaked GM, Shaked Y, Kariv-Inbal Z, et al. A protease-resistant prion protein isoform is present in urine of animals and humans affected with prion diseases. *J Biol Chem* 2001;276:31479-82

[138] Furukawa H, Doh-ura K, Okuwaki R, et al. A pitfall in diagnosis of human prion diseases using detection of protease-resistant prion protein in urine. Contamination with bacterial outer membrane proteins. *J Biol Chem* 2004;279:23661-7

[139] Serban A, Legname G, Hansen K, et al. Immunoglobulins in urine of hamsters with scrapie. *J Biol Chem* 2004;279:48817-20

[140] Gregori L, Kovacs GG, Alexeeva I, et al. Excretion of transmissible spongiform encephalopathy infectivity in urine. *Emerg Infect Dis* 2008;14:1406-12

[141] Seeger H, Heikenwalder M, Zeller N, et al. Coincident scrapie infection and nephritis lead to urinary prion excretion. *Science* 2005;310:324-6

[142] Gonzalez-Romero D, Barria MA, Leon P, et al. Detection of infectious prions in urine. *FEBS Lett* 2008;582:3161-6

[143] Dagdanova A, Ilchenko S, Notari S, et al. Characterization of the prion protein in human urine. *J Biol Chem* 2010;285:30489-95

[144] McKhann GM, Knopman DS, Chertkow H, et al. The diagnosis of dementia due to Alzheimer's disease: recommendations from the National Institute on Aging-Alzheimer's Association workgroups on diagnostic guidelines for Alzheimer's disease. *Alzheimers Dement.* 2011 May;7(3):263-9

[145] Mattsson N, Zetterberg H, Hansson O et al. CSF biomarkers and incipient Alzheimer disease in patients with mild cognitive impairment. *JAMA.* 2009 Jul 22;302(4):385-93.

[146] Albert MS, DeKosky ST, Dickson D. et al. The diagnosis of mild cognitive impairment due to Alzheimer's disease: Recommendations from the National Institute on Aging and Alzheimer's Association workgroup. *Alzheimer's & Dementia* - (2011) 1–10

[147] Kovacs GG, Botond G, Budka H. Protein coding of neurodegenerative dementias: the neuropathological basis of biomarker diagnostics. *Acta Neuropathol* 2010;119:389-408

[148] Head MW, Lowrie S, Chohan G, et al. Variably protease-sensitive prionopathy in a PRNP codon 129 heterozygous UK patient with co-existing tau, alpha synuclein and Abeta pathology. *Acta Neuropathol* 2010;120: 821-3

[149] Klunk, W.E., Engler H, Nordberg A. et al, Imaging brain amyloid in Alzheimer's disease with Pittsburgh Compound-B. *Ann Neurol* 2004; 55: 306-19

[150] Ishikawa K, Doh-ura K, Kudo Y, et al. Amyloid imaging probes are useful for detection of prion plaques and treatment of transmissible spongiform encephalopathies. *J Gen Virol* 2004; 85:1785-90

[151] Kepe V, Ghetti B, Farlow MR, et al. PET of brain prion protein amyloid in Gerstmann-Straussler-Scheinker disease. *Brain Pathol* 2010;20: 419-30

[152] Otto M, Wiltfang J, Cepek L, et al. Tau protein and 14-3-3 protein in the differential diagnosis of Creutzfeldt-Jakob disease. *Neurology* 2002; 58:192-7

[153] Van Everbroeck B, Quoilin S, Boons J, et al. A prospective study of CSF markers in 250 patients with possible Creutzfeldt-Jakob disease. *J Neurol Neurosurg Psychiatry* 2003; 74:1210-14

[154] Wang GR, Gao C, Shi Q, et al. Elevated levels of tau protein in cerebrospinal fluid of patients with probable Creutzfeldt-Jakob disease. *Am J Med Sci* 2010; 340: 291-5

[155] Riemenschneider M, Wagenpfeil S, Vanderstichele H, et al. Phospho-tau/ total tau ratio in cerebrospinal fluid discriminates Creutzfeldt-Jakob disease from other dementias. *Mol Psychiatry* 2003; 8:343-7
[156] Goodall CA, Head MW, Everington D, et al. Raised CSF phospho-tau concentrations in variant Creutzfeldt-Jakob disease: diagnostic and pathological implications. *J Neurol Neurosurg Psychiatry* 2006;77: 89-91
[157] Skinningsrud A, Stenset V, Gundersen AS, Fladby T. Cerebrospinal fluid markers in Creutzfeldt-Jakob disease. *Cerebrospinal Fluid Res* 2008;5:14
[158] Satoh K, Shirabe S, Eguchi H, et al. 14-3-3 protein, total tau and phosphorylated tau in cerebrospinal fluid of patients with Creutzfeldt-Jakob disease and neurodegenerative disease in Japan. *Cell Mol Neurobiol* 2006;26:45-52
[159] Baldeiras IE, Ribeiro MH, Pacheco P, et al. Diagnostic value of CSF protein profile in a portuguese population of sCJD patients. *J Neurol* 2009; 256: 1540-50
[160] Steinacker P, Rist W, Swiatek-de-Lange M, et al. Ubiquitin as potential cerebrospinal fluid marker of Creutzfeldt-Jakob disease. Proteomics 2010;10: 81-9
[161] Cairns NJ, Neumann M, Bigio EH et al. TDP-43 in familial and sporadic frontotemporal lobar degeneration with ubiquitin inclusions. *Am J Pathol.* 2007 Jul;171(1):227-40.
[162] Iqbal K, Flory M, Khatoon S, Soininen H et al. I.Subgroups of Alzheimers disease based on cerebrospinal fluid molecular markers. *Ann Neurol.* 2005 Nov;58(5):748-57.
[163] Jones M, Peden AH, Wight D, et al. Effects of human PrPSc type and PRNP genotype in an in-vitro conversion assay. *Neuroreport* 2008;19:1783-6
[164] Parchi P, Cescatti M, Notari S, et al. Agent strain variation in human prion disease: insights from a molecular and pathological review of the national institutes of health series of experimentally transmitted disease. *Brain* 2010;133:3030-42
[165] Pocchiari M, Puopolo M, Croes EA, et al. Predictors of survival in sporadic Creutzfeldt-Jakob disease and other human transmissible spongiform encephalopathies. Brain 2004; 127: 2348-59
[166] Kovacs GG, Budka H. Distribution of apoptosis-related proteins in sporadic Creutzfeldt-Jakob disease. Brain Res 2010; 1323:192-9

In: Prions and Prion Diseases: New Developments ISBN: 978-1-62100-027-3
Editor: Jean-Michel Verdier © 2012 Nova Science Publishers, Inc.

Chapter 9

ANTI-PRION STRATEGIES FOR IN VIVO GENE THERAPY ASSAYS

Véronique Perrier, Thibaut Imberdis and Adeline Ayrolles-Torro
Université Montpellier, Montpellier,
Montpellier, France; EPHE, Paris, France

ABSTRACT

Recent studies have reported variant Creutzfeldt-Jakob disease (vCJD) cases resulting from transfusion of prion-contaminated blood, raising concerns about the safety of blood product, as well as the possibility of a second epidemic of vCJD. Since classical drug therapies were unsuccessful to identify a treatment to cure prion diseases, the searches of radically different strategies were undertaken by many researchers. With the advent of the techniques of molecular biology and cell biology, several gene therapy approaches have been explored based on the use of siRNA to shut down PrP^{C} expression, or prion antagonists to block the conversion process, as well as anti-PrP antibodies exhibiting inhibitory effect. In this chapter book, we will summarize and compare the various *in vivo* assays that were recently published in the literature and will discuss the data. The scientific repercussions of these works will benefit to other neurodegenerative disorders including Alzheimer's, Huntington's and Parkinson's diseases which share many common features with prion diseases.

INTRODUCTION

Prion diseases are neurodegenerative disorders that have the unique particularity of being both sporadic, transmissible and inherited diseases through genetic mutation in the prion protein gene, *PRNP*. Clinically, patients are affected with dementia, ataxia, motor coordination troubles that invariably lead to death of affected persons. Pathologically, they are characterized by spongiform degeneration of the brain due to neuronal loss, astrocytic gliosis and abnormal PrP aggregates throughout the brain. The hallmark of prion diseases is the deposition in the brain of PrP^{Sc}, an abnormal β-sheet-rich form of the cellular PrP (PrP^{C}) [1]. Many lines of evidences suggest that these diseases are propagated by a misfolded conformer, PrP^{Sc} that can trigger the autocatalytic conversion of a normal prion protein PrP^{C} into PrP^{Sc}. This conversion process involves several PrP^{Sc} pre-amyloid intermediates, generated through a complex mechanism of oligomerization [2-4], followed by the self-assembling of PrP^{Sc} oligomers into proto-fibrils, which in turn grow into amyloid fibrils (Figure 1). The nature of the agent responsible of neurotoxicity in prion diseases is not clearly established. Currently the hypothesis is in favor of soluble PrP oligomers rather than amyloid fibrils, and this concept was largely extended to other neurodegenerative disorders (soluble Aβ oligomers). The different species implicated in the conversion process of prions can, therefore, be specific target for therapeutic interventions (Figure 1). From this point, few gene therapy approaches have been developed that target the different protagonists of the prion replication cycle. In this review, we will precisely describe the major experiments performed in the field and discuss the results.

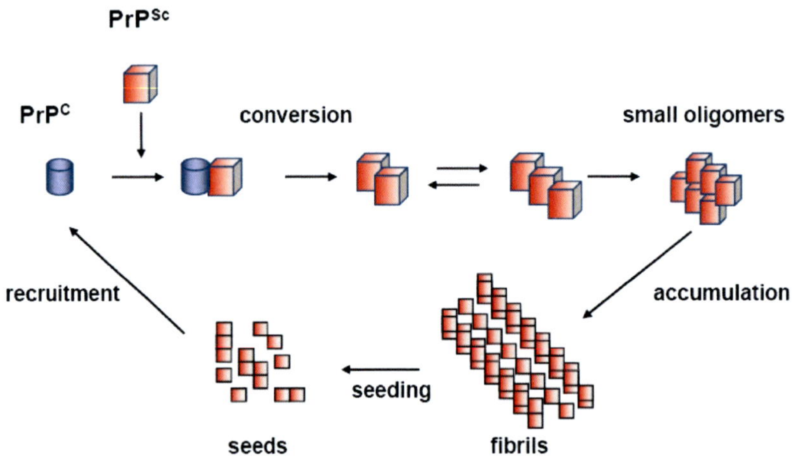

Figure 1.

Depleting PrP^{C} with siRNA: An Approach to Remove the Key Substrate Essential for Conversion and Formation of Neurotoxic Prion Species

One of the most obvious strategies in the gene therapy field has consisted to suppress the PrP^{C} protein, the essential provisioning source for prion replication and their propagation. Indeed, several studies performed on PrP knockout mice have demonstrated that those animals were resistant to prion disease and unable to replicate the infectious agent [5-7]. Besides, ablation of the *Prnp* gene in embryonic mice or adult-onset PrP knockout mice [8], is well tolerated *in vivo* and did not exhibit deleterious effects, suggesting that treatment based on suppression of the PrP^{C} function would not have deleterious effects. Studies of engraftment of $PrP^{+/+}$ neuronal tissue into the brain of $PrP^{0/0}$ mice have showed that only the graft is able to allow replication of prions, and exhibit PrP^{Sc} deposits [9]. Thus, PrP^{Sc} only produces toxicity and cell death, where PrP^C is also expressed. Altogether, these PrP shut down experiments have demonstrated the proof of principle in term of therapeutic potential, but the direct therapeutic effect was still not shown, until the studies conducted by White et al. [10].

In this article, bilateral hippocampal injections of LV-MW1 lentiviral vector expressing siRNA were performed into the brain of Tg37 mice. The tested protocol targets the asymptomatic phase of the disease, and especially a short therapeutic window spanning from 50-60 days where PrP^{Sc} deposits start to accumulate in the brain of Tg37 mice (Table 1). Mice treated with LV-MW1 expressing siRNA survived significantly longer (mean survival time 105 ± 4 days) compared to CTR group treated with empty virions LV-empty (mean 88 ± 3 days) or untreated prion-infected mice (mean 85 ± 3 days). This prolonged survival showed an increase of the survival time of about 23 % in ΨLV-MW1 treated mice compared with untreated animals (Table 1). Neuropathological examinations on brains from each group of mice selected when animals developed clinical signs at terminal stage of prion diseases revealed substantial differences in term of brain spongiosis and PrP^{Sc} deposition. In the hippocampus area, expression of RNAi consecutive to lentiviral injection is neuroprotective. Indeed, quantification based on systematic neuronal counts showed 60% more CA1 pyramidal cells in the brain of ΨLV-MW1 treated mice compared with ΨLV-empty treated animals. Animals withRNAi-mediated PrP knockdown exhibit a mild spongiosis in the hippocampus area whereas LV-Empty-treated mice showed with severe spongiosis. Hippocampal PrP^{Sc} accumulation was also reduced in LV-MW1-treated mice compared to control group treated with ΨLV-Empty virions. In summary, administration of virions expressing siRNA in both hippocampus, is enough to prolong the lifespan of prion-infected animals significantly and prevent the transduced neurons from neurodegeneration. In this article, the strategy aiming to slow down the rate of prion replication by reducing PrP^C levels, is thus valuable to limit prion propagation and neurodegeneration.

Prion Antagonists with Dominant Negative Effect to Inhibit Conversion Process: Natural Polymorphysm PrPQ167R and Soluble Dimeric PrP-Fc2

Natural Polymorphysms

Several audacious approaches were also developed in the gene therapy field that were based on the observation that "prion-resistant" polymorphysms naturally exist in sheep and humans. For instance, polymorphysm ARR/ARR at codon 136, 154 and 171 in sheep has a protective effect and prevent prion propagation in flocks, by opposition to ARQ/VRQ polymorphysm that favours prion infection [11, 12]. Humans heterozygous for a common polymorphysm at codon 129 are largely protected from CJD. In addition, the heterozygous polymorphism E/K at codon 218 in the Japanese population prevents from sporadic Creutzfeldt-Jacob disease [13]. Kaneko et al. (1997) introduced the Q171R sheep mutation and E219K human mutation in the mouse *Prnp* gene (MoPrPQ167R and MoPrPQ218K respectively). Molecular studies on prion-infected cells showed that these mutated PrPs could not be converted into the abnormal PrP^{Sc} isoforms and significantly, they also inhibit the conversion of wild-type (wt) PrP^C into PrP^{Sc} [14]. The substitution Q167R and Q218K in MoPrP were therefore described as "dominant negative" mutants because they block the replication of their wild-type counterparts. These dominant negative inhibition effects were analysed in transgenic mice by Perrier et al. [15]. Result showed that transgenic animals carrying PrP with Q167R or Q218K substitutions on a $Prnp^{-/-}$ background were unable to replicate and propagate prion diseases [15]. When wtPrP gene was re-inserted by back crossing in transgenic animals, the conversion of wt PrP^C into PrP^{Sc} was dramatically slowed down compared to non transgenic animals on a $Prnp^{+/+}$ background. The dominant negative effect seemed to depend on the ratio of the mutated PrP molecules produced by the transgene and the endogeneous wt PrP molecules. These transgenic experiments demonstrate the relevance of the dominant negative mutant but because they are not directly applicable in gene therapy, it was necessary to develop vectors for their in vivo delivery.

Table 1. Post-exposure prophylactic treatment using a lentiviral vector carrying shRNA. Treatment was administered in both hemispheres of mice, and during a short therapeutic window ranging from 52-58 days p.i. with prions (10)

Schema of the therapeutic protocol assayed in Tg37 mice

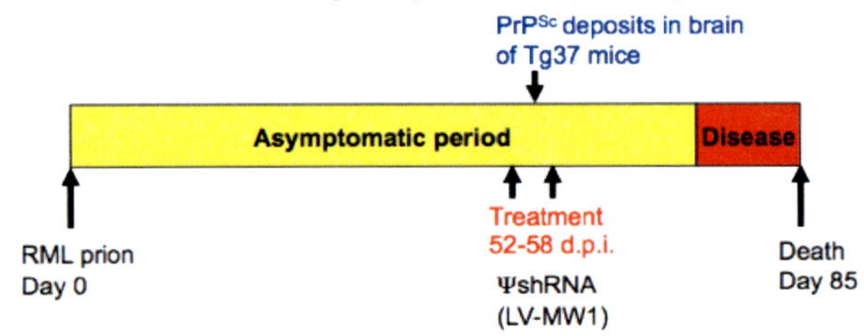

Prion antagonist	Vector and quantity	Animal model	Prion doses	Survival time versus CTR group (%)
-	-	Tg37 mice - CTR group (n=18)	RML prion strain	85 ± 3 days
LV-empty	Lentivirus : ΨGFP 2 x10^6 I.U. in 2 µl/side	Tg37 mice - CTR group (n=18)	RML prion strain	88 ± 3 days no delay
LV-MW1	Lentivirus : ΨshRNA 2 x10^6 I.U. in 2 µl/side	Tg37 mice treated group (n=22)	RML prion strain	105 ± 4 days +19% delay

Crozet et al. [16] were the first in the prion field to develop lentiviral gene transfer tools for their application in gene and cell therapy approaches to prion diseases [16]. Indeed, lentiviral vectors carrying the MoPrPQ167R or MoPrPQ218K mutants were able to abolish endogeneous $wtPrP^{Sc}$ replication in chronically prion-infected N2a58/22L cells. In addition, injection of virion preparations into mice by intracerebral route, demonstrate that the lentiviral vectors can transduce post-mitotic cells such as neurons mainly in the vicinity of the injection site. Following systemic lentiviral injections, expression of delivered genes was observed mainly in the blood vessels of the spleen, which is somehow pertinent since this structure is innervated by the peripheric autonomous nervous system implicated in the neuroinvasion process of prion agent [16].

Table 2. Post-exposure prophylatic treatment using a lentiviral vector carrying a prion antagonist, the PrPQ167R, administered at 35 or 105 days p.i. with prions (17)

Schema of the therapeutic protocol assayed in C57Bl/6 mice

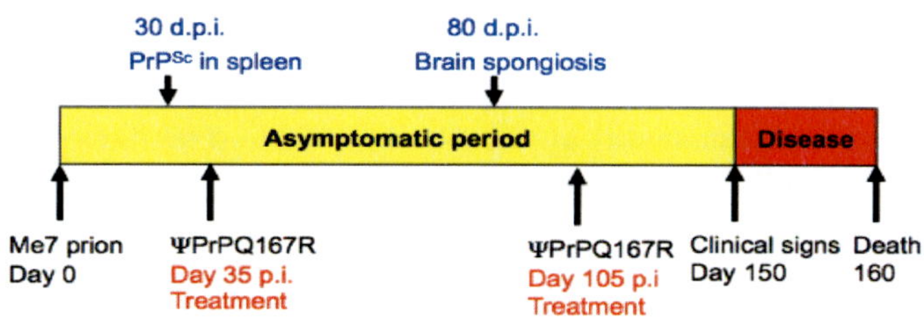

Prion antagonist	Vector and quantity	Animal model	Prion doses	Survival time versus CTR group (%)
- Single injection of lentivirus administered at 35 days post infection with prions				
PBS	-	C57BL/6 mice - CTR group (n=13)	Me7 prion strain 2.10^5 LD_{50}	157 ± 0.9 days
GFP	Lentivirus : ΨGFP 2 x10^5 I.U. in 5 μl	C57BL/6 mice - CTR group (n=5)	Me7 prion strain 2.10^5 LD_{50}	158 ± 0.9 days
PrPQ167R	Lentivirus : ΨPrPQ167R 2 x10^5 I.U. in 5 μl	C57BL/6 mice treated group (n=5)	Me7 prion strain 2.10^5 LD_{50}	176 ± 0.2 days +12% delay
- Single injection of lentivirus administered at 105 days post infection with prions				
PrPQ167R	Lentivirus : ΨPrPQ167R 2 x10^5 I.U. in 5 μl	C57BL/6 mice treated group (n=4)	Me7 prion strain 2.10^5 LD_{50}	166 ± 0.6 days +6% delay

To evaluate *in vivo* the possible therapeutic effect of dominant negative virions, Toupet *et al.* [17] have administered the treatment at two different stages: at 35 days post-infection (p.i.) with prions, which is the beginning of the neuroinvasion of the central nervous system (CNS), and at 105 days p.i., once the brain tissues are already damaged, corresponding to a very late treatment (Table 2). Mice treated with virions ΨPrPQ167R at 35 days p.i. exhibited an increase of the survival time of 12% which is statistically significant from the PBS or ΨGFP treated controls. Interestingly the group of mice treated at 105 days p.i. seemed also to have a delay of about 9 days (6%). To enhance protection, Toupet *et al.* [17] have implemented a system of guide cannula implantation to allow chronic injections into the brain (Table 3). Based on the previous assays with single injections, the chronic treatment was administered at 80 and 95 days p.i. both because: (*i*) it corresponds to the beginning of the spongiosis in mice brain; (ii) the expression of PrPQ167R protein after virions integration in cells is stable during 2 months, allowing the presence of the dominant negative molecules in the mice brain up to the terminal stage of the disease. After only 2 injections, the mean survival of the ΨPrPQ167R treated mice was extended by 30 days (20%), accompanied by substantial improvement in behaviour (Table 3). This delay was correlated with a strong reduction of spongiosis in the ipsilateral side of the brain compared to the contralateral side. Histological examinations of brain tissue sections of ΨPrPQ167R treated animals killed at the terminal stage of the disease, revealed that the number of vacuoles in the treated side was 3 times less important than in the contralateral side. Besides, the total vacuolar area was strongly reduced by a factor of 20. A remarkable decrease in astrocytic gliosis was also observed not only, in brain tissue sections close to the site of injection, but also in the contralateral side, suggesting that expression of the PrPQ167R proteins contribute to reduce the inflammation process in the brain. Together these results demonstrate that combination of dominant negative lentiviral vectors and chronic injections into mice brain allow partial neuroprotection and increase lifespan of animals.

Table 3. Lentiviral treatment was applied twice at 80 and 95 days p.i. with prions, via a cannula implanted into mice brain (17)

Schema of the therapeutic protocol assayed in C57Bl/6 mice

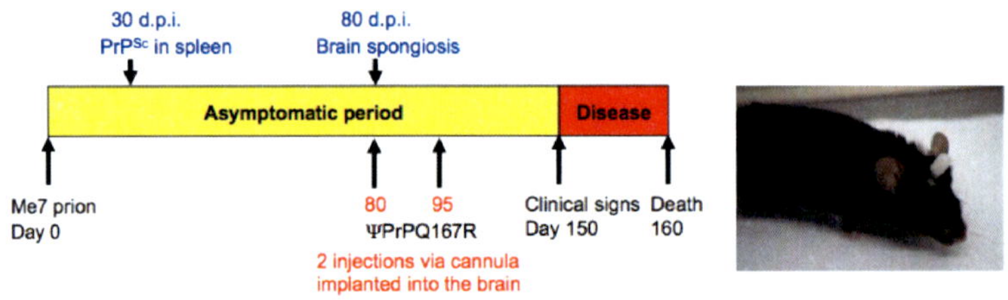

Prion antagonist	Vector and quantity	Animal model	Prion doses	Survival time versus CTR group (%)
PBS	-	C57BL/6 mice - CTR group (n=13)	Me7 prion strain 2.10^5 LD_{50}	157 ± 0.9 days
GFP	Lentivirus : 2 times ΨGFP 2 x10^5 I.U. in 5 μl	C57BL/6 mice - CTR group (n=5)	Me7 prion strain 2.10^5 LD_{50}	164 ± 3 days non significatif
PrPQ167R	Lentivirus : 2 times ΨPrPQ167R 2 x10^5 I.U. in 5 μl	C57BL/6 mice treated group (n=5)	Me7 prion strain 2.10^5 LD_{50}	187 ± 2 days +20% delay

Synthetic Antagonist with Dominant Negative Effect: PrP-Fc2

Another interesting gene therapy approach developed by Genoud et al. [18] was based on the generation of a synthetic antagonist named PrP-Fc2, corresponding to 2 PrP^C molecules fused by an immunoglobulin Fcγ domain. Initially the Fcγ tail served multiple purposes: (*i*) ligand dimerization which may enhance its avidity for interacting partner; (*ii*) a convenient tag for protein purification; and (*iii*) an increased stability in body fluids for active immunization or therapeutic purpose. Surprisingly, the PrP-Fc2 fusion protein exhibited a "dominant negative" inhibitory effect, by competing with PrP^C for PrP^{Sc} interaction. Transgenic animals expressing the PrP-Fc2 constructs survived longer to prion infection by increasing the asymptomatic phase of the disease [19]. The high solubility and stability of PrP-Fc2 construct, incited Genoud et al. [18] to clone it into a lentiviral vector, in order to investigate whether sustained intracerebral expression of PrP-Fc2 inhibit prion replication *in vivo*. Two protocols were conducted: (*i*) a pre-exposure assay where PrP-Fc2 were first injected to mice during 20 days before prion infection; and (*ii*) a post-exposure treatment where PrP-Fc2 was administered either at 30 or 121 days p.i. Best therapeutic effects were obtained with the pre-exposure prophylactic treatment where ΨPrP-Fc2-treated mice showed an increase of the survival time up to 40 % (Table 4). This remarkable effect seemed due to a combination of a lower dose of prion used for inoculation ($3x10^2$ LD_{50}, usually the dose is higher about $2x10^5$ LD_{50}), a tremendous dose of virions ($1.5x10^9$ T.U. compared to $2x10^5$ for the study by Toupet et al. [17], and $2x10^6$ for the study by White et al. [10]), and pre-exposure treatment. However, the enthusiasm for this result is diminished since one can regret the lack of a control group of mice injected with an equivalent dose of ΨGFP virions to evaluate the influence of such high dose on the progression of the prion disease (Table 4). In the experiments where mice were treated with ΨGFP after prion exposure, the high variations observed in the incubation time reinforce our interrogation on this particular point (Table 5).

In the post-exposure prophylactic assays, the protocol applied is comparable to the 2 other previous gene therapy strategies described above (Table1-3). Mice treated with ΨPrP-Fc2 at 30 days p.i. showed a moderate prolonged lifespan of 15%, although the quantity of virions administered is 1000-10000 times more important than in the 2 other studies described above (Table 5). The group of C57Bl/6 mice treated with ΨPrP-Fc2 at 121 days p.i. did not show any difference in their lifespan, compared to control group treated with ΨGFP (Table 5). Terminally sick mice from both groups showed similar PrP^{Sc} accumulation in their brains. Altogether these results showed that lentiviral vectors delivering soluble dimeric PrP-Fc2 antagonist are more efficient in pre-exposure than in post-exposure treatment, suggesting that a better neuroprotective effect is achieved when dimeric PrP-Fc2 is already present in the organism before prion replication.

Table 4. Pre-exposure prophylatic treatment using a lentiviral vector carrying a prion antagonist, the soluble dimeric PrP-Fc2 (18)

Schema of the therapeutic protocol assayed in C57Bl/6 mice

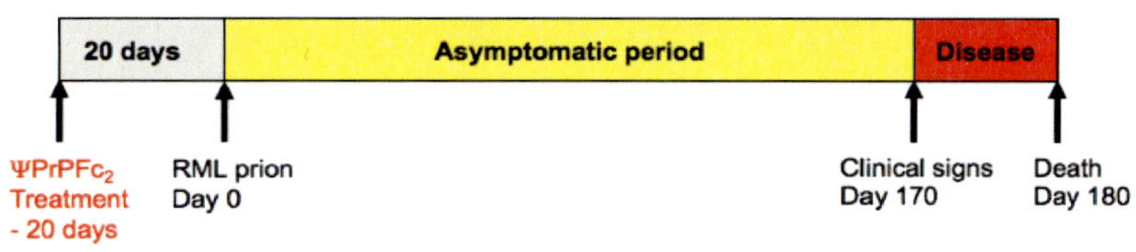

Prion antagonist	Vector and quantity	Animal model	Prion doses	Survival time versus CTR group (%)
PBS	-	C57BL/6 mice - CTR group (n=4)	RML prion strain 3.10^2 LD50	177 ± 8 days
Soluble dimeric PrP-Fc2	Lentivirus : ΨPrP-Fc2 $3x10^8$ I.U. in 5 μl	C57BL/6 mice - Treated group (n=4)	RML prion strain 3.10^2 LD50	213 ± 6 days +20% delay
Soluble dimeric PrP-Fc2	Lentivirus : ΨPrP-Fc2 $1.5x10^9$ I.U. in 30 μl	C57BL/6 mice - Treated group (n=3)	RML prion strain 3.10^2 LD50	247 ± 8 days +40% delay

Table 5. Post-exposure prophylatic treatment using a lentiviral vector carrying a prion antagonist, the soluble dimeric PrP-Fc2, administered at 30 or 121 days p.i. with prions (18)

Schema of the therapeutic protocol assayed in C57Bl/6 mice

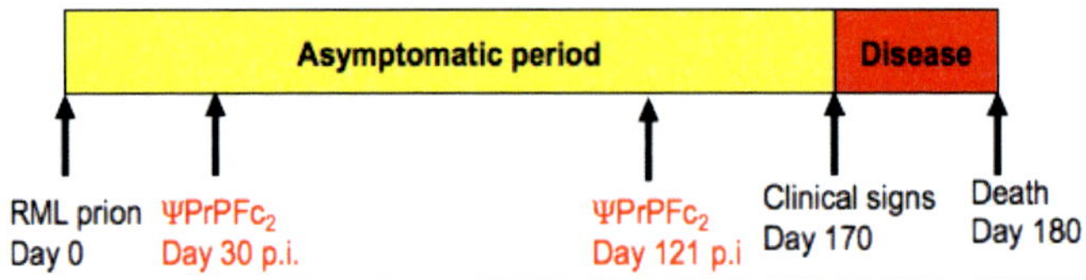

Prion antagonist	Vector and quantity	Animal model	Prion doses	Survival time versus CTR group (%)
- Lentivirus administered at 30 days post infection with prions				
GFP-Fc	Lentivirus : ΨGFP-Fc 0.8 x10^9 I.U. in 5 µl	C57BL/6 mice - CTR group (n=6)	RML prion strain 3.10^2 LD50	163 ± 4 days
Soluble dimeric PrP-Fc2	Lentivirus : ΨPrP-Fc2 1.5x10^9 I.U. in 30 µl	C57BL/6 mice treated group (n=7)	RML prion strain 3.10^2 LD50	188 ± 11 days +15% delay
- Lentivirus administered at 121 days post infection with prions				
GFP-Fc	Lentivirus : ΨGFP-Fc 0.8 x10^9 I.U. in 5 µl	C57BL/6 mice - CTR group (n=7)	RML prion strain 3.10^2 LD50	197 ± 17 days
Soluble dimeric PrP-Fc2	Lentivirus : ΨPrP-Fc2 1.5x10^9 I.U. in 30 µl	C57BL/6 mice treated group (n=8)	RML prion strain 3.10^2 LD50	197 ± 9 days no delay

Anti-PrP Antibodies with Anti-Prion Effects for Gene Therapy

The potential of therapeutic antibodies for the treatment or prevention of prion diseases has been intensively investigated the last 10 years. By preventing the binding of PrPC to molecules essential for the conversion process, Peretz et al. hypothesized that anti-PrP antibodies could inhibit prions replication. They identified two recombinant prion protein-specific Fabs, D18 and D13, which not only inhibit PrPSc formation but also clear ScN2a cells of their prion infectivity [20]. In the meantime, the monoclonal anti-PrP antibody 6H4 which recognized epitope 144-152 of PrP protein, also prevents infection of susceptible N2a cells [21]. Transgenic mice expressing anti-PrP antibody 6H4 in their spleen, prevent scrapie pathogenesis in vivo, sustaining the development of a vaccination strategy [22]. White et al. [23 also performed passive immunization experiments using two anti-PrP monoclonal antibodies, ICSM35 and ICSM18, which recognized residues (91-110) and (146-159) on PrP protein, respectively. Antibodies were administered in FVB mice challenged intraperitoneally with RML prions strain. Both antibodies, not only significantly reduced the splenic PrPSc levels in mice but also delayed the appearance of scrapie pathogenesis in treated animals.

However, the passive transfer of these anti-PrP antibodies had no effect late in the incubation time when clinical signs had developed and are not efficient if mice are challenged with prions intracerebrally. This is likely due to the low ability of the antibodies to cross the blood brain barrier. Altogether these studies have showed that 2 regions of the PrP protein, spanning residues (90-110) and residues (140-155), are essential to the replication process of the prion agent. It was suggested that anti-PrP antibodies bind specifically to PrPC molecules on the cell surface and thereby hindering the docking of PrPSc template for the conversion of PrPC into PrPSc. However, those in vivo studies have utilized full-length PrP specific antibodies, which are not easy to implement in a gene therapy strategy. In contrast single-chain fragment variable (scFv) antibodies are simplified version of full-length antibodies, allowing for the production of a single polyptide sequence that retains recognition of its cognate antigen. This technology combined to gene transfer vector, allows the evaluation of the in vivo therapeutic potential of anti-prion antibodies.

Table 6. Pre-exposure prophylatic treatment using recombinant adeno-associated virus (rAAV2) carrying single chain fragment variable antibodies directed against PrP^C (24)

Schema of the therapeutic protocol assayed in wt mice intraperitoneally challenged with prions

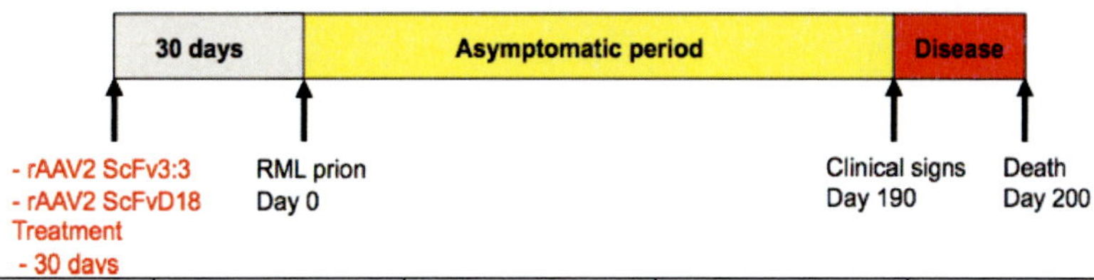

Antibodies	Vector and quantity	Animal model	Prion doses	Survival time versus CTR group (%)
CTR : anti Phenobarbital ScFvPhe	AAV2 scFvPhe $9x10^9$ I.U.	wt mice - CTR group (n=5)	RML prion strain $1x10^6$ LD_{50}	199 ± 1 days
Anti-PrP scFv3:3	AAV2 scFv3:3 $9x10^9$ I.U.	wt mice - Treated group (n=5)	RML prion strain $1x10^6$ LD_{50}	222± 13 days + 11% delay
Anti-PrP scFvD18	AAV2 scFvD18 $9x10^9$ I.U.	wt mice - Treated group (n=3)	RML prion strain $1x10^6$ LD_{50}	250 ± 8 days + 25% delay

In that purpose, Wuertzer et al. [24] have cloned several scFv anti-PrP antibodies in adeno-associated vector type 2 (AAV2) to evaluate the impact of scFv gene transfer on the course of the prion disease. Pre-exposure treatment were assayed on wt mice that received bilaterally in the striatum and thalamus, 9x109 IU of gene transfer vector either of: (i) rAAV2scFvPhe as a CTR; or (ii) rAAV2scFvD18; or (iii) rAAV2scFv3:3, (Table 6). One month later, at the time when rAAV2 transgene expression is optimal, mice were inoculated intraperitoneally with infectious prions. Mice in the control group treated with rAAV2scFvPhe died with a mean incubation time of 199 ± 1 days, whereas rAAV2 scFv3:3- and rAAV2 scFvD18-treated mice, showed an increase in their incubation time of 11% (222

± 13) and 25% (250 ± 8), respectively. Delays in incubation time were accompanied by a decrease in the PrPSc amyloid burden, as well as improvement of Rotarod performances.

CONCLUSION

From post-exposure prophylactic treatment described above using gene transfer technology to deliver different proteins of interest (siRNA, anti-PrP antibodies, natural or artificial dominant negative prion molecules), the results converged towards an increase in the incubation time of about 20% when optimal conditions are met (ranging from 15-23%). Although the lentiviral vectors delivered very different anti-prion molecules and the quantities of virions administered were quite different (ranging from $2x10^5$ to $1.5x10^9$), it is interesting to see that delays are equivalent (Tables 1, 3 and 5). Huge quantities of lentiviral vectors administered in the brain, even with empty virions ($0.8x10^9$ for GFP-Fc), may be detrimental since GFP treated animals exhibited shorter incubation time than PBS treated animals (177 ± 8 days for PBS-treated group, versus 163 ± 4 for GFP-Fc-treated group, Tables 2-3). Altogether, these results are very promising since the treatment have been applied relatively late during the course of the disease (between 30-121 days p.i.). These protocols are interesting since post-exposure treatment late in the incubation time of the disease can be transposed to human cases, by opposition to pre-exposure protocols.

Now the future goals are to develop strategies to improve these first results. One can imagine a tri-therapy assay combining a mixture of these different lentiviral vectors, such as siRNA to block PrP synthesis, anti-PrP antibodies to block PrP^C/PrP^{Sc} interactions and dominant negative prion proteins that could block interaction with prion partners, could be a good way to improve post-prophylactic treatment of prion diseases.

REFERENCES

[1] Prusiner, S. B. (1982) *Science.* 216(4542), 136-144

[2] Silveira, J. R., Raymond, G. J., Hughson, A. G., Race, R. E., Sim, V. L., Hayes, S. F., and Caughey, B. (2005) *Nature.* 437(7056), 257-261

[3] DeMarco, M. L., Silveira, J., Caughey, B., and Daggett, V. (2006) *Biochemistry.* 45(51), 15573-15582

[4] Stohr, J., Weinmann, N., Wille, H., Kaimann, T., Nagel-Steger, L., Birkmann, E., Panza, G., Prusiner, S. B., Eigen, M., and Riesner, D. (2008) *Proc. Natl. Acad. Sci. U. S. A.* 105(7), 2409-2414

[5] Bueler, H., Fischer, M., Lang, Y., Bluethmann, H., Lipp, H. P., DeArmond, S. J., Prusiner, S. B., Aguet, M., and Weissmann, C. (1992) *Nature.* 356(6370), 577-582

[6] Bueler, H., Aguzzi, A., Sailer, A., Greiner, R. A., Autenried, P., Aguet, M., and Weissmann, C. (1993) *Cell.* 73(7), 1339-1347

[7] Sailer, A., Bueler, H., Fischer, M., Aguzzi, A., and Weissmann, C. (1994) *Cell.* 77(7), 967-968

[8] Mallucci, G. R., Ratte, S., Asante, E. A., Linehan, J., Gowland, I., Jefferys, J. G., and Collinge, J. (2002) *Embo J.* 21(3), 202-210

[9] Brandner, S., Isenmann, S., Raeber, A., Fischer, M., Sailer, A., Kobayashi, Y., Marino, S., Weissmann, C., and Aguzzi, A. (1996) *Nature.* 379(6563), 339-343

[10] White, M. D., Farmer, M., Mirabile, I., Brandner, S., Collinge, J., and Mallucci, G. R. (2008) *Proc. Natl. Acad. Sci. U. S. A.* 105(29), 10238-10243

[11] Goldmann, W., Hunter, N., Smith, G., Foster, J., and Hope, J. (1994) *J Gen. Virol.* 75 (Pt 5), 989-995

[12] Bossers, A., Schreuder, B. E., Muileman, I. H., Belt, P. B., and Smits, M. A. (1996) *J. Gen. Virol.* 77 (Pt 10), 2669-2673

[13] Shibuya, S., Higuchi, J., Shin, R. W., Tateishi, J., and Kitamoto, T. (1998) *Lancet.* 351(9100), 419

[14] Kaneko, K., Zulianello, L., Scott, M., Cooper, C. M., Wallace, A. C., James, T. L., Cohen, F. E., and Prusiner, S. B. (1997) *Proc. Natl. Acad. Sci. U. S. A.* 94(19), 10069-10074

[15] Perrier, V., Kaneko, K., Safar, J., Vergara, J., Tremblay, P., DeArmond, S. J., Cohen, F. E., Prusiner, S. B., and Wallace, A. C. (2002) *Proc. Natl. Acad. Sci. U. S. A.* 99(20), 13079-13084

[16] Crozet, C., Lin, Y. L., Mettling, C., Mourton-Gilles, C., Corbeau, P., Lehmann, S., and Perrier, V. (2004) *J. Cell Sci..* 117(Pt 23), 5591-5597

[17] Toupet, K., Compan, V., Crozet, C., Mourton-Gilles, C., Mestre-Frances, N., Ibos, F., Corbeau, P., Verdier, J. M., and Perrier, V. (2008) *PLoS One.* 3(7), e2773

[18] Genoud, N., Ott, D., Braun, N., Prinz, M., Schwarz, P., Suter, U., Trono, D., and Aguzzi, A. (2008) *Am. J. Pathol.* 172(5), 1287-1296

[19] Meier, P., Genoud, N., Prinz, M., Maissen, M., Rulicke, T., Zurbriggen, A., Raeber, A. J., and Aguzzi, A. (2003) *Cell.* 113(1), 49-60

[20] Peretz, D., Williamson, R. A., Kaneko, K., Vergara, J., Leclerc, E., Schmitt-Ulms, G., Mehlhorn, I. R., Legname, G., Wormald, M. R., Rudd, P. M., Dwek, R. A., Burton, D. R., and Prusiner, S. B. (2001) *Nature.* 412(6848), 739-743

[21] Enari, M., Flechsig, E., and Weissmann, C. (2001) *Proc. Natl. Acad. Sci. U. S. A.* 98(16), 9295-9299

[22] Heppner, F. L., Musahl, C., Arrighi, I., Klein, M. A., Rulicke, T., Oesch, B., Zinkernagel, R. M., Kalinke, U., and Aguzzi, A. (2001) *Science.* 294(5540), 178-182

[23] White, A. R., Enever, P., Tayebi, M., Mushens, R., Linehan, J., Brandner, S., Anstee, D., Collinge, J., and Hawke, S. (2003) *Nature.* 422(6927), 80-83

[24] Wuertzer, C. A., Sullivan, M. A., Qiu, X., and Federoff, H. J. (2008) *Mol. Ther.* 16(3), 481-486

INDEX

C

H

I

N

Q

R

X

Y

Z